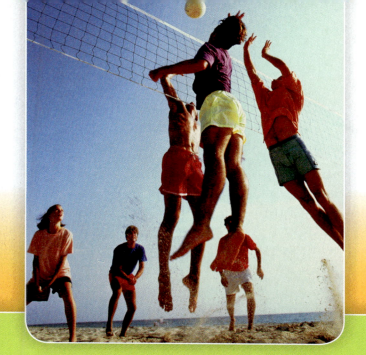

FIT & WELL

EIGHTH EDITION

Core Concepts and Labs in Physical Fitness and Wellness

Brief Edition

Thomas D. Fahey
California State University, Chico

Paul M. Insel
Stanford University

Walton T. Roth
Stanford University

McGraw-Hill
Higher Education

Boston   Burr Ridge, IL   Dubuque, IA   New York
San Francisco   St. Louis   Bangkok   Bogotá   Caracas   Kuala Lumpur
Lisbon   London   Madrid   Mexico City   Milan   Montreal   New Delhi
Santiago   Seoul   Singapore   Sydney   Taipei   Toronto

The McGraw·Hill Companies

McGraw-Hill
Higher Education

Published by McGraw-Hill, an imprint of The McGraw-Hill Companies, Inc., 1221 Avenue of the Americas, New York, NY 10020. Copyright © 2009. All rights reserved. No part of this publication may be reproduced or distributed in any form or by any means, or stored in a database or retrieval system, without the prior written consent of The McGraw-Hill Companies, Inc., including, but not limited to, in any network or other electronic storage or transmission, or broadcast for distance learning.

This book is printed on acid-free paper.

1 2 3 4 5 6 7 8 9 0 DOW/DOW 0 9 8

ISBN: 978-0-07-332565-1
MHID: 0-07-332565-1

Editor in Chief: *Michael J. Ryan*
Publisher: *William R. Glass*
Executive editor: *Christopher Johnson*
Executive marketing manager: *Nick Agnew*
Director of development: *Kathleen Engelberg*
Developmental editor: *Tim Huddleston, Docugistics, Inc.*
Developmental editor for technology: *Julia D. Akpan*
Editorial coordinator: *Sarah B. Hill*
Media Project Manager: *Ron Nelms, Jr.*
Production editor: *Chanda Feldman*
Manuscript Editor: *Thomas L. Briggs*
Art Director: *Jeanne M. Schreiber*
Design Manager: *Andrei Pasternak*
Text Designer: *Irene Morris*
Cover Designer: *Lisa Buckley*
Art Manager: *Robin Mouat*
Illustrators: *John and Judy Waller and Susan Seed*
Manager, Photo Research: *Brian J. Pecko*
Supplements Producer: *Alan Noyes*
Production Supervisor: *Randy Hurst*
Composition: *10.5/12 Berkeley Book by Aptara, Inc.*
Printing: *45# Pub Matte, R. R. Donnelley & Sons*
Cover: © Stockbyte/Getty Images

Library of Congress Cataloging-in-Publication Data

Fahey, Thomas D. (Thomas Davin), 1947-
Fit & well, brief: core concepts and labs in physical fitness and wellness / Thomas D. Fahey, Paul M. Insel, Walton T. Roth.—8th ed.
p. cm.
Includes bibliographical references and index.
ISBN-13: 978-0-07-332565-1 (alk. paper);
ISBN-10: 0-07-332565-1 (alk. paper)
1. Physical fitness. 2. Health. I. Title. II. title: Fit and well.
GV481.F26 2009
613.7'043—dc22   2008003396

The Internet addresses listed in the text were accurate at the time of publication. The inclusion of a Web site does not indicate an endorsement by the authors or McGraw-Hill, and McGraw-Hill does not guarantee the accuracy of the information presented at these sites.

Photo Credits

BRIEF CONTENTS

CONTENTS

BOXES

LABORATORY ACTIVITIES

PREFACE

For today's fitness-conscious student, *Fit and Well: Brief Edition* combines the best of two worlds. In the area of physical fitness, *Fit and Well* offers expert knowledge based on the latest findings in exercise physiology and sports medicine, along with tools for self-assessment and guidelines for becoming fit. In the area of wellness, it offers accurate, current information on today's most important health-related topics and issues, again with self-tests and guidelines for achieving wellness. To create this book, we have drawn on our combined expertise and experience in exercise physiology, athletic training, personal health, scientific research, and teaching.

OUR AIMS

Our aims in writing this book can be stated simply:

- To show students that becoming fit and well greatly improves the quality of their lives
- To show students how they can become fit and well
- To motivate students to make healthy choices and to provide them with tools for change

The first of these aims means helping students see how their lives can be enhanced by a fit and well lifestyle. This book offers convincing evidence of a simple truth: To look and feel our best, to protect ourselves from degenerative diseases, and to enjoy the highest quality of life, we need to place fitness and wellness among our top priorities. *Fit and Well* makes clear both the imprudence of our modern, sedentary lifestyle and the benefits of a wellness lifestyle.

Our second aim is to give students the tools and information they need to become fit and well. This book provides students with everything they need to create personalized fitness programs, including instructions for fitness tests, explanations of the components of fitness and guidelines for developing them, descriptions and illustrations of exercises, sample programs, and more. In addition, *Fit and Well* provides accurate, up-to-date, scientifically based information about other key topics in wellness, including nutrition, weight management, stress, cardiovascular health, cancer, drugs, alcohol, STDs, and a multitude of others.

In providing this material, we have pooled our efforts. Thomas Fahey has contributed his knowledge as an exercise physiologist, teacher, and author of numerous exercise science textbooks. Paul M. Insel and Walton T. Roth have contributed their knowledge of current topics in health as the authors of the leading personal health textbook *Core Concepts in Health*.

Because we know this expert knowledge can be overwhelming, we have balanced the coverage of complex topics with student-friendly features designed to make the book accessible. Written in a straightforward, easy-to-read style and presented in a colorful, open format, *Fit and Well* invites students to read, learn, and remember. Boxes, labs, tables, figures, artwork, photographs, and other features add interest to the text and highlight areas of special importance.

Our third aim is to involve students in taking responsibility for their health. *Fit and Well* makes use of interactive features to get students thinking about their current levels of physical fitness and wellness. We offer students assessment tools and laboratory activities to evaluate themselves in terms of each component of physical fitness and each major wellness area, ranging from cardiorespiratory endurance and muscular strength to heart disease, cancer, and STDs.

We also show students how they can make difficult lifestyle changes by using the principles of behavior change. Chapter 1 contains a step-by-step description of this simple but powerful tool for change. The chapter not only explains the five-step process but also offers a wealth of tips for ensuring success. Behavior management aids, including personal contracts, behavior checklists, and self-tests, appear throughout the book. *Fit and Well's* combined emphasis on self-assessment, self-development in each area of wellness, and behavior change ensures that students are inspired to become fit and well and also have the tools to do so.

When students use these tools to make significant lifestyle changes, they begin to realize that they are in charge of their health—and their lives. From this realization comes a sense of competence and personal power. Perhaps our overriding aim in writing *Fit and Well* is to convey the fact that virtually everyone has the ability to understand, monitor, and make changes in his or her levels of fitness and wellness. By making healthy choices from an early age, individuals may minimize the amount of professional medical care they will ever require. Our hope is that *Fit and Well* will help people make this exciting discovery: that they have the power to shape their future.

CONTENT AND ORGANIZATION OF THE EIGHTH EDITION

The content of *Fit and Well: Brief Edition* is organized into 8 chapters. Chapter 1 provides an introduction to fitness and wellness and explains the principles of behavior change. Chapters 2–7 focus on the various areas of fitness. Chapter 2 provides an overview, discussing the components of fitness, the principles of physical training, and the factors involved in designing a well-rounded, personalized exercise program. Chapter 3 provides basic information on how the cardiorespiratory system functions, how the body produces energy for exercise, and how individuals can create successful cardiorespiratory fitness programs. Chapters 4, 5, and 6 look at muscular strength and endurance, flexibility and low-back health, and body composition, respectively. Chapter 7 puts it all together, describing the nature of a complete program that develops all the components of fitness. This chapter also includes complete sample exercise programs. Finally, Chapter 8 treats the key wellness area of nutrition.

For the eighth edition, each chapter was carefully reviewed, revised, and updated. The latest information from scientific and wellness-related research is incorporated in the text, and newly emerging topics are discussed. The following list gives a sample of some of the new and updated material in the eighth edition:

- Physical activity guidelines from the CDC, ACSM, and other authorities
- Nutritional guidelines, including the 2005 Dietary Guidelines for Americans, MyPyramid, the DASH diet, and the Mediterranean diet
- Occupational and financial wellness as important aspects of wellness
- Benefits of exercise for all dimensions of wellness
- Top physical and emotional health issues facing college students today
- Common food allergens and food labeling, food safety and foodborne illness, top antioxidant-containing foods, organic food and farming, and cancer-fighting phytochemicals in foods
- Diabetes, pre-diabetes, insulin resistance, and metabolic syndrome
- Functional leg strength tests as a measure of muscular strength (Lab 4.1)
- Gender differences in muscular strength
- Performance-enhancing drugs, their supposed effects, and their side effects
- Buying and using heart rate monitors
- Calisthenics circuit training
- Yoga for relaxation and pain relief
- Correct body posture and hand position for a computer workstation
- Revised emergency care guidelines for someone who is choking or experiencing cardiac arrest
- Updated nutritional content of common foods and of popular items from fast-food restaurants

Research in the areas of health and wellness is ongoing, with new discoveries, advances, trends, and theories reported nearly every week. For this reason, no wellness book can claim to have the final word on every topic. Yet, within these limits, *Fit and Well* does present the latest available information and scientific thinking on important wellness topics. Taken together, the chapters of the book provide students with a complete, up-to-date guide to maximizing their well-being, now and throughout their lives.

To make sure that students have access to the most current information available, each chapter in the eighth edition is also closely tied to the Web site developed as a companion to the text. Boxes, illustrations, tables, terms, and sections of text marked with the World Wide Web icon have corresponding links and activities on the *Fit and Well* Online Learning Center (www.mhhe.com/fahey).

In addition, to help students make the best use of this text, we have updated the way much of the content is presented. We recognize that some students today may learn in different ways than students did in the past. The eighth edition offers a more streamlined approach to content, with more information "chunked" in lists and charts for greater accessibility and easier learning and retention. This edition also features a brighter, more open, and more eye-catching design to appeal to today's visually oriented student.

FEATURES OF THE EIGHTH EDITION

This edition of *Fit and Well* builds on the features that attracted and held our readers' interest in previous editions. These features are designed to help students increase their understanding of the core concepts of wellness and to make better use of the book.

Laboratory Activities

To help students apply the principles of fitness and wellness to their lives, *Fit and Well* includes **laboratory activities** for classroom use. These hands-on activities give students the opportunity to assess their current level of fitness and wellness, to create plans for changing their lifestyle to reach wellness, and to monitor their progress. They can assess their current lifestyle, for example, or their level of cardiorespiratory endurance; they can design a program to improve muscular strength or develop flexibility, and they can explore their risk of developing cardiovascular disease. Many labs end with a Using Your Results section, which guides students in evaluating their scores, setting goals for change, and moving forward. Labs are found at the end of each chapter; they are perforated for easy removal. For a complete list of laboratory activities, see p. vii in the table of contents.

Illustrated Exercise Sections

To ensure that students understand how to perform important exercises and stretches, *Fit and Well* includes three **illustrated exercise sections,** one in Chapter 4 and two in Chapter 5. The section in Chapter 4 covers exercises for developing muscular strength and endurance, as performed both with free weights and on weight machines. One section in Chapter 5 presents stretches for flexibility, and the other presents exercises to stretch and strengthen the lower back. Each exercise is illustrated with one or more full-color photographs showing proper technique. Digital video clips of the exercises from the text and key lab activities are found on the *Fit and Well* Online Learning Center. Look for the video icon in the text to find out when to look online for corresponding video clips.

Sample Programs

To help students get started, Chapter 7 offers seven complete **sample programs** designed to develop overall fitness. The programs are built around four cardiorespiratory endurance activities: walking/jogging/running, bicycling, swimming, and calisthenics circuit training. Each program includes detailed information and guidelines on equipment and technique; target intensity, duration, and frequency; calorie cost of the activity; record keeping; and adjustments to make as fitness improves. The chapter also includes general guidelines for putting together a personal fitness program: setting goals; selecting activities; setting targets for intensity, duration, and frequency; maintaining a commitment; and recording and assessing progress.

Boxes

Boxes are used in *Fit and Well* to explore a wide range of current topics in greater detail than is possible in the text itself. Boxes fall into five different categories, each marked with a special icon and label.

 Take Charge boxes distill from the text the practical advice students need to apply information to their lives. By referring to these boxes, students can easily find information about such topics as making time for physical activity, deciding between walking and running, varying their activities, stretching safely, reducing the saturated and trans fats in their diets, and many others.

 Critical Consumer boxes are designed to help students develop and apply critical thinking skills, thereby enabling them to make sound choices related to health and well-being. Critical Consumer boxes provide specific guidelines for choosing exercise footwear, heart rate monitors, and home exercise equipment; using food and dietary supplement labels; evaluating Web sites and other sources of health information; and more.

 Dimensions of Diversity boxes focus on the important theme of diversity. Most wellness issues are universal; we all need to exercise and eat well, for example. However, certain differences among people—based on gender, educational attainment, socioeconomic status, ethnicity, age, and other factors—do have important implications for

wellness. Dimensions of Diversity boxes give students opportunities to identify special wellness concerns that affect them because of who they are, as individuals or as members of a group. Topics of Dimensions of Diversity boxes include gender differences in muscular strength, fitness for people with disabilities, the healthiest ethnic foods, and others.

 Wellness Connection boxes highlight important links among the different dimensions of wellness—physical, emotional, social/interpersonal, intellectual, spiritual, and environmental—and emphasize that all the dimensions must be developed for an individual to achieve optimal health and well-being. Topics include the wellness benefits of exercise, occupational wellness, yoga for relaxation and pain relief, paths to spiritual wellness, and sleep.

 In Focus boxes highlight current topics and issues of particular interest to students. These boxes focus on such topics as the wellness concerns of college students, exercise safety, classification of activity levels, diabetes, and many others.

Vital Statistics

Vital Statistics tables and figures highlight important facts and figures in an accessible format. From tables and figures marked with the Vital Statistics label, students learn about such matters as the leading causes of death for Americans and the factors that play a part in each cause; the relationship between lifestyle and quality of life; public health achievements of the twentieth century; and a wealth of other information. For students who learn best when material is displayed graphically or numerically, Vital Statistics tables and figures offer a way to grasp information quickly and directly.

Common Questions Answered

Sections called **Common Questions Answered** appear at the ends of Chapters 2–8. In these student-friendly sections, the answers to frequently asked questions are presented in easy-to-understand terms. Included are such questions as, Do I need a special diet for my endurance exercise program? Will strength training improve my sports performance? Is stretching the same as warming up? Which should I eat—butter or margarine? Answers to many additional questions can be found on the Online Learning Center.

Motivation Booster

Motivation Booster sections provide strategies for beginning a behavior change program and maintaining healthy new habits over time. Motivation Booster strategies focus on such key aspects of behavior change as building self-efficacy, finding role models and social support, overcoming obstacles and lapses, changing environmental cues, giving

Questions for Critical Thinking and Reflection

New to the eighth edition, **Questions for Critical Thinking and Reflection** appear at appropriate points throughout the chapters. These questions are designed to prompt students to think critically about the content they have just read, relate it to their own lives, and probe a little more deeply into their own attitudes, values, and beliefs.

Tips for Today and the Future

Chapter-ending **Tips for Today and the Future** sections provide a brief distillation of the major message of each chapter, followed by suggestions for a few simple things that students can try right away and in the near future. Tips for Today and the Future are designed to encourage students and to build their confidence by giving them easy steps they can take immediately and in the next few days and weeks to improve their wellness.

Quick-Reference Appendixes

Included at the end of the book are four appendixes containing vital information in an easy-to-use format. **Appendix A, Injury Prevention and Personal Safety,** is a reference guide to preventing common injuries, whether at home, at work, at play, or on the road. It also provides information on emergency preparedness, and it includes the latest guidelines on giving emergency care when someone else's life is in danger.

Appendix B, Nutritional Content of Common Foods, allows students to assess their daily diet in terms of 11 nutrient categories, including protein, fat, saturated fat, fiber, cholesterol, and sodium. **Appendix C, Nutritional Content of Popular Items from Fast-Food Restaurants,** provides a breakdown of the nutritional content of commonly ordered menu items at popular fast-food restaurants.

Appendix D, Monitoring Your Progress, is a log that enables students to record and summarize the results of the assessment tests they complete as part of the laboratory activities. With space for preprogram and postprogram assessment results, the log provides an easy way to track the progress of a behavior change program.

OTHER FEATURES AND LEARNING AIDS

At the beginning of each chapter, under the heading **Looking Ahead,** five or six statements preview the main points of the chapter for students and serve as learning objectives. Each chapter also opens with **Test Your Knowledge**—three multiple-choice and true-false questions, with answers. These self-quizzes facilitate learning by emphasizing key points, highlighting common misconceptions, and sparking debate. Within each chapter, important terms appear in boldface type and are defined on the same or facing page of text in a **running glossary,** helping students handle new vocabulary.

Other features and learning aids are found at the end of each chapter. **Chapter summaries** offer students a concise review and a way to make sure they have grasped the most important concepts in the chapter. **For Further Exploration** sections list recommended books, newsletters, organizations, hotlines, and Web sites.

For more on the features of the book, refer to the illustrated **User's Guide to *Fit and Well*,** found on pp. xv–xviii.

TEACHING TOOLS

Available with the eighth edition of *Fit and Well* is a comprehensive package of supplementary materials designed to enhance teaching and learning.

Instructor's Media DVD (ISBN 0-07-332568-6)

The Instructor's Media DVD includes the major electronic resources offered with the eighth edition of *Fit and Well.*

- The **Course Integrator Guide** includes learning objectives, extended chapter outlines, lists of additional resources, and many other teaching tools. It also describes all the supplements available with the text and shows how to integrate them into lectures and assignments for each chapter. For the eighth edition, the guide was prepared by Julie Lombardi, Millersville University.

- The **test bank** includes more than 1500 true-false, multiple-choice, and essay questions. The questions are available as Word files and with the **EZ Test computerized testing software.** EZ Test provides a powerful, easy-to-use test maker to create printed quizzes and exams. For secure online testing, exams created in EZ Test can be exported to WebCT, Blackboard, PageOut, and EZ Test Online. EZ Test comes with a Quick Start Guide, and once the program is installed, users have access to a User's Manual and Flash tutorials. Additional help is available online at www.mhhe.com/eztest.

- The **PowerPoint slides** provide a lecture tool that you can alter or expand to meet the needs of your course. The slides include key lecture points and images from the text and other sources. For the eighth edition, the PowerPoint presentations were created by Andrew Shim, Indiana University of Pennsylvania. As an aid for instructors who wish to create their own presentations, a complete **image bank,** including all the illustrations from the text, is also available on the Instructor's Media DVD.

Primis Online
www.mhhe.com/primis/online

Primis Online is a database-driven publishing system that allows instructors to create customized textbooks, lab manuals, or readers for their courses directly from the Primis Web site. The custom text can be delivered in print or electronic (eBook) form. A Primis eBook is a digital version of the customized text sold directly to students as a file downloadable to their computer or accessed online by password. *Fit and Well* can be customized using Primis Online.

Digital Solutions

The *Fit and Well* Online Learning Center (**www.mhhe.com/fahey**) provides many resources for both instructors and students. Instructor tools include downloadable versions of the Course Integrator Guide, the PowerPoint slides, and the computerized test bank, as well as links to professional resources. For students, there are learning objectives, self-quizzes and glossary flashcards for review, interactive Internet activities, video clips of correct training techniques, and extensive links. The Online Learning Center also includes many tools for wellness behavior change, including a 15-activity Behavior Change Workbook.

Classroom Performance System (CPS) brings interactivity into the classroom or lecture hall. CPS is a wireless response system that gives instructors and students immediate feedback from the entire class. Each student uses a wireless response pad similar to a television remote to instantly respond to polling or quiz questions. Contact your local sales representative for more information about using CPS with *Fit and Well*.

PageOut (**www.pageout.net**) is a free, easy-to-use program that enables instructors to quickly develop Web sites for their courses. PageOut can be used to create a course home page, an instructor home page, an interactive syllabus that can be linked to elements in the Online Learning Center, Web links, online discussion areas, an online grade book, and much more. Instructors can combine Online Learning Center resources with popular **course-management systems.** For more information about McGraw-Hill's digital resources, including how to obtain passwords for PageOut, contact your local sales representative.

Student Resources Available with Fit and Well

In addition to the materials on the Online Learning Center, there are many resources available with *Fit and Well* designed to help students learn and apply key concepts.

- The **Daily Fitness and Nutrition Journal** (ISBN 0-07-332567-8) is a handy booklet that guides students in planning and tracking their fitness programs. It also helps students assess their current diet and make appropriate changes. It is available as an optional package with new copies of the text.

- The **Health and Fitness Pedometer** (ISBN 0-07-320933-3) can be packaged with copies of the text. It allows students to count their daily steps and track their level of physical activity.

- **NutritionCalc Plus** (ISBN 0-07-319532-4) is a dietary analysis program with an easy-to-use interface that allows users to track their nutrient and food group intakes, energy expenditures, and weight control goals. It generates a variety of reports and graphs for analysis, including comparisons with the Dietary Reference Intakes. The ESHA database includes thousands of ethnic foods, supplements, fast foods, and convenience foods; users can also add foods to the database. NutritionCalc Plus is available on CD-ROM (Windows only) or in an Internet version.

- **HealthQuest 4.2** (ISBN 0-07-295117-6) is an interactive CD-ROM that helps students explore their wellness behavior. It includes tutorials, assessments, and behavior change guidance in such key areas as stress, fitness, nutrition, communicable diseases, cardiovascular disease, cancer, tobacco, alcohol, and other drugs.

Additional supplements and many packaging options are available; check with your local sales representative.

A NOTE OF THANKS

Fit and Well has benefited from the thoughtful commentary, expert knowledge, and helpful suggestions of many people. We are deeply grateful for their participation in the project.

Academic Reviewers of the Eighth Edition

Kym Atwood, University of West Florida
Motier Becque, Southern Illinois University, Carbondale
Laura Blitzer, Florida International University, Miami
Robert "BC" Charles-Liscomb, Greensboro College
Lori Clark, Chemeketa Community College
Mary Ann Erickson, Fort Lewis College
Danny Essary, East Texas Baptist University
Megan Franks, North Harris College
Steven Frierman, Hofstra University
Charlie Goehl, Elmhurst College
Jeffrey S. Hallam, University of Mississippi
Kevin Harper, University of Texas, Arlington
Robert Hess, Community College of Baltimore County at Catonsville
Stacy J. Ingraham, University of Minnesota, Minneapolis
Wayne Jacobs, LeTourneau University
Linda Jenuwine, Macomb Community College
Joe Jones, Cameron University
Heather Krueger, Concordia University
Toni LaSala, William Paterson University
Raymond Leung, University of Southern Indiana
Rosemary Lindle, University of Maryland
Karen McConnell, Pacific Lutheran University
Kathleen Meyer, Clemson University
Michelle Miller, Indiana University, Bloomington
Cenell Munford-Clark, Mount Union College
Peggy Ondrea, Columbia College
Sara Parr, Madison Area Technical College

Tim Patrick, Furman University
Charles Pelitera, Canisius College
Katherine Poole, Radford University
Kelly Quick, University of Sioux Falls
Lindsey Reider, Onondaga Community College
Misti Reisman, Tarleton State University
Amy Ries, Northeast Community College
Natalie Rose, Kennesaw State University
Phil Ryan, State University of New York,
    Buffalo North Campus
Rich Schroeder, De Anza College
Paula Stauf, Emory University
Martha Stephenson, San Antonio College
McKinley Thomas, Augusta State University
Iva Toler, Prince George's Community College
Gerald Walker, Fort Valley State University
Mike Webster, University of Southern Mississippi,
    Hattiesburg
James Zarick, High Point University

Special thanks are due to Rich Schroeder, De Anza College, for hosting the photo and video shoots for several editions and to the many students at De Anza College and California State University, Chico, who have participated in these shoots. Special thanks also go to Gary Ligouri at North Dakota State University and to the NDSU students who participated in special fitness and wellness focus groups. We are also grateful to the *Fit and Well* book team at McGraw-Hill, without whose efforts the book could not have been published. Special thanks to Chris Johnson, sponsoring editor; Kirstan Price, long-time developmental editor of this text; Tim Huddleston, developmental editor of the eighth edition; Kate Engelberg, director of development; Julia D. Akpan, developmental editor for technology; Sarah Hill, editorial coordinator; Nick Agnew, marketing manager; Chanda Feldman, production editor; Randy Hurst, production supervisor; Andrei Pasternak, design manager; Robin Mouat, art manager; Brian J. Pecko, manager, photo research; and Marty Granahan, permissions editor.

Thomas D. Fahey
Paul M. Insel
Walton T. Roth

FIT & WELL

Are you looking for ways to improve your lifestyle and become fit and well? Do you need help finding reliable wellness resources online? Would you like to boost your grade? *Fit and Well* can help you do all this and much more!

LABORATORY ACTIVITIES

These hands-on self-assessments help you determine your current level of wellness and create plans for making positive changes in your lifestyle. Lab activities are included at the end of every chapter on easy-to-use perforated pages.

FIT AND WELL
ONLINE LEARNING CENTER
(WWW.MHHE.COM/FAHEY)

Look for the World Wide Web icon throughout the text. Elements marked with the icon have corresponding activities and links on the *Fit and Well* Online Learning Center.

A USER'S GUIDE TO
FIT & WELL

SAMPLE EXERCISE PROGRAMS

Illustrated exercise programs in Chapters 4 and 5 show proper technique for exercises and stretches that develop muscular strength and endurance, flexibility, and low-back health; video clips of the exercises can be found on the Online Learning Center. The complete sample fitness programs in Chapter 7 are built around popular endurance activities such as walking, jogging, cycling, and swimming.

TAKE CHARGE BOXES

Take Charge boxes, found throughout the text, provide practical advice that you can apply to your everyday life.

CRITICAL CONSUMER BOXES

Critical Consumer boxes help you develop and apply critical thinking skills so you can make sound choices related to wellness. Additional resources for each Critical Consumer topic are found on the Online Learning Center.

MOTIVATION BOOSTER

Motivation Booster sections provide strategies for beginning a behavior change program and maintaining new healthy habits over time.

QUESTIONS FOR CRITICAL THINKING AND REFLECTION

Questions for Critical Thinking and Reflection prompt you to think critically about the information you have read and consider how it relates to your own life and experience. Some questions also ask you to reflect on your values, beliefs, and attitudes.

TIPS FOR TODAY AND THE FUTURE

Tips for Today and the Future sections, found at the end of each chapter, provide a brief summary of the major message of the chapter, followed by suggestions for a few easy steps you can try right away and in the next few weeks and months to improve your level of wellness.

FOR FURTHER EXPLORATION

For Further Exploration sections at the end of each chapter describe books, newsletters, organizations, hotlines, and Web sites that you can turn to for additional information and advice.

A USER'S GUIDE TO
FIT & WELL

RUNNING GLOSSARY

Important terms appear in boldface type in the text and are defined in a running glossary on the same or facing page. A pronunciation guide to the glossary terms is found on the Online Learning Center.

BEHAVIOR CHANGE WORKBOOK

The Behavior Change Workbook takes you step-by-step through the process of behavior change. It helps you target a specific behavior, set goals, create a plan, and overcome common obstacles to change. The Workbook is available in an interactive format on the Online Learning Center, and a printed copy is included in the full and alternate editions of the text.

FIT&WELL

Core Concepts and Labs in Physical Fitness and Wellness

EIGHTH EDITION

Brief Edition

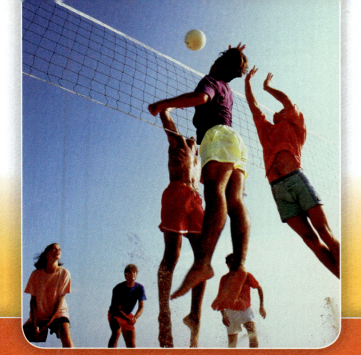

LOOKING AHEAD>>>>>

AFTER READING THIS CHAPTER, YOU SHOULD BE ABLE TO:

- Describe the dimensions of wellness
- Identify the major health problems in the United States today, and discuss their causes
- Describe the behaviors that are part of a fit and well lifestyle
- Explain the steps in creating a behavior management plan to change a wellness-related behavior
- Discuss the available sources of wellness information and how to think critically about them

INTRODUCTION TO
WELLNESS, FITNESS, AND LIFESTYLE MANAGEMENT

1

TEST YOUR KNOWLEDGE

1. **Which of the following lifestyle factors is the leading preventable cause of death for Americans?**
   a. excess alcohol consumption
   b. cigarette smoking
   c. obesity

2. **The terms *health* and *wellness* mean the same thing.**

   True or false?

3. **Which of the following health-related issues affects the greatest number of college students each year?**
   a. stress
   b. colds/flu/sore throat
   c. sleep problems
   d. concern for a friend or family member

ANSWERS

1. **b. Smoking** causes about 500,000 deaths per year; obesity is responsible for more than 100,000; and alcohol, as many as 85,000.

2. **FALSE.** Although the words are used interchangeably, they actually have different meanings. The term *health* refers to the overall condition of the body or mind and to the presence or absence of illness or injury. The term *wellness* refers to optimal health and vitality, encompassing six dimensions of well-being.

3. **a. About** 32% of college students suffer so much stress that it affects their academic performance. High stress levels affect overall health and wellness, making it important to learn effective stress-management techniques.

FIT AND WELL ONLINE LEARNING CENTER www.mhhe.com/fahey

Visit the *Fit and Well* Online Learning Center for resources that will help you get the most out of your course!
- Study and review aids include practice quizzes, glossary flashcards, chapter summaries, learning objectives, PowerPoint presentations, Common Questions Answered, student handouts, crossword puzzles, Internet activities, and links to wellness Web sites.
- Behavior change tools include a daily fitness and nutrition journal, a behavior change workbook, sample behavior change plans, and blank behavior change logs to print and use.

A college sophomore sets the following goals for herself:

- To join in new social circles and make new friends whenever possible
- To exercise every day
- To clean up trash and plant trees in blighted neighborhoods in her community

These goals may differ, but they have one thing in common. Each contributes, in its own way, to this student's health and well-being. Not satisfied merely to be free of illness, she wants more. She has decided to live actively and fully—not just to be healthy but to pursue a state of overall wellness.

WELLNESS: THE NEW HEALTH GOAL

Generations of people have viewed health simply as the absence of disease. That view largely prevails today; the word **health** typically refers to the overall condition of a person's body or mind and to the presence or absence of illness or injury. **Wellness** is a relatively new concept that expands our idea of health. Beyond the simple presence or absence of disease, wellness refers to optimal health and vitality—to living life to its fullest. Although we use the words *health* and *wellness* interchangeably, there are two important differences between them:

- Health—or some aspects of it—can be determined or influenced by factors beyond your control, such as your genes, age, and family history. For example, consider a 60-year-old man with a strong family history of prostate cancer. These factors place this man at a higher-than-average risk for developing prostate cancer himself.
- Wellness is largely determined by the decisions you make about how you live. That same 60-year-old man can reduce his risk of cancer by eating sensibly, exercising, and having regular screening tests. Even if he develops the disease, he may still rise above its effects to live a rich, meaningful life. This means

choosing not only to care for himself physically but to maintain a positive outlook, keep up his relationships with others, challenge himself intellectually, and nurture other aspects of his life.

Enhanced wellness, therefore, involves making conscious decisions to control **risk factors** that contribute to disease or injury. Age and family history are risk factors you cannot control. Behaviors such as smoking, exercising, and eating a healthy diet are well within your control.

The Dimensions of Wellness

Experts have defined six dimensions of wellness:

- Physical
- Emotional
- Intellectual
- Interpersonal
- Spiritual
- Environmental

These dimensions are interrelated; each has an effect on the others. Further, the process of achieving wellness is constant and dynamic (Figure 1.1), involving change and growth. Wellness is not static; ignoring any dimension of wellness can have harmful effects on your life. The following sections briefly introduce the dimensions of wellness. Table 1.1 lists some of the specific qualities and behaviors associated with each dimension.

Physical Wellness Your physical wellness includes not just your body's overall condition and the absence of disease but your fitness level and your ability to care for yourself. The higher your fitness level (which is discussed throughout this book), the higher your level of physical wellness will be. Similarly, as you develop the ability to take care of your own physical needs, you ensure a greater level of physical wellness. To achieve optimum physical wellness, you need to make choices that will help you avoid illnesses and injuries. The decisions you make now, and the habits you develop over

FIGURE 1.1 The wellness continuum. The concept of wellness includes vitality in six interrelated dimensions, all of which contribute to overall wellness.

Table 1.1	Examples of Qualities and Behaviors Associated with the Dimensions of Wellness				
Physical	**Emotional**	**Intellectual**	**Interpersonal**	**Spiritual**	**Environmental**
• Eating well	• Optimism	• Openness to new ideas	• Communication skills	• Capacity for love	• Having abundant, clean natural resources
• Exercising	• Trust	• Capacity to question	• Capacity for intimacy	• Compassion	• Maintaining sustainable development
• Avoiding harmful habits	• Self-esteem	• Ability to think critically	• Ability to establish and maintain satisfying relationships	• Forgiveness	• Recycling whenever possible
• Practicing safer sex	• Self-acceptance	• Motivation to master new skills	• Ability to cultivate support system of friends and family	• Altruism	• Reducing pollution and waste
• Recognizing symptoms of disease	• Self-confidence	• Sense of humor		• Joy	
• Getting regular checkups	• Ability to understand and accept one's feelings	• Creativity		• Fulfillment	
• Avoiding injuries	• Ability to share feelings with others	• Curiosity		• Caring for others	
		• Lifelong learning		• Sense of meaning and purpose	
				• Sense of belonging to something greater than oneself	

your lifetime, will largely determine the length and quality of your life.

Emotional Wellness   Your emotional wellness reflects your ability to understand and deal with your feelings. Emotional wellness involves attending to your own thoughts and feelings, monitoring your reactions, and identifying obstacles to emotional stability. Achieving this type of wellness means finding solutions to emotional problems, with professional help if necessary.

Intellectual Wellness   Those who enjoy intellectual (or mental) wellness constantly challenge their minds. An active mind is essential to wellness because it detects problems, finds solutions, and directs behavior. People who enjoy intellectual wellness never stop learning; they continue trying to learn new things throughout their lifetime. They seek out and relish new experiences and challenges.

Interpersonal Wellness   Your interpersonal (or social) wellness is defined by your ability to develop and maintain satisfying and supportive relationships. Such relationships are essential to physical and emotional health. Social wellness requires participating in and contributing to your community, country, and world.

Spiritual Wellness   To enjoy spiritual wellness is to possess a set of guiding beliefs, principles, or values that give meaning and purpose to your life, especially in difficult times. The spiritually well person focuses on the positive aspects of life and finds spirituality to be an antidote for negative feelings such as cynicism, anger, and pessimism. Organized religions help many people develop spiritual health. Religion, however, is not the only source or form of spiritual wellness. Many people find meaning and purpose in their lives on their own—through nature, art, meditation, or good works—or with their loved ones.

Environmental Wellness   Your environmental wellness is defined by the livability of your surroundings. Personal health depends on the health of the planet—from the safety of the food supply to the degree of violence in society. Your physical environment either supports your wellness or diminishes it. To improve your environmental wellness, you can learn about and protect yourself against hazards in your surroundings and work to make your world a cleaner and safer place.

Lab 1.1 will help you learn what wellness means to you and where you fall on the wellness continuum. In addition, see the box "Occupational Wellness" (p. 4) to learn about another important aspect of wellness.

New Opportunities, New Responsibilities

Wellness is a fairly new concept. A century ago, Americans considered themselves lucky just to survive to adulthood (Figure 1.2, p. 5). A child born in 1900, for example, could expect to live only about 47 years. Many people died from common **infectious diseases** (such as pneumonia, tuberculosis, or diarrhea) and poor environmental conditions (such as water pollution and poor sanitation). Since 1900, however, life expectancy has nearly doubled, due largely to the development of vaccines and

health   The overall condition of body or mind and the presence or absence of illness or injury.

wellness   Optimal health and vitality, encompassing the six dimensions of well-being.

risk factor   A condition that increases one's chances of disease or injury.

infectious disease   A disease that can spread from person to person; caused by microorganisms such as bacteria and viruses.

TERMS WEB

Occupational Wellness

Many experts contend that occupational (or career) wellness is a seventh dimension of wellness, in addition to the six dimensions described in this chapter. Whether or not occupational wellness appears on every list of wellness dimensions, a growing body of evidence suggests that our daily work has a considerable effect on our overall wellness.

Defining Occupational Wellness

The term *occupational wellness* refers to the level of happiness and fulfillment you gain through your work. Although high salaries and prestigious titles are nice, they alone generally do not bring about occupational wellness. An occupationally well person truly likes his or her work, feels a connection to others in the workplace, and has opportunities to learn and be challenged.

Key aspects of occupational wellness include the following:

- Enjoyable work
- Job satisfaction
- Recognition and acknowledgment from managers and colleagues
- Feelings of achievement
- Opportunities to learn and grow

An ideal job draws on your passions and interests, as well as your vocational skills, and allows you to feel that you are contributing to society in your everyday work.

Financial Wellness

Another important facet of occupational wellness is financial wellness. A person's economic situation is a key factor in his or her overall well-being. People with low socioeconomic status have higher rates of death, injury, and disease; are less likely to have access to preventive health services; and are more likely to engage in unhealthy habits.

Although money and possessions in themselves won't necessarily make you happy, financial security can contribute to your peace of mind. If you are financially secure, you can worry less about daily expenses and focus on personal interests and your future. On the other hand, money problems are a source of stress for individuals and families and are a contributing factor in many divorces and suicides.

You don't need to be rich to achieve financial wellness. Instead, you need to be comfortable with your financial situation. Financially well people understand the limits of their income and live within their means by keeping expenses in check. They know how to balance a checkbook and interpret their bank statements. The financially well person may not strive to be wealthy but at least tries to save money for the future.

Achieving Occupational Wellness

How do you achieve such wellness? Career experts suggest setting career goals that reflect your personal values. For example, a career in sales may be a good way to earn a high income but may not be a good career choice for someone whose highest values involve service to others. Such a person might find more personal satisfaction in teaching or nursing.

Aside from career choices, education is a critical factor in occupational and financial wellness. For starters, learn to manage money *before* you start making it. Classes on personal money management are available through many sources and can help you on your way to financial security, whether you dream of being wealthy or not.

---

antibiotics to fight infections and to public health measures to improve living conditions. Today, a different set of diseases has emerged as our major health threat, and heart disease, cancer, and stroke are now the three leading causes of death for Americans. Treating such **chronic diseases** is costly and difficult.

The good news is that people have some control over whether they develop chronic diseases. People make choices every day that increase or decrease their risks for such diseases. These **lifestyle choices** include behaviors such as smoking, diet, exercise, and alcohol use. As Tables 1.2 and 1.3 (p. 6) make clear, lifestyle factors contribute to many deaths in the United States, and people can influence their own health risks.

The global toll of preventable chronic diseases is high. The World Health Organization (WHO) reports that 4.9 million people die annually from tobacco use, 2.6 million from obesity, 4.4 million from high cholesterol, and 7.1 million from high blood pressure.

The Healthy People Initiative

Wellness is a personal concern, but the U.S. government has financial and humanitarian interests in it, too. A

TERMS

chronic disease A disease that develops and continues over a long period of time, such as heart disease or cancer.

lifestyle choice A conscious behavior that can increase or decrease a person's risk of disease or injury; such behaviors include smoking, exercising, eating a healthy diet, and others.

VITAL STATISTICS

FIGURE 1.2   Public health achievements of the twentieth century. During the twentieth century, public health achievements greatly improved the quality of life for Americans. A shift in the leading causes of death also occurred, with deaths from infectious diseases declining from 33% of all deaths to just 2%. Heart disease, cancer, and stroke are now responsible for more than half of all deaths among Americans.

SOURCE: National Center for Health Statistics; Centers for Disease Control and Prevention. 1999. Ten great public health achievements—United States, 1900–1999. *Morbidity and Mortality Weekly Report* 48(50): 1141.

 VITAL STATISTICS

Table 1.2	Leading Causes of Death in the United States				
Rank	**Cause of Death**	**Number of Deaths**	**Percent of Total Deaths**	**Male/Female Ratio***	**Lifestyle Factors**
1	Heart disease	652,486	27.2	1.5	D I S A
2	Cancer	553,888	23.1	1.4	D I S A
3	Stroke	150,074	6.3	1.0	D I S A
4	Chronic lower respiratory disease	121,987	5.1	1.4	S
5	Unintentional injuries (accidents)	112,012	4.7	2.1	I S A
6	Diabetes mellitus	73,138	3.1	1.3	D I S
7	Alzheimer's disease	65,965	2.8	0.7	
8	Influenza and pneumonia	59,664	2.5	1.4	S
9	Kidney disease	42,480	1.8	1.4	D I S A
10	Septicemia (systemic blood infection)	33,373	1.4	1.2	A
11	Intentional self-harm (suicide)	32,439	1.4	4.0	A
12	Chronic liver disease and cirrhosis	27,013	1.1	2.2	A
13	Hypertension (high blood pressure)	23,076	1.0	1.0	D I S A
14	Parkinson's disease	17,989	0.8	2.3	
15	Homicide	17,357	0.7	3.7	A
	All causes	2,397,615			

Key	D	Diet plays a part	S	Smoking plays a part
	I	Inactive lifestyle plays a part	A	Excessive alcohol consumption plays a part

NOTE: Although not among the overall top 15 causes of death, HIV/AIDS (approximately 13,000 deaths) is a major killer. HIV/AIDS is among the 10 leading causes of death among Americans age 15–44.

*Ratio of males to females who died of each cause. For example, for each woman who died of heart disease, 1.5 men died from the same cause.

SOURCE: National Center for Health Statistics. 2007. Deaths: Final data for 2004. *National Vital Statistics Report* 55 (19).

| Table 1.3 | Actual Causes of Death Among Americans* |

	Number of Deaths per Year	Percentage of Total Deaths per Year
Tobacco	440,000	18.1
Obesity**	112,000	4.6
Alcohol consumption	85,000	3.5
Microbial agents	75,000	3.1
Toxic agents	55,000	2.3
Motor vehicles	43,000	1.8
Firearms	29,000	1.2
Sexual behavior	20,000	0.8
Illicit drug use	17,000	0.7

*NOTE: Actual causes of death are defined as lifestyle and environmental factors that contribute to the leading killers of Americans. Microbial agents include bacterial and viral infections like influenza and pneumonia; toxic agents include environmental pollutants and chemical agents such as asbestos.

**The number of deaths due to obesity is an area of ongoing controversy and research. Recent estimates have ranged from 112,000 to 365,000.

SOURCES: Centers for Disease Control and Prevention. 2005. *Frequently Asked Questions About Calculating Obesity-Related Risk* (http://www.cdc.gov/PDF/Frequently_Asked_Questions_About_Calculating_Obesity-Related_Risk.pdf; retrieved December 6, 2007). Mokdad, A. H., et al. 2005. Correction: Actual causes of death in the United States, 2000. *Journal of the American Medical Association* 293(3): 293–294. Mokdad, A. H., et al. 2004. Actual causes of death in the United States, 2000. *Journal of the American Medical Association* 291(10): 1238–1245.

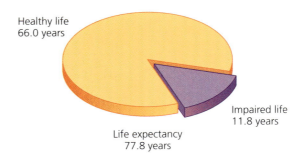

Healthy life 66.0 years

Impaired life 11.8 years

Life expectancy 77.8 years

FIGURE 1.3 Quantity of life versus quality of life. Years of healthy life as a proportion of life expectancy in the U.S. population.

SOURCES: National Center for Health Statistics. 2007. Deaths: Final data for 2004. *National Vital Statistics Reports.* 55(19). National Center for Health Statistics. *Healthy People* 2010; Midcourse Review. Hyattsville, Md.: Public Health Service.

healthy population is the nation's source of vitality, creativity, and wealth. Poor health drains the nation's resources and raises health care costs for all.

The national Healthy People initiative aims to prevent disease and improve Americans' quality of life. Healthy People reports, published each decade since 1980, set national health goals based on 10-year agendas.

The latest report, *Healthy People 2010,* proposes two broad national goals:

• **Increase quality and years of healthy life.** One way to measure quality of life is to count the number of "sick days" people endure—days they can't function due to illness. About 18% of Americans take 14 or more sick days each year, a number that continually rises. Along those same lines, Americans increasingly describe their health as fair or poor rather than excellent or very good. Further, although the life expectancy of Americans has increased significantly in the past century, people can expect poor health to limit their

activities and cause distress during the last 15% of their lives (Figure 1.3).

• **Eliminate health disparities among Americans.** Many health problems today disproportionately affect certain American populations (see the box "Wellness Issues for Diverse Populations" on p. 8). *Healthy People 2010* calls for eliminating disparities in health status, health risks, and use of preventive services among all population groups within the next decade.

Examples of individual health promotion objectives from *Healthy People 2010,* as well as estimates of how we are tracking toward the goals, appear in Table 1.4.

Behaviors That Contribute to Wellness

A lifestyle based on good choices and healthy behaviors maximizes quality of life. It helps people avoid disease, remain strong and fit, and maintain their physical and mental health as long as they live. Figure 1.4 highlights the results of just two of the research studies that have found clear links between lifestyle behaviors and the risk of developing and dying from chronic disease. The most important behaviors and habits are introduced briefly here and described in detail in later chapters.

Be Physically Active The human body is designed to work best when it is active. It readily adapts to nearly any level of activity and exertion; in fact, **physical fitness** is defined as a set of physical attributes that allow the body to respond or adapt to the demands and stress of physical effort. The more we ask of our bodies, the stronger and more fit they become. When our bodies are not kept active, however, they deteriorate. Bones lose their density, joints stiffen, muscles become weak, and cellular energy systems begin to degenerate. To be truly well, human beings must be active. Unfortunately, a **sedentary** lifestyle is common among Americans today: About one-half

TERMS

physical fitness A set of physical attributes that allow the body to respond or adapt to the demands and stress of physical effort.

sedentary Physically inactive; literally, "sitting."

Table 1.4	Selected *Healthy People 2010* Objectives		
Objective		**Estimate of Current Status (%)**	**Goal (%)**
Increase the proportion of people age 18 and older who engage regularly in moderate physical activity.		30	50
Increase the proportion of people age 2 and older who consume at least 3 daily servings of vegetables, with at least one-third being dark-green or orange vegetables.		3	50
Increase the prevalence of healthy weight among people age 20 and older.		32	60
Reduce the proportion of adults 18 and older who use cigarettes.		21	12
Reduce the proportion of college students reporting binge drinking during the past 2 weeks.		39	20
Increase the proportion of adults who take protective measures to reduce the risk of skin cancer (sunscreens, sun-protective clothing, and so on).		71	85
Increase the use of safety belts by motor vehicle occupants.		82	92
Increase the number of residences with a functioning smoke alarm on every floor.		90	100
Increase the proportion of persons with health insurance.		84	100

SOURCE: National Center for Health Statistics. 2007. *DATA 2010: The Healthy People 2010 Database, October 2007 Edition* (http://wonder.cdc.gov/data2010/obj.htm; retrieved December 6, 2007).

of Americans are not regularly physically active, and about 15% are not active at all.

The benefits of physical activity are both physical and mental, immediate and long-term (Figure 1.5, p. 8). In the short term, being physically fit makes it easier to do everyday tasks, such as lifting; it provides reserve strength for emergencies; and it helps people look and feel good. In the long term, being physically fit confers protection against chronic diseases and lowers the risk of dying prematurely. Physically active individuals are less likely to develop or die from heart disease, respiratory disease, high blood pressure, cancer, osteoporosis, and type 2 diabetes (the most common form of diabetes). As they get older, they may be able to avoid weight gain, muscle and bone loss, fatigue, and other problems associated with aging.

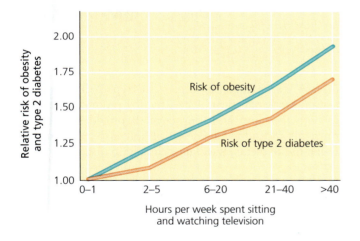

(a) Sedentary lifestyle and risk of obesity and type 2 diabetes

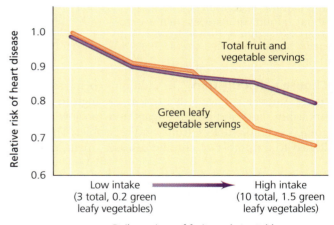

(b) Fruit and vegetable intake and risk of heart disease

 VITAL STATISTICS

FIGURE 1.4 Lifestyle and risk of chronic disease. Many research studies have found links between lifestyle behaviors and risk of chronic disease. The results of just two such studies are shown here. They indicate that (a) people who spend more time watching television are more likely to be obese and to develop type 2 diabetes and (b) people who consume more fruits and vegetables, especially leafy green vegetables, have a lower risk of heart disease.

SOURCES: (a) Hu, F. B., et al. 2003. Television watching and other sedentary behaviors in relation to risk of obesity and type 2 diabetes mellitus in women. *Journal of the American Medical Association* 289(14): 1785–1791. (b) Joshipura, K. J., et al. 2001. The effect of fruit and vegetable intake on risk for coronary heart disease. *Annals of Internal Medicine* 134(12): 1106–1114.

Wellness Issues for Diverse Populations

When it comes to striving for wellness, most differences among people are insignificant. We all need to exercise, eat well, and manage stress. We all need to know how to protect ourselves from heart disease, cancer, sexually transmitted diseases, and injuries.

But some of our differences—both as individuals and as members of groups—do have implications for wellness. Some of us, for example, have grown up with eating habits that increase our risk of obesity or heart disease. Some of us have inherited predispositions for certain health problems, such as osteoporosis or high cholesterol levels. These health-related differences among individuals and groups can be biological—determined genetically—or cultural—acquired as patterns of behavior through daily interactions with family, community, and society. Many health conditions are a function of biology and culture combined.

Every person is an individual with her or his own unique genetic endowment as well as unique experiences in life. However, many of these influences are shared with others of similar genetic and cultural backgrounds. Information about group similarities relating to wellness issues can be useful; for example, it can alert people to areas that may be of special concern for them and their families.

Wellness-related differences among groups can be described along several dimensions, including:

- **Gender.** Men and women have different life expectancies and different incidences of many diseases, including heart disease, cancer, and osteoporosis. Men have higher rates of death from injuries, suicide, and homicide; women are at greater risk for Alzheimer's disease and depression. Men and women also differ in body composition and certain aspects of physical performance.

- **Race and ethnicity.** A genetic predisposition for a particular health problem can be linked to race or ethnicity as a result of each group's relatively distinct history. Diabetes is more prevalent among individuals of Native American or Latino heritage, for example, and African Americans have higher rates of hypertension. Racial or ethnic groups may also vary in other ways that relate to wellness: traditional diets; patterns of family and interpersonal relationships; and attitudes toward using tobacco, alcohol, and other drugs, to name just a few.

- **Income and education.** Inequalities in income and education underlie many of the health disparities among Americans. People with low incomes (low *socioeconomic status*, or *SES*) and less education have higher rates of injury and many diseases, are more likely to smoke, and have less access to health care. Poverty and low educational attainment are far more important predictors of poor health than any racial or ethnic factor.

These are just some of the "dimensions of diversity"—differences among people and groups that are associated with different wellness concerns. Other factors, too, such as age, geographic location, sexual orientation, and disability, can present challenges as an individual strives for wellness. In this text, topics related to wellness and diversity are given special consideration in boxes labeled Dimensions of Diversity.

Choose a Healthy Diet In addition to being sedentary, many Americans have a diet that is too high in calories, unhealthy fats, and added sugars and too low in fiber, complex carbohydrates, fruits, and vegetables. This diet is linked to a number of chronic diseases, including heart disease, stroke, high blood pressure, type 2 diabetes, and certain kinds of cancer. A healthy diet promotes wellness in both the short and long term. It provides necessary nutrients and sufficient energy without also providing too much of the dietary substances linked to diseases.

- Increased endurance, strength, and flexibility
- Healthier muscles, bones, and joints
- Increased energy (calorie) expenditure
- Improved body composition
- More energy
- Improved ability to cope with stress
- Improved mood, higher self-esteem, and greater sense of well-being
- Improved ability to fall asleep and sleep well

- Reduced risk of dying prematurely from all causes
- Reduced risk of developing and/or dying from heart disease, diabetes, high blood pressure, and colon cancer
- Reduced risk of becoming obese
- Reduced anxiety, tension, and depression
- Reduced risk of falls and fractures
- Reduced spending for health care

FIGURE 1.5 Benefits of regular physical activity.

Maintain a Healthy Body Weight Overweight and obesity are associated with a number of disabling and potentially fatal conditions and diseases, including heart disease, cancer, and type 2 diabetes. The Centers for Disease Control and Prevention (CDC) estimates that obesity kills 112,000 Americans each year. Healthy body weight is an important part of wellness—but short-term dieting is not part of fitness or wellness. Maintaining a healthy body weight requires a lifelong commitment to regular exercise, a healthy diet, and effective stress management.

Manage Stress Effectively Many people cope with stress by eating, drinking, or smoking too much. Others don't deal with it at all. In the short term, inappropriate stress management can lead to fatigue, sleep disturbances, and other unpleasant symptoms. Over longer periods of time, poor management of stress can lead to less efficient functioning of the immune system and increased susceptibility to disease. There *are* effective ways to handle stress, and learning to incorporate them into daily life is an important part of a fit and well lifestyle.

Avoid Tobacco and Drug Use and Limit Alcohol Consumption Tobacco use is associated with 8 of the top 10 causes of death in the United States; it kills about 440,000 Americans each year, more than any other behavioral or environmental factor. With nearly 21% of adult Americans smoking, lung cancer is the most common cause of cancer death among both men and women and one of the leading causes of death overall. The direct health care costs associated with smoking exceed $75 billion per year. If the cost of lost productivity from sickness, disability, and premature death is included, the total is closer to $157 billion.

Excessive alcohol consumption is linked to 6 of the top 10 causes of death and results in about 85,000 deaths a year in the United States. The social, economic, and medical costs of alcohol abuse are estimated at over $180 billion per year. Alcohol or drug intoxication is an especially notable factor in the death and disability of young people, particularly through **unintentional injuries** (such as drownings and car crashes caused by drunken driving) and violence. Unintentional injuries, homicide, and suicide are the top three leading causes of death for 15- to 24-year-olds.

Protect Yourself from Disease and Injury The most effective way of dealing with disease and injury is to prevent them. Many of the lifestyle strategies discussed here—being physically active, managing body weight, and so on—help protect you against chronic illnesses. In addition, you can take specific steps to avoid infectious diseases, particularly those that are sexually transmitted.

Take Other Steps Toward Wellness Other important behaviors contribute to wellness, including these:

- Developing meaningful relationships
- Planning for successful aging

- Learning about the health care system
- Acting responsibly toward the environment

Lab 1.2 will help you evaluate your behaviors as they relate to wellness.

The Role of Other Factors in Wellness

Heredity, the environment, and adequate health care are other important influences on health. These factors can interact in ways that raise or lower the quality of a person's life and the risk of developing particular diseases. For example, a sedentary lifestyle combined with a genetic predisposition for diabetes can greatly increase a person's risk for developing the disease. If this person also lacks adequate health care, he or she is much more likely to suffer dangerous complications from diabetes.

MOTIVATION BOOSTER
Chart your family health history. Learning about the diseases and health conditions that run in your family can help you start improving your lifestyle. Such knowledge helps you understand the health risks you may face in the future. It can also help motivate you to keep a behavior change program on track. Put together a simple family health tree by plugging key health information on your close relatives—siblings, parents, aunts and uncles, grandparents—into a family tree format. Don't focus only on causes of death. Look at all chronic conditions and health-related behaviors that affect both quality and quantity of life—alcoholism, diabetes, high blood pressure, high cholesterol, obesity, osteoporosis, depression, and so on. What patterns do you see? Visit the U.S. Surgeon General's Family History Initiative Web site (www.hhs.gov/familyhistory) for more information and a sample family health tree form.

QUESTIONS FOR CRITICAL THINKING AND REFLECTION
How often do you feel exuberant? Vital? Joyful? What makes you feel that way? Conversely, how often do you feel downhearted, de-energized, or depressed? What makes you feel that way? Have you ever thought about how you might increase experiences of vitality and decrease experiences of discouragement?

unintentional injury An injury that occurs without harm being intended.

But in many cases, behavior can tip the balance toward health even if heredity or environment is a negative factor. Breast cancer, for example, can run in families, but it is also associated with overweight and a sedentary lifestyle. A woman with a family history of breast cancer is less likely to die from the disease if she controls her weight, exercises, performs regular breast self-exams, and consults with her physician about mammograms.

REACHING WELLNESS THROUGH LIFESTYLE MANAGEMENT

As you consider this description of behaviors that contribute to wellness—being physically active, choosing a healthy diet, and so on—you may be doing a mental comparison with your own behaviors. If you are like most young adults, you probably have some healthy habits and some habits that place your health at risk. For example, you may be physically active and have a healthy diet but indulge in binge drinking on weekends. You may be careful to wear your seat belt in your car but smoke cigarettes or use chewing tobacco. Moving in the direction of wellness means cultivating healthy behaviors and working to overcome unhealthy ones. This approach to lifestyle management is sometimes called **behavior change.**

As you may already know from experience, changing an unhealthy habit can be harder than it looks. When you embark on a behavior change plan, it may seem like too much work at first. But as you make progress, you will gain confidence in your ability to take charge of your life. You will also experience the benefits of wellness—more energy, greater vitality, deeper feelings of appreciation and curiosity, and a higher quality of life.

In the rest of this chapter, we outline a general process for changing unhealthy behaviors that is backed by research and that has worked for many people. We also offer many specific strategies and tips for change. For additional support, work through the activities in the Behavior Change Workbook at the end of the text and on the Online Learning Center.

Getting Serious About Your Health

Before you can start changing a wellness-related behavior, you have to know that the behavior is problematic and that you *can* change it. To make good decisions, you need information about relevant topics and issues, including what resources are available to help you change.

Examine Your Current Health Habits   Have you considered how your current lifestyle is affecting your health today and how it will affect your health in the future? Do you know which of your current habits enhance your health and which detract from it? Begin your journey toward wellness with self-assessment: Think about your own behavior, complete the self-assessment in Lab 1.2, and talk with friends and family members about what they've noticed about your lifestyle and your health. Challenge any unrealistically optimistic attitudes or ideas you may hold—for example, "To protect my health, I don't need to worry about quitting smoking until I'm 40 years old," or "Being overweight won't put *me* at risk for diabetes." Health risks are very real, and health habits throughout life are important.

Many people start to consider changing a behavior when friends or family members express concern, when a landmark event occurs (such as turning 30), or when new information raises their awareness of risk. If you find yourself reevaluating some of your behaviors as you read this text, take advantage of the opportunity to make a change in a structured way.

Choose a Target Behavior   Changing any behavior can be demanding. This is why it's a good idea to start small, by choosing one behavior you want to change—called a **target behavior**—and working on it until you succeed. Your chances of success will be greater if your first goal is simple, such as resisting the urge to snack between classes. As you change one behavior, make your next goal a little more significant, and build on your success.

Learn About Your Target Behavior   Once you've chosen a target behavior, you need to learn its risks and benefits for you—both now and in the future. Ask these questions:

- How is your target behavior affecting your level of wellness today?
- What diseases or conditions does this behavior place you at risk for?
- What effect would changing your behavior have on your health?

As a starting point, use this text and the resources listed in the For Further Exploration section at the end of each chapter; see the box "Evaluating Sources of Health Information" for additional guidelines.

Find Help   Have you identified a particularly challenging target behavior or mood, something like alcohol addiction, binge eating, or depression, that interferes with your ability to function or places you at a serious health risk? Help may be needed to change behaviors or conditions that are too deeply rooted or too serious for self-management. Don't be stopped by the seriousness of the

CRITICAL CONSUMER

Evaluating Sources of Health Information

Believability of Health Information Sources

A 2006 survey conducted by the American College Health Association indicated that college students are smart about evaluating health information. They trust the health information they receive from health professionals and educators and are skeptical about popular information sources.

Rank	Source	Rank	Source
1	Health center staff	7	Campus peer educators
2	Health educators	8	Resident assistants/ advisers
3	Faculty/coursework	9	Friends
4	Parents	10	Religious centers
5	Leaflets, pamphlets, flyers	11	Internet/Web
6	Campus newspaper articles	12	Magazines
		13	Television

How smart are you about evaluating health information? Here are some tips.

General Strategies

Whenever you encounter health-related information, take the following steps to make sure it is credible:

• *Go to the original source.* Media reports often simplify the results of medical research. Find out for yourself what a study really reported, and determine whether it was based on good science. What type of study was it? Was it published in a recognized medical journal? Was it an animal study or did it involve people? Did the study include a large number of people? What did the authors of the study actually report?

• *Watch for misleading language.* Reports that tout "breakthroughs" or "dramatic proof" are probably hype. A study may state that a behavior "contributes to" or is "associated with" an outcome; this does not prove a cause-and-effect relationship.

• *Distinguish between research reports and public health advice.* Do not change your behavior based on the results of a single report or study. If an agency such as the National Cancer Institute urges a behavior change, however, you should follow its advice. Large, publicly funded organizations issue such advice based on many studies, not a single report.

• *Remember that anecdotes are not facts.* A friend may tell you he lost weight on some new diet, but individual success stories do not mean the plan is truly safe or effective. Check with your doctor before making any serious lifestyle changes.

• *Be skeptical.* If a report seems too good to be true, it probably is. Be wary of information contained in advertisements. An ad's goal is to sell a product, even if there is no need for it.

• *Make choices that are right for you.* Friends and family members can be a great source of ideas and inspiration, but you need to make health-related choices that work best for you.

Internet Resources

Online sources pose special challenges; when reviewing a health-related Web site, ask these questions:

• *What is the source of the information?* Web sites maintained by government agencies, professional associations, or established academic or medical institutions are likely to present trustworthy information. Many other groups and individuals post accurate information, but it is important to look at the qualifications of the people who are behind the site. (Check the home page or click the "About Us" link.)

• *How often is the site updated?* Look for sites that are updated frequently. Check the "last modified" date of any Web page.

• *Is the site promotional?* Be wary of information from sites that sell specific products, use testimonials as evidence, appear to have a social or political agenda, or ask for money.

• *What do other sources say about a topic?* Be cautious of claims or information that appear at only one site or come from a chat room, bulletin board, or blog.

• *Does the site conform to any set of guidelines or criteria for quality and accuracy?* Look for sites that identify themselves as conforming to some code or set of principles, such as those set forth by the Health on the Net Foundation or the American Medical Association. These codes include criteria such as use of information from respected sources and disclosure of the site's sponsors.

problem; many resources are available to help you solve it. On campus, the student health center or campus counseling center can provide assistance. To locate community resources, consult the yellow pages, your physician, or the Internet.

Building Motivation to Change

Knowledge is necessary for behavior change, but it isn't usually enough to make people act. Millions of people have sedentary lifestyles, for example, even though they know it's bad for their health. This is particularly true of young adults, who may not be motivated to change because they feel healthy in spite of their unhealthy

behaviors (see the box "Wellness Matters for College Students" on p. 12). To succeed at behavior change, you need strong motivation.

Examine the Pros and Cons of Change Health behaviors have short-term and long-term benefits and costs. Consider the benefits and costs of an inactive lifestyle:

• Short-term, such a lifestyle allows you more time to watch TV and hang out with friends, but it leaves you less physically fit and less able to participate in recreational activities.

• Long-term, it increases the risk of heart disease, cancer, stroke, and premature death.

Wellness Matters for College Students

If you are like most college students, you probably feel pretty good about your health right now. Most college students are in their late teens or early twenties, lead active lives, have plenty of friends, and look forward to a future filled with opportunity. With all these things going for you, why shouldn't you feel good?

A Closer Look

Although most college-age people look healthy, appearances can be deceiving. Each year, thousands of students lose productive academic time to physical and emotional health problems—some of which can continue to plague them for life.

The following table shows the top 10 health issues affecting students' academic performance, according to the 2006 National College Health Assessment.

Health Issue	Students Affected (%)
Stress	32.0
Cold/flu/sore throat	26.0
Sleep problems	23.9
Concern for a friend or family member	18.0
Depression/anxiety	15.7
Relationship problems	15.6
Internet/computer game use	15.4
Death of friend or family member	8.5
Sinus infection/ear infection/ bronchitis/strep throat	8.3
Alcohol use	7.3

Each of these issues is related to one or more of the six dimensions of wellness, and most can be influenced by choices students make daily. Although some troubles—such as the death of a friend—cannot be controlled, other physical and emotional concerns can be minimized by choosing healthy behaviors. For example, there are many ways to manage stress, the top health issue affecting students. By reducing unhealthy choices (such as using alcohol to relax) and by increasing healthy choices (such as using time management techniques), even busy students can reduce the impact of stress on their life.

The survey also estimated that, based on students' reporting of their height and weight, more than 30% of college students are either over-weight or obese. Although heredity plays a role in determining one's weight, lifestyle is also a factor in weight and weight management. In many studies over the past few decades, a large percentage of students have reported behaviors such as these:

- Overeating
- Snacking on junk food
- Frequently eating high-fat foods
- Using alcohol and binge drinking

Clearly, eating behaviors are often a matter of choice. Although students may not see (or feel) the effects of their dietary habits today, the long-term health risks are significant. Overweight and obese persons run a higher-than-normal risk of developing diabetes, heart disease, and cancer later in life. We now know with certainty that improving one's eating habits, even a little, can lead to weight loss and improved overall health.

Other Choices, Other Problems

Students commonly make other unhealthy choices. Here are some examples from the 2006 National College Health Assessment:

- Nearly 50% of students reported that they did not use a condom the last time they had vaginal intercourse.
- About 25% of students had as many as 8 drinks the last time they partied.
- Almost 18% of students had used tobacco at least once during the past month.

What choices do you make in these situations? Remember: It's never too late to change. The sooner you trade an unhealthy behavior for a healthy one, the longer you'll be around to enjoy the benefits.

To successfully change your behavior, you must believe that the benefits of change outweigh the costs.

Carefully examine the pros and cons of continuing your current behavior and of changing to a healthier one. Focus on the effects that are most meaningful to you, including those that are tied to your personal identity and values. For example, if you see yourself as an active person who is a good role model for others, then adopting behaviors such as engaging in regular physical activity and getting adequate sleep will support your personal identity. If you value independence and control over your life, then quitting smoking will be consistent with your values and goals. To complete your analysis, ask friends and family members about the effects of your behavior on them. For example, a younger sister may tell you that your smoking habit influenced her decision to take up smoking.

The short-term benefits of behavior change can be an important motivating force. Although some people are motivated by long-term goals, such as avoiding a disease that may hit them in 30 years, most are more likely to be moved to action by shorter-term, more personal goals. Feeling better, doing better in school, improving at a sport, reducing stress, and increasing self-esteem are common short-term benefits of health behavior change. Many wellness behaviors are associated with immediate improvements in quality of life. For example, surveys of Americans have found that nonsmokers feel healthy and full of energy more days each month than do smokers, and they report fewer days of sadness and troubled sleep; the same is true when physically active people are compared with sedentary people. Over time, these types of differences add up to a substantially higher quality of life for people who engage in healthy behaviors.

You can further strengthen your motivation by raising your consciousness about your problem behavior. This will enable you to focus on the negatives of the behavior and imagine the consequences if you don't make a change. At the same time, you can visualize the positive results of changing your behavior. Ask yourself, "What do I want for myself, now and in the future?"

Boost Self-Efficacy   When you start thinking about changing a health behavior, a big factor in your eventual success is whether you have confidence in yourself and in your ability to change. **Self-efficacy** refers to your belief in your ability to successfully take action and perform a specific task. Strategies for boosting self-efficacy include developing an internal locus of control, using visualization and self-talk, and obtaining encouragement from supportive people.

LOCUS OF CONTROL   Who do you believe is controlling your life? Is it your parents, friends, or school? Is it "fate"? Or is it you? **Locus of control** refers to the figurative "place" a person designates as the source of responsibility for the events in his or her life. People who believe they are in control of their own lives are said to have an internal locus of control. Those who believe that factors beyond their control determine the course of their lives are said to have an external locus of control.

For lifestyle management, an internal locus of control is an advantage because it reinforces motivation and commitment. An external locus of control can sabotage efforts to change behavior. For example, if you believe that you are destined to die of breast cancer because your mother died from the disease, you may view monthly breast self-exams and regular checkups as a waste of time. In contrast, if you believe that you can take action to reduce your risk of breast cancer in spite of hereditary factors, you will be motivated to follow guidelines for early detection of the disease.

If you find yourself attributing too much influence to outside forces, gather more information about your wellness-related behaviors. List all the ways that making lifestyle changes will improve your health. If you believe you'll succeed, and if you recognize that you are in charge of your life, you're on your way to wellness.

VISUALIZATION AND SELF-TALK   One of the best ways to boost your confidence and self-efficacy is to visualize yourself successfully engaging in a new, healthier behavior. Imagine yourself going for an afternoon run 3 days a week or no longer smoking cigarettes. Also visualize yourself enjoying all the short-term and long-term benefits that your lifestyle change will bring. Create a new self-image: What will you and your life be like when you become a regular exerciser or a nonsmoker?

You can also use self-talk, the internal dialogue you carry on with yourself, to increase your confidence in your ability to change. Counter any self-defeating patterns of thought with more positive or realistic thoughts:

"I am a strong, capable person, and I can maintain my commitment to change." See Chapter 10 for more on self-talk.

ROLE MODELS AND OTHER SUPPORTIVE INDIVIDUALS   Social support can make a big difference in your level of motivation and your chances of success. Perhaps you know people who have reached the goal you are striving for; they could be role models or mentors for you, providing information and support for your efforts. Gain strength from their experiences, and tell yourself, "If they can do it, so can I." In addition, find a buddy who wants to make the same changes you do and who can take an active role in your behavior change program. For example, an exercise buddy can provide companionship and encouragement when you might be tempted to skip your workout.

MOTIVATION BOOSTER

Find a role model. It can be motivating to observe people who have successfully changed their behavior. For example, watch physically active people; note what they're doing and when. If you know people who are successfully managing their weight, note their eating habits, such as food choices and portion sizes. In general, try to observe people who are similar to you in age, sex, and fitness level.

Identify and Overcome Barriers to Change   Don't let past failures at behavior change discourage you; they can be a great source of information you can use to boost your chances of future success. Make a list of the problems and challenges you faced in any previous behavior change attempts; to this, add the short-term costs of behavior change that you identified in your analysis of the pros and cons of change. Once you've listed these key barriers to change, develop a practical plan for overcoming each one. For example, if you always smoke when you're with certain friends, decide in advance how you will turn down the next cigarette you are offered.

Enhancing Your Readiness to Change

The transtheoretical, or "stages of change," model has been shown to be an effective approach to lifestyle self-management. According to this model, you move through distinct stages as you work to change your target behavior.

self-efficacy   The belief in one's ability to take action and perform a specific task.

locus of control   The figurative "place" a person designates as the source of responsibility for the events in his or her life.

Tips for Moving Forward in the Cycle of Behavior Change

PRECONTEMPLATION

- **Raise your awareness.** Research your target behavior and its effects.
- **Be self-aware.** Look at the mechanisms you use to resist change, such as denial or rationalization. Find ways to counteract these mechanisms.
- **Seek social support.** Friends and family members can help you identify target behaviors and understand their impact on the people around you.
- **Identify helpful resources.** These might include exercise classes or stress-management workshops offered by your school.

CONTEMPLATION

- **Keep a journal.** A record of your target behavior and the circumstances that elicit the behavior can help you plan a change program.
- **Do a cost-benefit analysis.** Identify the costs and benefits (both current and future) of maintaining your behavior and of changing it. Costs can be monetary, social, emotional, and so on.
- **Identify barriers to change.** Knowing these obstacles can help you overcome them.
- **Engage your emotions.** Watch movies or read books about people with your target behavior. Imagine what your life will be like if you don't change.
- **Create a new self-image.** Imagine what you'll be like after changing your target behavior. Try to think of yourself in new terms right now.
- **Think before you act.** Learn why you engage in the target behavior. Determine what "sets you off," and train yourself not to act reflexively.

PREPARATION

- **Create a plan.** Include a start date, goals, rewards, and specific steps you will take to change your behavior.
- **Make change a priority.** Create and sign a contract with yourself.
- **Practice visualization and self-talk.** These techniques can help prepare you mentally for challenging situations.
- **Take short steps.** Successfully practicing your new behavior for a short time—even a single day—can boost your confidence and motivation.

ACTION

- **Monitor your progress.** Keep up with your journal entries.
- **Change your environment.** Make changes that will discourage the target behavior—for example, getting rid of snack foods or not stocking the refrigerator with beer.
- **Find alternatives to your target behavior.** Make a list of things you can do to replace the behavior.
- **Reward yourself.** Rewards should be identified in your change plan. Give yourself lots of praise, and focus on your success.
- **Involve your friends.** Tell them you want to change, and ask for their help.
- **Don't get discouraged.** Real change is difficult.

MAINTENANCE

- **Keep going.** Continue using the positive strategies that worked in earlier stages.
- **Be prepared for lapses.** Don't let slip-ups set you back.
- **Be a role model.** Once you have successfully changed your behavior, you may be able to help someone else do the same thing.

It is important to determine what stage you are in now so that you can choose appropriate strategies for progressing through the cycle of change. This approach can help you enhance your readiness and intention to change. Read the following sections to determine what stage you are in for your target behavior. For ideas on changing stages, see the box "Tips for Moving Forward in the Cycle of Behavior Change."

Precontemplation People at this stage do not think they have a problem and do not intend to change their behavior. They may be unaware of the risks associated with their behavior or may deny them. They may have tried unsuccessfully to change in the past and may now think the situation is hopeless. They may also blame other people or external factors for their problems. People in the precontemplation stage believe that there are more reasons or more important reasons not to change than there are reasons to change.

Contemplation People at this stage know they have a problem and intend to take action within 6 months. They acknowledge the benefits of behavior change but are also aware of the costs of changing—to be successful, people must believe that the benefits of change outweigh the costs. People in the contemplation stage wonder about possible courses of action but don't know how to proceed. There may also be specific barriers to change that appear too difficult to overcome.

Preparation People at this stage plan to take action within a month or may already have begun to make small changes in their behavior. They may be engaging in their new, healthier behavior but not yet regularly or consistently.

They may have created a plan for change but may be worried about failing.

Action   During the action stage, people outwardly modify their behavior and their environment. The action stage requires the greatest commitment of time and energy, and people in this stage are at risk for reverting to old, unhealthy patterns of behavior.

Maintenance   People at this stage have maintained their new, healthier lifestyle for at least 6 months. Lapses may have occurred, but people in maintenance have been successful in quickly reestablishing the desired behavior. The maintenance stage can be as short as 6 months or as long as 5 years or more.

Termination   For some behaviors, a person may reach the sixth and final stage of termination. People at this stage have exited the cycle of change and are no longer tempted to lapse back into their old behavior. They have a new self-image and total self-efficacy with regard to their target behavior.

Dealing with Relapse

People seldom progress through the stages of change in a straightforward, linear way; rather, they tend to move to a certain stage and then slip back to a previous stage before resuming their forward progress. Research suggests that most people make several attempts before they successfully change a behavior; four out of five people experience some degree of backsliding. For this reason, the stages of change are best conceptualized as a spiral, in which people cycle back through previous stages but are further along in the process each time they renew their commitment (Figure 1.6).

If you experience a lapse—a single slip—or a relapse—a return to old habits—don't give up. Relapse can be demoralizing, but it is not the same as failure; failure means stopping before you reach your goal and never changing your target behavior. During the early stages of the change process, it's a good idea to plan for relapse so you can avoid guilt and self-blame and get back on track quickly. Follow these steps:

1. *Forgive yourself.* A single setback isn't the end of the world, but abandoning your efforts to change could have negative effects on your life.

2. *Give yourself credit for the progress you have already made.* You can use that success as motivation to continue.

3. *Move on.* You can learn from a relapse and use that knowledge to deal with potential setbacks in the future.

If relapses keep occurring or if you can't seem to control them, you may need to return to a previous stage of the behavior change process. If this is necessary, reevaluate your goals and your strategy. A different or less stressful approach may help you avoid setbacks when you try again.

Developing Skills for Change: Creating a Personalized Plan

Once you are committed to making a change, it's time to put together a plan of action. Your key to success is a well-thought-out plan that sets goals, anticipates problems, and includes rewards.

1. Monitor Your Behavior and Gather Data   Keep a record of your target behavior and the circumstances surrounding it. Record this information for at least a week or

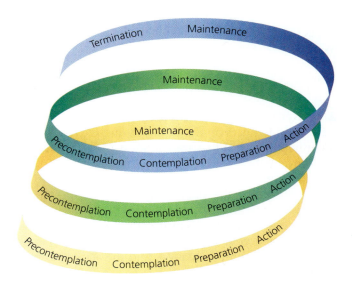

FIGURE 1.6   The stages of change: A spiral model.

SOURCE: Adapted from Prochaska, J. O., C. C. Diclemente, and J. C. Norcross. 1992. In search of how people change. *American Psychologist* 47(9): 1102–1114.

Date	November 5				Day	M	TU	W	TH	F	SA	SU		

Time of day	M/S	Food eaten	Cals.	H	Where did you eat?	What else were you doing?	How did someone else influence you?	What made you want to eat what you did?	Emotions and feelings?	Thoughts and concerns?
7:30	M	1 C Crispix cereal 1/2 C skim milk coffee, black 1 C orange juice	110 40 — 120	3	home	reading newspaper	alone	I always eat cereal in the morning	a little keyed up & worried	thinking about quiz in class today
10:30	S	1 apple	90	1	hall outside classroom	studying	alone	felt tired & wanted to wake up	tired	worried about next class
12:30	M	1 C chili 1 roll 1 pat butter 1 orange, 2 oatmeal cookies 1 soda	290 120 35 60 120 150	2	campus food court	talking	eating w/ friends; we decided to eat at the food court	wanted to be part of group	excited and happy	interested in hearing everyone's plans for the weekend
	M/S = Meal or snack				H = Hunger rating (0–3)					

FIGURE 1.7 Sample health journal entries. Visit the Online Learning Center for examples of health journal formats focusing on other target behaviors.

two. Keep your notes in a health journal or notebook or on your computer (see the sample journal entries in Figure 1.7). Record each occurrence of your behavior, noting the following:

- What the activity was
- When and where it happened
- What you were doing
- How you felt at that time

If your goal is to start an exercise program, track your activities to determine how to make time for workouts. A blank log is provided in Activity 3 in the Behavior Change Workbook at the end of this text, and sample logs for a variety of target behaviors can be found on the Online Learning Center.

2. Analyze the Data and Identify Patterns After you have collected data on the behavior, analyze the data to identify patterns. When are you most likely to overeat? What events trigger your appetite? Perhaps you are especially hungry at midmorning or when you put off eating dinner until 9:00. Perhaps you overindulge in food and drink when you go to a particular restaurant or when you're with certain friends. Note the connections between your feelings and such external cues as time of day, location, situation, and the actions of others around you.

3. Be "SMART" About Setting Goals If your goals are too challenging, you will have trouble making steady progress and will be more likely to give up altogether. If,

for example, you are in poor physical condition, it will not make sense to set a goal of being ready to run a marathon within 2 months. If you set goals you can live with, it will be easier to stick with your behavior change plan and be successful.

Experts suggest that your goals meet the "SMART" criteria; that is, your behavior change goals should be:

- *Specific:* Avoid vague goals like "eat more fruits and vegetables." Instead, state your objectives in specific terms, such as "eat 2 cups of fruit and 3 cups of vegetables every day."

- *Measurable.* Recognize that your progress will be easier to track if your goals are quantifiable, so give your goal a number. You might measure your goal in terms of time (such as "walk briskly for 20 minutes a day"), distance ("run 2 miles, 3 days per week"), or some other amount ("drink 8 glasses of water every day").

- *Attainable.* Set goals that are within your physical limits. For example, if you are a poor swimmer, it might not be possible for you to meet a short-term fitness goal by swimming laps. Walking or biking might be better options.

- *Realistic.* Manage your expectations when you set goals. For example, it may not be possible for a long-time smoker to quit cold turkey. A more realistic approach might be to use nicotine-replacement patches or gum for several weeks while getting help from a support group.

- *Time frame–specific.* Give yourself a reasonable amount of time to reach your goal, state the time frame in your behavior change plan, and set your agenda to meet the goal within the given time frame.

Using these criteria, a sedentary person who wanted to improve his health and build fitness might set a goal of being able to run 3 miles in 30 minutes, to be achieved within a time frame of 6 months. To work toward that goal, he might set a number of smaller, intermediate goals that are easier to achieve. For example, his list of goals might look like this:

Week	Frequency (days/week)	Activity	Duration (minutes)
1	3	Walk < 1 mile	10–15
2	3	Walk 1 mile	15–20
3	4	Walk 1–2 miles	20–25
4	4	Walk 2–3 miles	25–30
5–7	3–4	Walk/run 1 mile	15–20
⋮			
21–24	4–5	Run 2–3 miles	25–30

Your environment contains powerful cues for both positive and negative lifestyle choices. Identifying and using the healthier options available to you throughout the day is a key part of a successful behavior change program.

Of course, it may not be possible to meet these goals, but you never know until you try. As you work toward meeting your long-term goal, you may find it necessary to adjust your short-term goals. For example, you may find that you can start running sooner than you thought, or you may be able to run farther than you originally estimated. In such cases, it may be reasonable to make your goals more challenging. Otherwise, you may want to make them easier in order to stay motivated.

For some goals and situations, it may make more sense to focus on something other than your outcome goal. If you are in an early stage of change, for example, your goal may be to learn more about the risks associated with your target behavior or to complete a cost-benefit analysis. If your goal involves a long-term lifestyle change, such as reaching a healthy weight, it is better to focus on developing healthy habits than to target a specific weight loss. Your goal in this case might be exercising for 30 minutes every day, reducing portion sizes, or eliminating late-night snacks.

4. Devise a Plan of Action

Develop a strategy that will support your efforts to change. Your plan of action should include the following steps:

• **Get what you need.** Identify resources that can help you. For example, you can join a community walking club or sign up for smoking cessation program. You may also need to buy some new running shoes or nicotine-replacement patches. Get the items you need right away; waiting can delay your progress.

• **Modify your environment.** If there are cues in your environment that trigger your target behavior, try to control them. For example, if you normally have alcohol at home, getting rid of it can help prevent you from indulging. If you usually study with a group of friends in an environment that allows smoking, try moving to a nonsmoking area. If you always buy a snack at a certain vending machine, change your route so you don't pass by it.

• **Control related habits.** You may have habits that contribute to your target behavior; modifying these habits can help change the behavior. For example, if you usually plop down on the sofa while watching TV, try putting an exercise bike in front of the set so you can burn calories while watching your favorite programs.

• **Reward yourself.** Giving yourself instant, real rewards for good behavior will reinforce your efforts. Plan your rewards; decide in advance what each one will be and how you will earn it. Tie rewards to achieving specific goals or subgoals. For example, you might treat yourself to a movie after a week of avoiding snacks. Make a list of items or events to use as rewards; they should be special to you and preferably unrelated to food or alcohol.

• **Involve the people around you.** Tell family and friends about your plan, and ask them to help. To help them respond appropriately to your needs, create a specific list of dos and don'ts. For example, ask them to support you when you set aside time to exercise or avoid second helpings at dinner.

• **Plan for challenges.** Think about situations and people that might derail your program, and develop ways to cope with them. For example, if you think it will be hard to stick to your usual exercise program during exams, schedule short bouts of physical activity (such as a brisk walk) as stress-reducing study breaks.

5. Make a Personal Contract A serious personal contract—one that commits you to your word—can result in a higher chance of follow-through than a casual, offhand promise. Your contract can help prevent procrastination by specifying important dates and can also serve as a reminder of your personal commitment to change.

Your contract should include a statement of your goal and your commitment to reaching it. The contract should also include details, such as the following:

- The date you will start
- The steps you will take to measure your progress
- The strategies you plan to use to promote change
- The date you expect to reach your final goal

Have someone—preferably someone who will be actively helping you with your program—sign your contract as a witness.

Figure 1.8 shows a sample behavior change contract for someone who is committing to eating more fruit every day. Additional sample plans and contracts for other target behaviors can be found on the *Fit and Well* Online Learning Center, and a blank contract is included as Activity 8 in the Behavior Change Workbook and on the Online Learning Center.

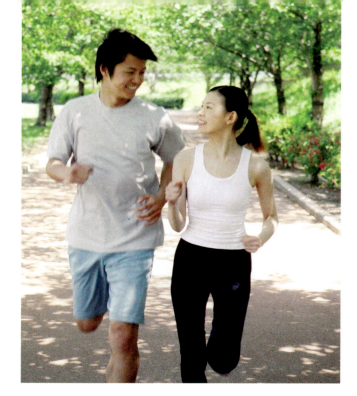

A beautiful setting and a friendly companion help make exercise a satisfying and pleasurable experience. Choosing the right activity and doing it the right way are important elements in a successful behavior change program.

Behavior Change Contract

1. I, _Tammy Lau_, agree to _increase my consumption of fruit from 1 cup per week to 2 cups per day._
2. I will begin on ___10/5___ and plan to reach my goal of _2 cups of fruit per day_ by _12/7_
3. To reach my final goal, I have devised the following schedule of mini-goals. For each step in my program, I will give myself the reward listed.

   I will begin to have ½ cup of fruit with breakfast ___10/5___ _see movie_

   I will begin to have ½ cup of fruit with lunch ___10/26___ _new cd_

   I will begin to substitute fruit juice for soda 1 time per day ___11/16___ _concert_

   My overall reward for reaching my goal will be _trip to beach_
4. I have gathered and analyzed data on my target behavior and have identified the following strategies for changing my behavior: _Keep the fridge stocked with easy-to-carry fruit. Pack fruit in my backpack every day. Buy lunch at place that serves fruit._
5. I will use the following tools to monitor my progress toward my final goal: _Chart on fridge door_ _Health journal_

   I sign this contract as an indication of my personal commitment to reach my goal: _Tammy Lau_ _9/28_

   I have recruited a helper who will witness my contract and _also increase his consumption of fruit; eat lunch with me twice a week._ _Eric March_ _9/28_

FIGURE 1.8 A sample behavior change contract.

Putting Your Plan into Action

The starting date has arrived, and you are ready to put your plan into action. This stage requires commitment, the resolve to stick with the plan no matter what temptations you encounter. Remember all the reasons you have to make the change—and remember that *you* are the boss. Use all your strategies to make your plan work. Make sure your environment is change-friendly, and get as much support and encouragement from others as possible. Keep track of your progress in your health journal, and give yourself regular rewards. And don't forget to give yourself a pat on the back—congratulate yourself, notice how much better you look or feel, and feel good about how far you've come and how you've gained control of your behavior.

Staying with It

As you continue with your program, don't be surprised when you run up against obstacles; they're inevitable. In fact, it's a good idea to expect problems and give yourself time to step back, see how you're doing, and make some changes before going on. If your program is grinding to a halt, identify what is blocking your progress. It may come from one of the sources described in the following sections.

Social Influences Take a hard look at the reactions of the people you're counting on, and see if they're really supporting you. If they come up short, connect with others who will be more supportive.

A related trap is trying to get your friends or family members to change *their* behaviors. The decision to make a major behavior change is something people come to only after intensive self-examination. You may be able to influence someone by tactfully providing facts or support, but that's all. Focus on yourself. When you succeed, you may become a role model for others.

Levels of Motivation and Commitment You won't make real progress until an inner drive leads you to the stage of change at which you are ready to make a personal commitment to the goal. If commitment is your problem, you may need to wait until the behavior you're dealing with makes you unhappier or unhealthier; then your desire to change it will be stronger. Or you may find that changing your goal will inspire you to keep going. For more ideas, refer to the box "Motivation Booster" and to Activity 9 in the Behavior Change Workbook.

Choice of Techniques and Level of Effort If your plan is not working as well as you thought it would, make changes where you're having the most trouble. If you've lagged on your running schedule, for example, maybe it's because you don't like running. An aerobics class might suit you better. There are many ways to move toward your goal. Or you may not be trying hard enough. You do have to push toward your goal. If it were easy, you wouldn't need a plan.

> ### ! MOTIVATION BOOSTER
>
> *Be patient with yourself.* Behavior change is like many other challenges you'll encounter at school and work—it requires that you develop certain skills. Just as when you take a course in an unfamiliar subject, you shouldn't expect to master everything in your behavior change program quickly and easily or to achieve perfection. But with consistent effort, you can build your skills and achieve your goals. Think of obstacles as challenges to your skills that require effort to address but that are within your ability to manage. Thinking of behavior change in this way will help you tolerate mistakes and lapses, remain motivated, and see your behavior change program as an opportunity for personal growth and improvement.

Stress Barrier If you hit a wall in your program, look at the sources of stress in your life. If the stress is temporary, such as catching a cold or having a term paper due, you may want to wait until it passes before strengthening your efforts. If the stress is ongoing, find healthy ways to manage it (see Chapter 10). You may even want to make stress management your highest priority for behavior change.

Procrastinating, Rationalizing, and Blaming Be alert to games you might be playing with yourself, so you can stop them. Such games include the following:

- *Procrastinating.* If you tell yourself, "It's Friday already; I might as well wait until Monday to start," you're procrastinating. Break your plan into smaller steps that you can accomplish one day at a time.
- *Rationalizing.* If you tell yourself, "I wanted to go swimming today but wouldn't have had time to wash my hair afterward," you're making excuses. When you "win" by deceiving yourself, it isn't much of a victory.
- *Blaming.* If you tell yourself, "I couldn't exercise because Dave was hogging the elliptical trainer," you're blaming others for your own failure to follow through. Blaming is a way of taking your focus off the real problem and denying responsibility for your own actions.

Being Fit and Well for Life

Your first attempts at making behavior changes may never go beyond the contemplation or preparation stage. Those that do may not all succeed. But as you experience some success, you'll start to have more positive feelings about yourself. You may discover new physical activities and sports you enjoy; you may encounter new situations and meet new people. Perhaps you'll surprise yourself by accomplishing things you didn't think were possible—breaking a long-standing nicotine habit, competing in a race, climbing a mountain, or developing a lean, muscular body. Most of all, you'll discover the feeling of empowerment that comes from taking charge of your health. Being healthy takes extra effort, but the paybacks in energy and vitality are priceless.

Once you've started, don't stop. Assume that health improvement is forever. Take on the easier problems first, and then use what you learn to tackle more difficult problems later. When you feel challenged, remind yourself that you are creating a lifestyle that minimizes your health risks and maximizes your enjoyment of life. You *can* take charge of your health in a dramatic and meaningful way. *Fit and Well* will show you how.

> ### QUESTIONS FOR CRITICAL THINKING AND REFLECTION
>
>
> Think about the last time you made an unhealthy choice instead of a healthy one. How could you have changed the situation, the people in the situation, or your own thoughts, feelings, or intentions to avoid making that choice? What can you do in similar situations in the future to produce a different outcome?

TIPS FOR TODAY AND THE FUTURE

You are in charge of your health. Many of the decisions you make every day have an impact on the quality of your life, both now and in the future. By making positive choices, large and small, you help ensure a lifetime of wellness.

RIGHT NOW YOU CAN

- Go for a 15-minute walk.
- Have an orange, a nectarine, or a plum for a snack.
- Call a friend and arrange for a time to catch up with each other.
- Start thinking about whether you have a health behavior you'd like to change. If you do, consider the elements of a behavior change strategy. For example, begin a mental list of the pros and cons of the behavior, or talk to someone who can support you in your attempts to change.

IN THE FUTURE YOU CAN

- Stay current on health- and wellness-related news and issues.
- Participate in health awareness and promotion campaigns in your community—for example, support smoking restrictions in local venues.
- Be a role model for someone else who is working on a health behavior you have successfully changed.

SUMMARY

- Wellness is the ability to live life fully, with vitality and meaning. Wellness is dynamic and multidimensional; it incorporates physical, emotional, intellectual, spiritual, interpersonal, and environmental dimensions.

- People today have greater control over and greater responsibility for their health than ever before.

- Behaviors that promote wellness include being physically active; choosing a healthy diet; maintaining a healthy body weight; managing stress effectively; avoiding tobacco and limiting alcohol use; and protecting yourself from disease and injury.

- Although heredity, environment, and health care all play roles in wellness and disease, behavior can mitigate their effects.

- To make lifestyle changes, you need information about yourself, your health habits, and resources available to help you change.

- You can increase your motivation for behavior change by examining the benefits and costs of change, boosting self-efficacy, and identifying and overcoming key barriers to change.

- The stages-of-change model describes six stages that people may move through as they try to change their behavior: precontemplation, contemplation, preparation, action, maintenance, and termination.

- A specific plan for change can be developed by (1) collecting data on your behavior and recording it in a journal; (2) analyzing the recorded data; (3) setting specific goals; (4) devising strategies for obtaining information, modifying the environment, rewarding yourself, involving others, and planning ahead; and (5) making a personal contract.

- To start and maintain a behavior change program, you need commitment, a well-developed and manageable plan, social support, and strong stress-management techniques. It is also important to monitor the progress of your program, revising it as necessary.

FOR FURTHER EXPLORATION

BOOKS

American Medical Association. 2006. *American Medical Association Concise Medical Encyclopedia.* New York: Random House. *Includes more than 3000 entries on health and wellness topics, symptoms, conditions, and treatments.*

Elghoroury, M. 2006. *How to Get the Most from Your Doctor's Visit.* Charleston, S.C.: BookSurge. *A doctor's advice for getting the greatest benefit from time spent with a physician, including visits for both sickness and wellness.*

Komaroff, A. L., ed. 2005. *Harvard Medical School Family Health Guide.* New York: Free Press. *Provides consumer-oriented advice for the prevention and treatment of common health concerns.*

Krueger, H., et al. 2007. *The Health Impact of Smoking and Obesity and What to Do About It.* Toronto: University of Toronto Press. *Examines the effects of smoking and sedentary lifestyle, the costs to individuals and society, and strategies for overcoming these behaviors.*

Prochaska, J. O., J. C. Norcross, and C. C. DiClemente. 1994. *Changing for Good: The Revolutionary Program That Explains the Six Stages of Change and Teaches You How to Free Yourself from Bad Habits.* New York: Morrow. *Outlines the authors' model of behavior change and offers suggestions and advice for each stage of change.*

Smith P. B., M. MacFarlane, and E. Kalnitsky. 2002. *The Complete Idiot's Guide to Wellness.* Indianapolis, Ind.: Alpha Books. *A concise guide to healthy habits, including physical activity, nutrition, and stress management.*

U.S. Government. 2007. *2007 American Health and Medical Encyclopedia: Authoritative, Practical Guide to Health and Wellness. FDA, CDC, NIH, Surgeon General Publications (CD-ROM).* Washington, D.C.: Progressive Management. *Contains thousands of documents from various federal agencies on myriad health issues, as well as links to dozens of health- and wellness-related Web sites.*

NEWSLETTERS

Center for Science in the Public Interest Nutrition Action Health Letter (http://www.cspinet.org/nah/index.htm)

Consumer Reports on Health (800-234-2188;
  http://www.consumerreports.org/oh/index.htm)
Harvard Health Letter (877-649-9457;
  http://www.health.harvard.edu)
Harvard Men's Health Watch (877-649-9457)
Harvard Women's Health Watch (877-649-9457)
Mayo Clinic Housecall;
  http://www.mayoclinic.com/health/housecall/HouseCall)
Tufts University Health & Nutrition Newsletter (800-274-7581;
  http://healthletter.tufts.edu)
University of California at Berkeley Wellness Letter (800-829-9170;
  http://www.wellnessletter.com)

ORGANIZATIONS, HOTLINES, AND WEB SITES

The Internet addresses listed here were accurate at the time of publication. Up-to-date links to these and many other wellness-oriented Web sites are provided on the links page of the *Fit and Well* Online Learning Center (http://www.mhhe.com/fahey).

Centers for Disease Control and Prevention. Provides a wide variety of health information.
  800-311-3435
  http://www.cdc.gov

Many other government sites provide health-related materials:
  Federal Trade Commission: Consumer Protection—Diet, Health, and Fitness:
    http://www.ftc.gov/bcp/menus/consumer/health.shtm
  First Gov for Consumers—Health:
    http://www.consumer.gov/health.htm
  MedlinePlus: http://www.medlineplus.gov
  National Institutes of Health: http://www.nih.gov

Go Ask Alice. Sponsored by the Columbia University Health Service; provides answers to student questions about stress, sexuality, fitness, and many other wellness topics.
  http://www.goaskalice.columbia.edu

Healthfinder. A gateway to online publications, Web sites, support and self-help groups, and agencies and organizations that produce reliable health information.
  http://www.healthfinder.gov

Healthy People 2010. Provides information on Healthy People objectives and priority areas.
  http://www.healthypeople.gov

MedlinePlus: Evaluating Health Information. Provides background information and links to sites with guidelines for finding and evaluating health information on the Web.
  http://www.nlm.nih.gov/medlineplus/
  evaluatinghealthinformation.html

National Health Information Center (NHIC). Puts consumers in touch with the organizations that are best able to provide answers to health-related questions.
  800-336-4797
  http://www.health.gov/nhic

National Women's Health Information Center. Provides information and answers to frequently asked questions.
  800-994-9662
  http://www.4woman.gov

Student Counseling Virtual Pamphlet Collection. Provides links to more than 400 pamphlets produced by different student counseling centers on a variety of wellness topics.
  http://counseling.uchicago.edu/vpc

World Health Organization (WHO). Provides information about health topics and issues affecting people around the world.
  http://www.who.int

The following are just a few of the many sites that provide consumer-oriented information on a variety of health issues:
  Family Doctor.Org: http://www.familydoctor.org
  InteliHealth: http://www.intelihealth.com
  Mayo Clinic: http://www.mayoclinic.com
  WebMD: http://webmd.com

The following sites provide daily health news updates:
  CNN Health: http://www.cnn.com/health
  MedlinePlus News: http://www.nlm.nih.gov/medlineplus/
    newsbydate.html
  Yahoo Health News: http://news.yahoo.com/i/751

SELECTED BIBLIOGRAPHY

American Cancer Society. 2007. *Cancer Facts and Figures 2007.* Atlanta: American Cancer Society.

American College Health Association. 2007. American College Health Association National College Health Assessment Spring 2006 Reference Group Data Report (Abridged). *Journal of American College Health* 55(4): 198.

American Heart Association. 2007. *2007 Heart and Stroke Statistical Update.* Dallas: American Heart Association.

Calle, E. E., et al. 2003. Overweight, obesity, and mortality from cancer in a prospectively studied cohort of U.S. adults. *New England Journal of Medicine* 348(17): 1625–1638.

Centers for Disease Control and Prevention. 2007. Prevalence of fruit and vegetable consumption and physical activity by race/ethnicity—United States, 2005, *Morbidity and Mortality Weekly Report* 56(13): 301–304.

Centers for Disease Control and Prevention. 2007. Prevalence of heart disease—United States, 2005. *Morbidity and Mortality Weekly Report* 56(6): 113–118.

Centers for Disease Control and Prevention. 2007. QuickStats: Prevalence of selected unhealthy behavior characteristics among adults Aged ≥ 18 years, by race—National Health Interview Survey, United States, 2002–2004. *Morbidity and Mortality Weekly Report* 56(04): 79.

Centers for Disease Control and Prevention. 2005. Annual smoking-attributable mortality, years of potential life lost, and productivity losses—United States, 1997–2001. *Morbidity and Mortality Weekly Report* 54(5): 113–117.

Centers for Disease Control and Prevention. 2005. Racial/ethnic and socioeconomic disparities in multiple risk factors for heart disease and stroke, United States, 2003. *Morbidity and Mortality Weekly Report* 54(5): 113–117.

Centers for Disease Control and Prevention. 2005. Trends in leisure-time physical inactivity by age, sex, and race/ethnicity—United States, 1994–2004. *Morbidity and Mortality Weekly Report* 54(39): 991–994.

Centers for Disease Control and Prevention. 2006. Health behaviors of adults: United States, 2002–2004. *Vital and Health Statistics* 10(230).

Centers for Disease Control and Prevention, Division of Nutrition and Physical Activity. 1999. *Promoting Physical Activity: A Guide for Community Action.* Champaign, Ill.: Human Kinetics.

Douglas, K. A., et al. 1997. Results from the 1995 National College Health Risk Behavior Survey. *Journal of American College Health* 46(2): 55–56.

Gallagher, K. I., and J. M. Jakicic. 2002. Overcoming barriers to effective exercise programming. *ACSM's Health and Fitness Journal,* November/December.

Glanz, K., B. K. Rimer, and F. M. Lewis, eds. 2002. *Health Behavior and Health Education: Theory, Research, and Practice,* 3rd ed. San Francisco: Jossey-Bass.

Marcus, B. H., and L. H. Forsyth. 2003. *Motivating People to Be Physically Active.* Champaign, Ill.: Human Kinetics.

McCracken, M., et al. 2007. Health behaviors of the young adult U.S. population: Behavioral risk factor surveillance system, 2003. *Preventing Chronic Disease* 4(2): A25.

Mokdad, A. H., et al. 2005. Correction: Actual causes of death in the United States, 2000. *Journal of the American Medical Association* 293(3): 293–294.

Ritchie, S. A., and J. M. Connell. 2007. The link between abdominal obesity, metabolic syndrome and cardiovascular disease. *Nutrition, Metabolism, and Cardiovascular Diseases* 17(4): 319–326.

Seals, J. G. 2007. Integrating the transtheoretical model into the management of overweight and obese adults. *Journal of the American Academy of Nurse Practitioners* 19(2): 63–71

Sillence, E., et al. 2007. How do patients evaluate and make use of online health information? *Social Science and Medicine* 64(9): 1853–1862.

Smith, S. C. 2007. Multiple risk factors for cardiovascular disease and diabetes mellitus. *The American Journal of Medicine* 120(3 Suppl. 1): S3–S11.

National Center for Health Statistics. 2007. *Health, United States, 2006.* Hyattsville, Md.: Public Health Service.

U.S. Department of Health and Human Services. 2000. *Healthy People 2010,* 2nd ed. Washington, D.C.: DHHS.

LAB 1.1 Your Wellness Profile

Consider how your lifestyle, attitudes, and characteristics relate to each of the six dimensions of wellness. Fill in your strengths for each dimension (examples of strengths are listed with each dimension). Once you've completed your lists, choose what you believe are your five most important strengths, and circle them.

Physical wellness: To maintain overall physical health and engage in appropriate physical activity (e.g., stamina, strength, flexibility, healthy body composition).

_____

_____

_____

Emotional wellness: To have a positive self-concept, deal constructively with your feelings, and develop positive qualities (e.g., optimism, trust, self-confidence, determination, persistence, dedication).

_____

_____

_____

Intellectual wellness: To pursue and retain knowledge, think critically about issues, make sound decisions, identify problems, and find solutions (e.g., common sense, creativity, curiosity).

_____

_____

_____

Spiritual wellness: To develop a set of beliefs, principles, or values that gives meaning or purpose to your life; to develop faith in something beyond yourself (e.g., religious faith, service to others).

_____

_____

_____

Interpersonal/social wellness: To develop and maintain meaningful relationships with a network of friends and family members, and to contribute to your community (e.g., friendly, good-natured, compassionate, supportive, good listener).

_____

_____

_____

Environmental wellness: To protect yourself from environmental hazards and to minimize the negative impact of your behavior on the environment (e.g., carpooling, recycling).

_____

_____

_____

Next, think about where you fall on the wellness continuum for each of the dimensions of wellness. Indicate your placement for each—physical, emotional, intellectual, spiritual, interpersonal/social, and environmental—by placing Xs on the continuum below.

| Low level of wellness | Physical, psychological, emotional symptoms | Change and growth | High level of wellness |

LABORATORY ACTIVITIES

LABORATORY ACTIVITIES

Based on both your current lifestyle and your goals for the future, what do you think your placement on the wellness continuum will be in 10 years? What new health behaviors will you have to adopt to achieve your goals? Which of your current behaviors will you need to change to maintain or improve your level of wellness in the future?

Does the description of wellness given in this chapter encompass everything you believe is part of wellness for you? Write your own definition of wellness, including any additional dimensions that are important to you. Then rate your level of wellness based on your own definition.

Using Your Results

How did you score? Are you satisfied with your current level of wellness—overall and in each dimension? In which dimension(s) would you most like to increase your level of wellness?

What should you do next? As you consider possible target behaviors for a behavior change program, choose things that will maintain or increase your level of wellness in one of the dimensions you listed as an area of concern. Remember to consider health behaviors such as smoking or eating a high-fat diet that may threaten your level of wellness in the future. Below, list several possible target behaviors and the wellness dimensions that they influence.

For additional guidance in choosing a target behavior, complete the lifestyle self-assessment in Lab 1.2.

LAB 1.2 Lifestyle Evaluation

How does your current lifestyle compare with the lifestyle recommended for wellness? For each question, choose the answer that best describes your behavior; then add up your score for each section.

Exercise/Fitness

	Almost Always	Sometimes	Never
1. I engage in moderate exercise, such as brisk walking or swimming, for 20–60 minutes, three to five times a week.	4	1	0
2. I do exercises to develop muscular strength and endurance at least twice a week.	2	1	0
3. I spend some of my leisure time participating in individual, family, or team activities, such as gardening, bowling, or softball.	2	1	0
4. I maintain a healthy body weight, avoiding overweight and underweight.	2	1	0

Exercise/Fitness Score: _____

Nutrition

	Almost Always	Sometimes	Never
1. I eat a variety of foods each day, including seven or more servings of fruits and/or vegetables.	3	1	0
2. I limit the amount of total fat and saturated and trans fat in my diet.	3	1	0
3. I avoid skipping meals.	2	1	0
4. I limit the amount of salt and sugar I eat.	2	1	0

Nutrition Score: _____

Tobacco Use

If you never or no longer use tobacco, enter a score of 10 for this section and go to the next section.

	Almost Always	Sometimes	Never
1. I avoid using tobacco.	2	1	0
2. I smoke only low-tar-and-nicotine cigarettes, *or* I smoke a pipe or cigars, *or* I use smokeless tobacco.	2	1	0

Tobacco Use Score: _____

Alcohol and Drugs

	Almost Always	Sometimes	Never
1. I avoid alcohol, or I drink no more than one (women) or two (men) drinks a day.	4	1	0
2. I avoid using alcohol or other drugs as a way of handling stressful situations or the problems in my life.	2	1	0
3. I am careful not to drink alcohol when taking medications (such as cold or allergy medications) or when pregnant.	2	1	0
4. I read and follow the label directions when using prescribed and over-the-counter drugs.	2	1	0

Alcohol and Drugs Score: _____

Emotional Health

	Almost Always	Sometimes	Never
1. I enjoy being a student, and I have a job or do other work that I enjoy.	2	1	0
2. I find it easy to relax and express my feelings freely.	2	1	0
3. I manage stress well.	2	1	0
4. I have close friends, relatives, or others whom I can talk to about personal matters and call on for help when needed.	2	1	0
5. I participate in group activities (such as community or church organizations) or hobbies that I enjoy.	2	1	0

Emotional Health Score: _____

Safety

1. I wear a safety belt while riding in a car.	2	1	0
2. I avoid driving while under the influence of alcohol or other drugs.	2	1	0
3. I obey traffic rules and the speed limit when driving.	2	1	0
4. I read and follow instructions on the labels of potentially harmful products or substances, such as household cleaners, poisons, and electrical appliances.	2	1	0
5. I avoid smoking in bed.	2	1	0

Safety Score: _____

Disease Prevention

1. I know the warning signs of cancer, heart attack, and stroke.	2	1	0
2. I avoid overexposure to the sun and use sunscreen.	2	1	0
3. I get recommended medical screening tests (such as blood pressure and cholesterol checks and Pap tests), immunizations, and booster shots.	2	1	0
4. I practice monthly skin and breast/testicle self-exams.	2	1	0
5. I am not sexually active, *or* I have sex with only one mutually faithful, uninfected partner, *or* I always engage in safer sex (using condoms), *and* I do not share needles to inject drugs.	2	1	0

Disease Prevention Score: _____

Scores of 9 and 10 Excellent! Your answers show that you are aware of the importance of this area to your health. More important, you are putting your knowledge to work for you by practicing good health habits. As long as you continue to do so, this area should not pose a serious health risk.

Scores of 6 to 8 Your health practices in this area are good, but there is room for improvement.

Scores of 3 to 5 Your health risks are showing.

Scores of 0 to 2 You may be taking serious and unnecessary risks with your health.

Using Your Results

How did you score? In which areas did you score the lowest? Are you satisfied with your scores in each area? In which areas would you most like to improve your scores?

What should you do next? To improve your scores, look closely at any item to which you answered "sometimes" or "never." Identify and list at least three possible targets for a health behavior change program. (If you are aware of other risky health behaviors you currently engage in, but which were not covered by this assessment, you may include those in your list.) For each item on your list, identify your current "stage of change" and one strategy you could adopt to move forward (see pp. 13–15). Possible strategies might be obtaining information about the behavior, completing an analysis of the pros and cons of change, or beginning a written record of your target behavior.

Behavior	Stage	Strategy
1. _____	_____	_____
2. _____	_____	_____
3. _____	_____	_____

SOURCE: Adapted from *Healthstyle: A Self-Test,* developed by the U.S. Public Health Service. The behaviors covered in this test are recommended for most Americans, but some may not apply to people with certain chronic diseases or disabilities or to pregnant women, who may require special advice from their physician.

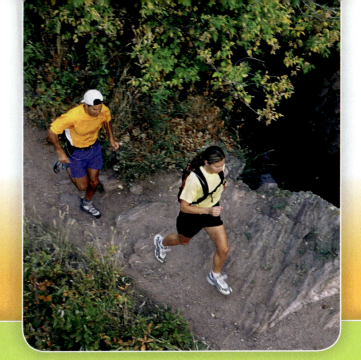

LOOKING AHEAD >>>>>

**AFTER READING THIS CHAPTER,
YOU SHOULD BE ABLE TO:**

- Describe how much physical activity is recommended for developing health and fitness
- Identify the components of physical fitness and the way each component affects wellness
- Explain the goal of physical training and the basic principles of training
- Describe the principles involved in designing a well-rounded exercise program
- Discuss the steps that can be taken to make an exercise program safe, effective, and successful

PRINCIPLES OF PHYSICAL FITNESS

2

TEST YOUR KNOWLEDGE

1. **To improve your health, you must exercise vigorously for at least 30 minutes straight, 5 or more days per week.**

   True or false?

2. **Among American adults, about what percentage of trips of less than 1 mile long are made by walking?**

   a. 15%
   b. 25%
   c. 50%

3. **If all inactive American adults became physically active, the savings in direct costs for medical care would be about _____ per year.**

   a. $75 million
   b. $7.5 billion
   c. $75 billion

ANSWERS

1. **FALSE.** Experts recommend about 30 minutes of moderate physical activity 5 or more days per week, but activity can be done in short bouts—10-minute sessions, for example—spread out over the course of the day.

2. **a.** The vast majority of short trips are made in cars. On average, Americans spend 100 minutes per day driving and 170 minutes per day watching television. Most people have many opportunities to incorporate more moderate physical activity into their daily routine.

3. **c.** People who engage in regular physical activity make fewer physician visits, use less medication, and have fewer hospital stays than physically inactive people. Nearly 25% of health care charges are linked to physical inactivity and obesity.

FIT AND WELL ONLINE LEARNING CENTER www.mhhe.com/fahey

Visit the *Fit and Well* Online Learning Center for resources that will help you get the most out of your course!
- Study and review aids include practice quizzes, glossary flashcards, chapter summaries, learning objectives, PowerPoint presentations, Common Questions Answered, student handouts, crossword puzzles, Internet activities, and links to wellness Web sites.
- Behavior change tools include a daily fitness and nutrition journal, a behavior change workbook, sample behavior change plans, and blank behavior change logs to print and use.

A ny list of the benefits of physical activity is impressive. Although people vary greatly in the levels of physical fitness and performance they can ultimately achieve, the benefits of regular physical activity are available to everyone. (For more on the benefits of exercise, see the box "Exercise and Total Wellness.")

This chapter provides an overview of physical fitness. It explains how lifestyle physical activity and more formal exercise programs contribute to wellness. It also describes the components of fitness, the basic principles of physical training, and the essential elements of a well-rounded exercise program. Chapters 3–6 provide an in-depth look at each of the elements of a fitness program; Chapter 7 will help you put all these elements together into a complete, personalized program.

PHYSICAL ACTIVITY AND EXERCISE FOR HEALTH AND FITNESS

Despite the many benefits of an active lifestyle, levels of physical activity remain low for all populations of Americans (Figure 2.1). The Centers for Disease Control and Prevention (CDC) recently reported the following statistics about the physical activity levels of adult Americans:

- About 48% participate in some leisure-time physical activity, including 50% of men and 47% of women.

- Between 2001 and 2005, physical activity levels increased slightly among all age and ethnic groups, with the exception of Hispanic males.

The study also shows that education is an important factor in activity levels. For example, 54% of college graduates report doing some type of physical activity compared to 37% of high school dropouts.

Other studies show that only about 12% of Americans exercise intensively at least five times per week, and 25% do some leisure-time strength training.

Why aren't more Americans active? Possible barriers include lack of time and resources, social and environmental influences, and—most important—lack of motivation and commitment (see Lab 2.2 for more on barriers). Some people also fear injury. Although physical activity does carry some risks, the risks of inactivity are far greater. Evidence is growing that for most Americans, becoming more physically active may be the single most important lifestyle change for promoting health and well-being.

Physical Activity on a Continuum

Physical activity is any body movement carried out by the skeletal muscles and requiring energy. Different types of physical activity can be arranged on a continuum based on the amount of energy they require. Quick, easy movements such as standing up or walking down a hallway

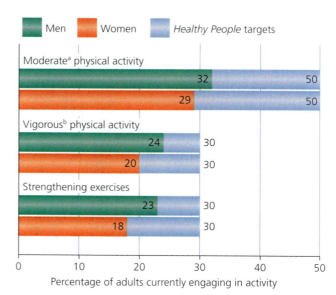

VITAL STATISTICS

FIGURE 2.1   Current levels of physical activity among American adults.

SOURCES: National Center for Health Statistics. 2007. *DATA2010: The Healthy People 2010 Database*, October 2007 Edition (http://wonder.cdc.gov/data2010; retrieved November 5, 2007). National Center for Health Statistics. 2006. Health Behavior of Adults: United States, 2002–04. *Vital and Health Statistics* 10 (230).

require little energy or effort; more intense, sustained activities such as cycling 5 miles or running in a race require considerably more.

Exercise refers to a subset of physical activity—planned, structured, repetitive movement of the body intended specifically to improve or maintain physical fitness. As discussed in Chapter 1, physical fitness is a set of physical attributes that allows the body to respond or adapt to the demands and stress of physical effort—to perform moderate-to-vigorous levels of physical activity without becoming overly tired. Levels of fitness depend on such physiological factors as the heart's ability to pump blood and the size of muscle fibers. These factors are a function both of genetics—a person's inborn potential for physical fitness—and of behavior—the amount of exercise a person does to improve fitness. To develop fitness, a person must perform enough physical activity to stress the body and cause long-term physiological changes.

Physical activity is essential to health and confers wide-ranging health benefits, but exercise is necessary to significantly improve physical fitness. This important distinction between physical activity, which improves health and wellness, and exercise, which improves fitness, is a key concept in understanding the guidelines discussed in this section.

Increasing Physical Activity to Improve Health and Wellness   In 1996, the U.S. Surgeon General issued

Exercise and Total Wellness

As you will see throughout this chapter, an active lifestyle provides a multitude of benefits. For example, physically active adults live from 2 to 4 years longer, on average, than do sedentary adults. The benefits of regular physical activity, however, go beyond longevity. They impact quality of life across multiple dimensions of wellness.

Physical Wellness

In terms of general health, exercise increases your physical capacity so that you are better able to meet the challenges of daily life with energy and vigor. Physical activity can help you do the following:

- Generate more energy.
- Increase your stamina.
- Control your weight.
- Manage stress.
- Boost your immune system.

Over the long term, even moderate physical activity can help you avoid illnesses such as heart disease, diabetes, high blood pressure, depression, osteoporosis, and some cancers. Evidence shows that exercise can even prevent premature death from several causes.

Emotional Wellness

Exercise provides psychological and emotional benefits, contributing to your sense of competence and well-being. People who focus on staying active can also enjoy an improved self-

image and a higher level of self-confidence. Such healthy self-esteem can positively affect other aspects of your life, as well. For example, a good self-image can be helpful when dealing with others or when competing.

Intellectual Wellness

Recent studies indicate that regular exercise is good for the brain—literally. One study shows that brain volume actually increases in adults who exercise regularly. Such gains in brain mass (growth or replenishment of brain matter) can improve cognitive functions and the overall health of the nervous system. Additionally, the process of mastering physical challenges—such as learning a proper golf swing—can boost intellectual fitness in the same manner as solving puzzles or engaging in other learning experiences.

Interpersonal Wellness

Joining in physical activity with a friend or a group can be a boon to your interpersonal or social wellness, too. By sharing physical challenges with others, you can make new friends, deepen your existing relationships, and build a stronger overall network of support.

Physical Activity and Health, a landmark report designed to encourage Americans to become more active. One of its findings was that people can obtain significant health benefits by including a moderate amount of physical activity on most, if not all, days of the week. This finding was echoed in the 2005 Dietary Guidelines for Americans, which recommended that all adults engage in at least 30 minutes of moderate-intensity physical activity, beyond usual activity, on most days of the week, in order to improve health. The recommendation was further refined in the publication *Physical Activity and Public Health: Updated Recommendations for Adults*, published jointly by the American College of Sports Medicine (ACSM) and the American Heart Association (AHA) in 2007. This report stated that, to promote and maintain health, adults need a minimum of 30 minutes of moderate-intensity aerobic (endurance) physical activity 5 days per week or 20 minutes of vigorous-intensity aerobic physical activity 3 days per week. Research shows that these levels of physical activity promote health and wellness in specific ways: by lowering the risk of high blood pressure, stroke, heart disease, type 2 diabetes, colon cancer, and osteoporosis and by reducing feelings of mild-to-moderate depression and anxiety.

What exactly is moderate physical activity? Activities such as brisk walking, dancing, swimming, cycling, and yard work can all count toward the daily total. The Surgeon General's report defines a moderate amount of activity as activity that uses about 150 calories of energy. Examples of activities that use about 150 calories are shown in Figure 2.2 (p. 30). You can burn the same number of calories by doing a lower-intensity activity for a longer time or higher-intensity activity for a shorter time. For more examples of light, moderate, and vigorous activities, see the box "Classifying Activity Levels" (p. 31).

The 2007 ACSM/AHA report defines moderate-intensity physical activity as activity that causes a noticeable increase in heart rate, such as a brisk walk. The report defines vigorous-intensity physical activity as activity that causes rapid breathing and a substantial increase in heart rate, as exemplified by jogging. Both the Surgeon General's report and

physical activity Any body movement carried out by the skeletal muscles and requiring energy.

exercise Planned, structured, repetitive movement of the body intended to improve or maintain physical fitness.

www.mhhe.com/fahey   PHYSICAL ACTIVITY AND EXERCISE FOR HEALTH AND FITNESS   **29**

Activity	Duration (min.)	
Washing a car	45–60	**Less Vigorous, More Time**
Washing windows or floors	45–60	
Volleyball	45	
Touch football	30–45	
Gardening	30–45	
Wheeling self in wheelchair	30–40	
Walking 1¾ miles	35 (20 min/mile)	
Shooting a basketball	30	
Bicycling 5 miles	30 (6 min/mile)	
Dancing fast	30	
Pushing a stroller 1½ miles	30	
Raking leaves	30	
Walking 2 miles	30 (15 min/mile)	
Water aerobics	30	
Swimming laps	20	
Wheelchair basketball	20	
Playing a game of basketball	15–20	
Bicycling 4 miles	15 (3¾ min/mile)	
Jumping rope	15	
Running 1½ miles	15 (10 min/mile)	
Shoveling snow	15	**More Vigorous, Less Time**
Stairwalking	15	

FIGURE 2.2 Examples of moderate amounts of physical activity. Each example uses about 150 calories.

SOURCE: Department of Health and Human Services. 1996. *Physical Activity and Health: A Report of the Surgeon General.* Atlanta: DHHS.

the ACSM/AHA report also recommend that people perform strength training exercises at least twice a week to build and maintain muscular strength and endurance.

The daily total of physical activity can be accumulated in multiple bouts of 10 or more minutes—for example, two 10-minute bike rides to and from class and a brisk 10-minute walk to the store. In this lifestyle approach to physical activity, people can choose activities that they find enjoyable and that fit into their daily routine; everyday tasks at school, work, and home can be structured to contribute to the daily activity total (see the box "Making Time for Physical Activity" on p. 32). If all Americans who are currently sedentary were to increase their lifestyle physical activity to 30 minutes per day, there would be an enormous benefit to public health and to individual well-being.

Increasing Physical Activity to Manage Weight   Because two-thirds of Americans are overweight, government agencies and health organizations have also published physical activity guidelines focusing on weight management. These guidelines call for higher daily physical activity goals than the guidelines designed for more general health promotion. Table 2.1 lists recommendations for promoting health and managing weight from just a few of these organizations.

Table 2.1	Summary of Physical Activity Recommendations from Selected Leading Health Organizations	
Organization	**Recommendation**	**Purpose**
Centers for Disease Control and Prevention	A minimum of 30 minutes of moderate-intensity physical activity on 5 or more days of the week	Promote health and prevent chronic disease
American College of Sports Medicine	A minimum of 30 minutes of moderate activity 5 days per week or 20 minutes of vigorous activity 3 days per week. (*The ACSM has separate guidelines for exercise programs to develop fitness; see pp. 38–41 and Table 2.2.*)	Promote health and prevent chronic disease
U.S. Surgeon General: Report on Physical Activity and Health	A minimum of 150 calories per day expended in moderate physical activity (the equivalent of about 30 minutes of brisk walking); resistance training twice a week	Promote health and prevent chronic disease
U.S. Department of Health and Human Services and U.S. Department of Agriculture: 2005 Dietary Guidelines for Americans	30 minutes of moderate-intensity exercise on most days of the week	Reduce the risk of chronic disease
	60 minutes of moderate-to-vigorous-intensity exercise on most days of the week	Manage body weight and prevent unhealthy weight gain
	60–90 minutes of moderate-intensity exercise per day	Sustain weight loss
Healthy People 2010	At least 30 minutes of moderate physical activity 5 or more days per week	Promote health and prevent chronic disease
Institute of Medicine, National Academies	At least 60 minutes of moderate physical activity per day	Promote health, prevent chronic disease, and control weight
International Association for the Study of Obesity	45–60 minutes of moderate physical activity per day	Prevent weight gain
	60–90 minutes of moderate physical activity per day	Maintain weight loss
World Health Organization	At least 30 minutes of moderate physical activity per day	Promote health, prevent chronic disease, and control weight

NOTE: See Chapter 7 for activity and exercise guidelines for people with special health concerns.

Classifying Activity Levels

Assessing your physical activity level is easier if you know how to classify different kinds of activities. Fitness experts categorize activities into the following three levels:

• *Light activity* includes the routine tasks associated with typical day-to-day life, such as vacuuming or walking to class. You probably perform dozens of light activities every day without even thinking about it. You can gain signifi-

cant health benefits by turning light activities into moderate activities—by walking briskly instead of slowly, for example.

• *Moderate activity* causes your breathing and heart rate to accelerate but still allows for comfortable conversation, such as walking at 3–4 miles per hour. It is sometimes described as activity that can be performed comfortably for about 45 minutes. Raking leaves is an example

of moderate physical activity, as are most occupational tasks that involve extended periods of moderate effort.

• *Vigorous activity* elevates your heart rate considerably and has other physical effects that improve your fitness level. During vigorous activity you are breathing too heavily to hold a conversation very easily. An example is walking faster than 4 miles per hour.

Here are some examples:

Light	Moderate	Vigorous
Walking slowly	Walking briskly	Walking briskly uphill
Routine tasks:	Cycling moderately on level terrain	Cycling on steep uphill terrain
• Cooking	Social dancing	Heavy housework:
• Shopping	Moderate housework:	• Moving furniture
Light housework:	• Scrubbing floors	• Carrying heavy objects upstairs
• Ironing	• Washing windows	Vigorous yard work or home activities:
• Dusting	Moderate yard work or home activities:	• Shoveling snow
• Washing dishes	• Planting	• Trimming trees
Light yard work or home activities:	• Raking	• Doing construction work
• Pruning	• Painting	• Digging
• Weeding	• Washing car	Fitness activities requiring vigorous effort:
• Plumbing	Fitness activities requiring moderate effort:	• Running
Light fitness activities:	• Doing low-impact aerobics	• Doing high-impact aerobics
• Light stretching or warm-up	• Playing Frisbee	• Doing circuit weight training
• Swimming, slow treading	• Swimming	• Swimming laps
	• Playing tennis, doubles	• Playing most competitive sports

These guidelines do not conflict with those from the Surgeon General, but they do have a different emphasis. They recognize that for people who need to prevent weight gain, lose weight, or maintain weight loss, 30 minutes per day of physical activity may not be enough. Instead, they recommend 45–90 or more minutes per day of physical activity. For example, the Dietary Guidelines recommend 60 minutes of daily physical activity to manage body weight and prevent unhealthy weight gain and 60–90 minutes of daily activity to sustain weight loss. The different recommendations may seem confusing, but all major health organizations have the same message: People can improve their health by becoming more active.

Exercising to Improve Physical Fitness As mentioned earlier, moderate physical activity confers significant health and wellness benefits, especially for those who are currently sedentary and become moderately active. The Surgeon General's report, the Dietary Guidelines for Americans, and the ACSM/AHA report all conclude that people can obtain even greater health and wellness benefits by increasing the duration and intensity of physical activity. With increased activity, they will see more

improvements in quality of life and greater reductions in disease and mortality risk.

More vigorous activity, as in a structured, systematic exercise program, is also needed to improve physical fitness; moderate physical activity alone is not enough. Physical fitness requires more intense movement that poses a substantially greater challenge to the body. The ACSM issued separate guidelines in 2006 for creating a formal exercise program that will develop physical fitness. These guidelines are described in detail later in the chapter.

How Much Physical Activity Is Enough?

Some experts feel that people get most of the health benefits of an exercise program simply by becoming more active over the course of the day; the amount of activity needed depends on an individual's health status and goals. Other experts feel that the activity goal set by the lifestyle approach is too low; they argue that people should exercise long enough and intensely enough to improve their body's capacity for exercise—that is, to improve physical fitness. More research is needed to clarify the health effects of different amounts of lifestyle physical activity, of

Making Time for Physical Activity

"Too little time" is a common excuse for not being physically active. Learning to manage your time successfully is crucial if you are to maintain a wellness lifestyle. You can begin by keeping a record of how you are currently spending your time; in your health journal, use a grid broken into blocks of 15, 20, or 30 minutes to track your daily activities. (See Activity 10 in the Behavior Change Workbook at the end of this text for a blank grid.) Then analyze your record: List each type of activity and the total time you engaged in it on a given day—for example, sleeping, 7 hours; eating, 1.5 hours; studying, 3 hours; and so on. Take a close look at your list of activities, and prioritize them according to how important they are to you, from essential to somewhat important to not important at all.

Based on the priorities you set, make changes in your daily schedule by subtracting time from some activities in order to make time for physical activity. Look particularly carefully at your leisure-time activities and your methods of transportation; these are areas where it is easy to build in physical activity. Make changes using a system of trade-offs. For example, you may choose to reduce the total amount of time you spend playing computer games, listening to the radio, and chatting on the phone in order to make time for an after-dinner bike ride or a walk with a friend. You may decide to watch 10 fewer minutes of television in the morning in order to change your 5-minute drive to class into a 15-minute walk. In making these kinds of changes in your schedule, don't feel that you have to miss out on anything you enjoy. You can get more from less time by focusing on what you are doing and by combining activities.

The following are just a few ways to incorporate more physical activity into your daily routine:

- Take the stairs instead of the elevator or escalator.
- Walk to the mailbox, post office, store, bank, or library whenever possible.
- Park your car a mile or even just a few blocks from your destination, and walk briskly.
- Do at least one chore every day that requires physical activity: Wash the windows or your car, clean your room or house, mow the lawn, or rake the leaves.
- Take study or work breaks to avoid sitting for more than 30 minutes at a time. Get up and walk around the library, your office, or your home or dorm; go up and down a flight of stairs.
- Stretch when you stand in line or watch TV.
- When you take public transportation, get off one stop early and walk to your destination.
- Go dancing instead of to a movie.
- Walk to visit a neighbor or friend rather than calling him or her on the phone. Go for a walk while you chat.
- Put your remote controls in storage; when you want to change TV or radio stations, get up and do it by hand.
- Take the dog for a walk (or an extra walk) every day.
- Play actively with children.
- If weather or neighborhood safety rule out walking outside, look for alternate locations—an indoor track, an enclosed shopping mall, or even a long hallway. Look for locations near or on the way to your campus, workplace, or residence.
- Remember, being busy isn't the same as being active. Seize every opportunity to get up and walk around. Move more and sit less.

Visit the U.S. Department of Health and Human Services Small Step Web site (www.smallstep.gov) for more ideas.

---

moderate-intensity versus high-intensity exercise, and of continuous versus intermittent exercise. However, there is probably some truth in both of these positions.

Regular physical activity, regardless of the intensity, makes you healthier and can help protect you from many chronic diseases. Although you get many of the health benefits of exercise simply by being more active, you obtain even more benefits when you are physically fit. In addition to long-term health benefits, fitness also significantly

QUESTIONS FOR CRITICAL THINKING AND REFLECTION

Does your current lifestyle include enough physical activity—30 minutes of moderate-intensity activity 5 or more days a week—to support health and wellness? Does your lifestyle go beyond this level to include enough vigorous physical activity and exercise to build physical fitness? What changes could you make in your lifestyle to start developing physical fitness?

contributes to quality of life. Fitness can give you freedom—freedom to move your body the way you want. Fit people have more energy and better body control. They can enjoy a more active lifestyle—cycling, hiking, skiing, and so on—than their more sedentary counterparts. Even if you don't like sports, you need physical energy and stamina in your daily life and for many nonsport leisure activities—visiting museums, playing with children, gardening, and so on.

Where does this leave you? Most experts agree that some physical activity is better than none, but that more—as long as it does not result in injury—is better than some. To set a personal goal for physical activity and exercise, consider your current activity level, your health status, and your overall goals. At the very least, strive to become more active and meet the goal set by the Surgeon General's report of using about 150 calories a day in physical activity—the equivalent of about 30 minutes of moderate-intensity activity. Choose to be active whenever you can. If weight management is a concern for you, begin by achieving the goal of 30 minutes of activity per day and then try to raise your activity level further, to

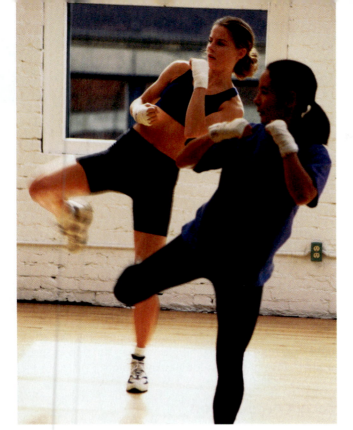

Cardiorespiratory endurance is a key component of health-related fitness. These participants in a kickboxing class are conditioning their hearts and lungs as well as gaining many other health benefits.

45–90 minutes per day or more. For even better health and well-being, participate in a structured exercise program that develops physical fitness. Any increase in physical activity will contribute to your health and well-being, now and in the future.

HEALTH-RELATED COMPONENTS OF PHYSICAL FITNESS

Some components of fitness are related to specific activities, and others relate to general health. **Health-related fitness** includes the following components:

- Cardiorespiratory endurance
- Muscular strength
- Muscular endurance
- Flexibility
- Body composition

Health-related fitness helps you withstand physical challenges and protects you from diseases.

Cardiorespiratory Endurance

Cardiorespiratory endurance is the ability to perform prolonged, large-muscle, dynamic exercise at moderate-to-high levels of intensity. It depends on such factors as the ability of

the lungs to deliver oxygen from the environment to the bloodstream, the capacity of the heart to pump blood, the ability of the nervous system and blood vessels to regulate blood flow, and the capability of the body's chemical systems to use oxygen and process fuels for exercise.

When cardiorespiratory fitness is low, the heart has to work hard during normal daily activities and may not be able to work hard enough to sustain high-intensity physical activity in an emergency. As cardiorespiratory fitness improves, related physical functions also improve. For example:

- The heart pumps more blood per heartbeat.
- Resting heart rate slows.
- Blood volume increases.
- Blood supply to tissues improves.
- The body can cool itself better.
- Resting blood pressure decreases.

A healthy heart can better withstand the strains of everyday life, the stress of occasional emergencies, and the wear and tear of time.

Endurance training also improves the functioning of the chemical systems, particularly in the muscles and liver, thereby enhancing the body's ability to use energy supplied by food and to do more exercise with less effort from the oxygen transport system.

Cardiorespiratory endurance is a central component of health-related fitness because the functioning of the heart and lungs is so essential to overall good health. A person can't live very long or very well without a healthy heart. Poor cardiorespiratory fitness is linked with heart disease,

health-related fitness   Physical capacities that contribute to health: cardiorespiratory endurance, muscular strength, muscular endurance, flexibility, and body composition.

cardiorespiratory endurance   The ability of the body to perform prolonged, large-muscle, dynamic exercise at moderate-to-high levels of intensity.

type 2 diabetes, colon cancer, stroke, depression, and anxiety. A moderate level of cardiorespiratory fitness can help compensate for certain health risks, including excess body fat: People who are lean but who have low cardiorespiratory fitness have been found to have higher death rates than people with higher levels of body fat who are otherwise fit. You can develop cardiorespiratory endurance through activities that involve continuous, rhythmic movements of large-muscle groups, such as the legs. Such activities include walking, jogging, cycling, and aerobic dancing.

Muscular Strength

Muscular strength is the amount of force a muscle can produce with a single maximum effort. It depends on such factors as the size of muscle cells and the ability of nerves to activate muscle cells. Strong muscles are important for everyday activities, such as climbing stairs, as well as for emergency situations. They help keep the skeleton in proper alignment, preventing back and leg pain and providing the support necessary for good posture. Muscular strength has obvious importance in recreational activities. Strong people can hit a tennis ball harder, kick a soccer ball farther, and ride a bicycle uphill more easily.

Muscle tissue is an important element of overall body composition. Greater muscle mass means a higher rate of **metabolism** and faster energy use. Training to build muscular strength can also help people manage stress and boost their self-confidence.

Maintaining strength and muscle mass is vital for healthy aging. Older people tend to experience a decrease in both number and size of muscle cells—a condition called *sarcopenia*. Many of the muscle cells that remain become slower, and some become nonfunctional because they lose their attachment to the nervous system. Strength training helps maintain muscle mass and function and possibly helps decrease the risk of osteoporosis (bone loss) in older people, which greatly enhances their quality of life and prevents life-threatening injuries.

Muscular Endurance

Muscular endurance is the ability to resist fatigue and sustain a given level of muscle tension—that is, to hold a muscle contraction for a long time or to contract a muscle over and over again. It depends on such factors as the size of muscle cells, the ability of muscles to store fuel, and the blood supply to muscles.

Muscular endurance is important for good posture and for injury prevention. For example, if abdominal and back muscles can't hold the spine correctly, the chances of low-back pain and back injury are increased. Good muscular endurance in the trunk muscles is more important than muscular strength for preventing back pain. Muscular endurance helps people cope with the physical demands of everyday life and enhances performance in sports and work.

QUESTIONS FOR CRITICAL THINKING AND REFLECTION
When you think about exercise, do you think of only one or two of the five components of health-related fitness, such as muscular strength or body composition? If so, where do you think your ideas come from? What role do the media play in shaping your ideas about fitness?

Flexibility

Flexibility is the ability to move the joints through their full range of motion. It depends on joint structure, the length and elasticity of connective tissue, and nervous system activity. Flexible, pain-free joints are important for good health and well-being. Inactivity causes the joints to become stiffer with age. Stiffness, in turn, often causes older people to assume unnatural body postures that can stress joints and muscles. Stretching exercises can help ensure a healthy range of motion for all major joints.

Body Composition

Body composition refers to the proportion of fat and **fat-free mass** (muscle, bone, and water) in the body. Healthy body composition involves a high proportion of fat-free mass and an acceptably low level of body fat, adjusted for age and gender. A person with excessive body fat—especially excess fat in the abdomen—is more likely to experience health problems, including heart disease, insulin resistance, high blood pressure, stroke, joint problems, type 2 diabetes, gallbladder disease, blood vessel inflammation, some types of cancer, and back pain.

The best way to lose fat is through a lifestyle that includes a sensible diet and exercise. The best way to add muscle mass is through resistance training, also known as strength training or, when weights are used, weight training. Large changes in body composition aren't necessary to improve health; even a small increase in physical activity and a small decrease in body fat can lead to substantial health improvements.

Skill-Related Components of Fitness

In addition to the five health-related components of physical fitness, the ability to perform a particular sport or activity may depend on **skill-related fitness** components such as the following:

- *Speed*—the ability to perform a movement in a short period of time
- *Power*—the ability to exert force rapidly, based on a combination of strength and speed
- *Agility*—the ability to change the position of the body quickly and accurately

- *Balance*—the ability to maintain equilibrium while moving or while stationary
- *Coordination*—the ability to perform motor tasks accurately and smoothly using body movements and the senses
- *Reaction and movement time*—the ability to respond and react quickly to a stimulus

Skill-related fitness tends to be sport-specific and is best developed through practice. For example, the speed, coordination, and agility needed to play basketball can be developed by playing basketball. Some fitness experts contend that some sports don't contribute to all the health-related components of physical fitness. However, engaging in sports is fun and can help you build fitness and contribute to other areas of wellness.

PRINCIPLES OF PHYSICAL TRAINING: ADAPTATION TO STRESS

The human body is very adaptable. The greater the demands made on it, the more it adjusts to meet those demands. Over time, immediate, short-term adjustments translate into long-term changes and improvements. When breathing and heart rate increase during exercise, for example, the heart gradually develops the ability to pump more blood with each beat. Then, during exercise, it doesn't have to beat as fast to meet the cells' demands for oxygen. The goal of **physical training** is to produce these long-term changes and improvements in the body's functioning. Although people differ in the maximum levels of physical fitness and performance they can achieve through training, the wellness benefits of exercise are available to everyone (see the box "Fitness and Disability" on p. 36).

Particular types and amounts of exercise are most effective in developing the various components of fitness. To put together an effective exercise program, you should first understand the basic principles of physical training, including the following:

- Specificity
- Progressive overload
- Reversibility
- Individual differences

All of these rest on the larger principle of adaptation.

Specificity—Adapting to Type of Training

To develop a particular fitness component, you must perform exercises that are specifically designed for that component. This is the principle of **specificity**. Weight training, for example, develops muscular strength but is less effective for developing cardiorespiratory endurance or flexibility. Specificity also applies to the skill-related fitness components—to improve at tennis, you must practice tennis—and to the different parts of the body—to develop stronger arms, you must exercise your arms. A well-rounded exercise program includes exercises geared to each component of fitness, to different parts of the body, and to specific activities or sports.

Progressive Overload—Adapting to Amount of Training and the FITT Principle

The body adapts to the demands of exercise by improving its functioning. When the amount of exercise (also called *overload* or *stress*) is progressively increased, fitness continues to improve. This is the principle of **progressive overload**.

The amount of overload is important. Too little exercise will have no effect on fitness (although it may improve health); too much may cause injury and problems with the body's immune system and hormone levels. The point at which exercise becomes excessive is highly individual—it occurs at a much higher level in an Olympic athlete than in a sedentary person. For every type of exercise, there is a training threshold at which fitness benefits begin to occur, a zone within which maximum fitness benefits occur, and an upper limit of safe training.

muscular strength   The amount of force a muscle can produce with a single maximum effort.

metabolism   The sum of all the vital processes by which food energy and nutrients are made available to and used by the body.

muscular endurance   The ability of a muscle to remain contracted or to contract repeatedly for a long period of time.

flexibility   The ability to move joints through their full range of motion.

body composition   The proportion of fat and fat-free mass (muscle, bone, and water) in the body.

fat-free mass   The nonfat component of the human body, consisting of skeletal muscle, bone, and water.

skill-related fitness   Physical capacities that contribute to performance in a sport or activity: speed, power, agility, balance, coordination, and reaction time.

physical training   The performance of different types of activities that cause the body to adapt and improve its level of fitness.

specificity   The training principle that the body adapts to the particular type and amount of stress placed on it.

progressive overload   The training principle that placing increasing amounts of stress on the body causes adaptations that improve fitness.

Fitness and Disability

Physical fitness and athletic achievement are not limited to the able-bodied. People with disabilities can also attain high levels of fitness and performance, as shown by the elite athletes who compete in the Paralympics. The premier event for athletes with disabilities, the Paralympics are held in the same year and city as the Olympics. The performance of these skilled athletes makes it clear that people with disabilities can be active, healthy, and extraordinarily fit; just like able-bodied athletes, athletes with disabilities strive for excellence and can serve as role models.

According to the U.S. Census Bureau, about 51 million Americans have some type of chronic disability. Some disabilities are the result of injury, such as spinal cord injuries sustained in car crashes. Other disabilities result from illness, such as the blindness that sometimes occurs as a complication of diabetes or the joint stiffness that accompanies arthritis. And some disabilities are present at birth, as in the case of congenital limb deformities or cerebral palsy.

Exercise and physical activity are as important for people with disabilities as for able-bodied individuals—if not *more* important. Being active helps prevent secondary conditions that may result from prolonged inactivity, such as circulatory or muscular problems. Currently, about 18% of people with disabilities engage in regular moderate activity.

People with disabilities don't have to be elite athletes to participate in sports and lead an active life. Some health clubs and fitness centers offer activities and events geared for people of all ages and types of disabilities. They may have modified aerobics classes, special weight training machines, classes involving mild

exercise in warm water, and other activities adapted for people with disabilities. Popular sports and recreational activities include adapted horseback riding, golf, swimming, and skiing. Competitive sports are also available—for example, there are wheelchair versions of billiards, tennis, hockey, and basketball, as well as sports for people with hearing, visual, or mental impairments. For those who prefer to get their exercise at home, special videos are available geared to individuals who use wheelchairs or who have arthritis, hearing impairments, or many other disabilities.

If you have a disability and want to be more active, check with your physician about what's appropriate for you. Call your local community center, YMCA/YWCA, independent living center, or fitness center to locate facilities; look for a facility with experienced personnel and appropriate adaptive equipment. For specialized videos, check with hospitals and health associations that are geared to specific disabilities, such as the Arthritis Foundation.

SOURCES: National Center for Health Statistics. 2007. *DATA 2010: The Healthy People 2010 Database, October, 2007 Edition* (http://wonder.cdc.gov/data2010/; retrieved November 5, 2007). Steinmetz, E. 2006. *Americans with Disabilities: 2002.* Washington, D.C.: U.S. Census Bureau.

The amount of exercise needed depends on the individual's current level of fitness, the person's genetically determined capacity to adapt to training, his or her fitness goals, and the component being developed. A novice, for example, might experience fitness benefits from jogging a mile in 10 minutes, but this level of exercise would cause no physical adaptations in a trained distance runner. Beginners should start at the lower end of the fitness benefit zone; fitter individuals will make more rapid gains by exercising at the higher end of the fitness benefit zone. Progression is critical because fitness increases only if the volume and intensity of workouts increase. Exercising at the same intensity every training session will maintain fitness but will not increase it, because the training stress is below the threshold to produce adaptation.

The amount of overload needed to maintain or improve a particular level of fitness for a particular fitness component is determined through four dimensions, represented by the acronym FITT:

- *Frequency*—how often
- *Intensity*—how hard
- *Time*—how long (duration)
- *Type*—mode of activity

Chapters 3, 4, and 5 show you how to apply the FITT principle to exercise programs for cardiorespiratory endurance, muscular strength and endurance, and flexibility, respectively.

Frequency Developing fitness requires regular exercise. Optimum exercise frequency, expressed in number of days per week, varies with the component being developed and the individual's fitness goals. For most people, a frequency of 3–5 days per week for cardiorespiratory endurance exercise and 2 or more days per week for resistance and flexibility training is appropriate for a general fitness program.

An important consideration in determining appropriate exercise frequency is recovery time, which is also highly individual and depends on factors such as training experience, age, and intensity of training. For example, 24 hours of rest between highly intensive workouts that involve heavy weights or track sprints is not enough recovery time for safe and effective training; intense workouts need to be spaced out during the week to allow for sufficient recovery time. On the other hand, you can exercise every day if your program consists of moderate-intensity walking or cycling. Learn to "listen to your body"

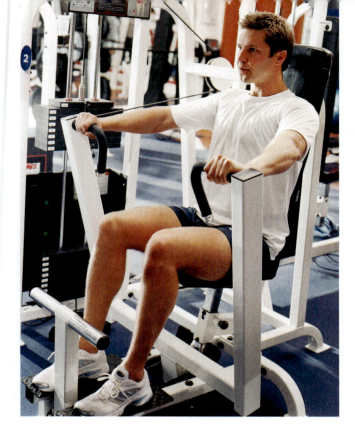

To safely and effectively develop strength, this exerciser must overload his muscles with enough weight that his body's functioning improves but not so much weight that he becomes injured.

to get enough rest between workouts. Chapters 3–5 provide more detailed information about training techniques and recovery periods for workouts focused on different fitness components.

Intensity Fitness benefits occur when a person exercises harder than his or her normal level of activity. The appropriate exercise intensity varies with each fitness component. To develop cardiorespiratory endurance, for example, you must raise your heart rate above normal; to develop muscular strength, you must lift a heavier weight than normal; to develop flexibility, you must stretch muscles beyond their normal length.

Time (Duration) Fitness benefits occur when you exercise for an extended period of time. For cardiorespiratory

endurance exercise, 20–60 minutes is recommended; exercise can take place in a single session or in several sessions of 10 or more minutes. The greater the intensity of exercise, the less time needed to obtain fitness benefits. For high-intensity exercise, such as running, 20–30 minutes is appropriate. For moderate-intensity exercise, such as walking, 45–60 minutes may be needed. High-intensity exercise poses a greater risk of injury than low-intensity exercise, so if you are a nonathletic adult, it's probably best to emphasize low- to moderate-intensity activity of longer duration.

To build muscular strength, muscular endurance, and flexibility, similar amounts of time are advisable, but these exercises are more commonly organized in terms of a specific number of repetitions of particular exercises. For resistance training, for example, a recommended program includes one or more sets of 8–12 repetitions of 8–10 different exercises that work the major muscle groups.

Type (Mode of Activity) The type of exercise in which you should engage varies with each fitness component and with your personal fitness goals. To develop cardiorespiratory endurance, you need to engage in continuous activities involving large-muscle groups—walking, jogging, cycling, or swimming, for example. Resistive exercises develop muscular strength and endurance, while stretching exercises build flexibility. The frequency, intensity, and time of the exercise will be different for each type of activity. (See pp. 38–41 for more on choosing appropriate activities for your fitness program.)

Reversibility—Adapting to a Reduction in Training

Fitness is a reversible adaptation. The body adjusts to lower levels of physical activity the same way it adjusts to higher levels. This is the principle of **reversibility.** When a person stops exercising, up to 50% of fitness improvements are lost within 2 months. However, not all fitness levels reverse at the same rate. Strength fitness is very resilient, so a person can maintain strength fitness by doing resistive exercise as infrequently as once a week. On the other hand, cardiovascular and cellular fitness reverse themselves more quickly—sometimes within just a few days or weeks. If you must temporarily curtail your training, you can maintain your fitness improvements by keeping the intensity of your workouts constant while reducing their frequency or duration.

QUESTIONS FOR CRITICAL THINKING AND REFLECTION
Many people who play sports have had the experience of realizing that they are not as physically gifted as a teammate or that they are never going to be in the Olympics. What can you say to encourage someone who is discouraged by this realization? What benefits of physical activity, exercise, and sports might you point out?

reversibility   The training principle that fitness improvements are lost when demands on the body are lowered.

Individual Differences—Limits on Adaptability

Anyone watching the Olympics can see that, from a physical standpoint, we are not all created equal. There are large individual differences in our ability to improve fitness, achieve a desirable body composition, and learn and perform sports skills. Some people are able to run longer distances, or lift more weight, or kick a soccer ball more skillfully than others will ever be able to, no matter how much they train. Each person responds to training at different rates; a program that works for one person may not be right for another person. There are limits on the adaptability—the potential for improvement—of any human body. The body's ability to transport and use oxygen, for example, can be improved by only about 15–30% through training. An endurance athlete must therefore inherit a large metabolic capacity in order to reach competitive performance levels. In the past few years, scientists have identified specific genes that influence body fat, strength, and endurance.

However, physical training improves fitness regardless of heredity. For the average person, the body's adaptability is enough to achieve reasonable fitness goals.

DESIGNING YOUR OWN EXERCISE PROGRAM

Physical training works best when you have a plan. A plan helps you make gradual but steady progress toward your goals. Once you've determined that exercise is safe for you, planning for physical fitness consists of assessing how fit you are now, determining where you want to be, and choosing the right activities to help you get there.

Getting Medical Clearance

People of any age who are not at high risk for serious health problems can safely exercise at a moderate intensity (60% or less of maximum heart rate) without a prior medical evaluation (see Chapter 3 for a discussion of maximum heart rate). Likewise, if you are male and under 40 or female and under 50 and in good health, exercise is probably safe for you. If you do not fit into these age groups or if you have health problems—especially high blood pressure, heart disease, muscle or

joint problems, or obesity—see your physician before starting a vigorous exercise program. The Canadian Society for Exercise Physiology has developed the Physical Activity Readiness Questionnaire (PAR-Q) to help evaluate exercise safety; it is included in Lab 2.1. Completing it should alert you to any potential problems you may have. If a physician isn't sure whether exercise is safe for you, she or he may recommend an **exercise stress test** or a **graded exercise test (GXT)** to see whether you show symptoms of heart disease during exercise. For most people, however, it's far safer to exercise than to remain sedentary. For more information, see the box "Is Exercise Safe?"

Assessing Yourself

The first step in creating a successful fitness program is to assess your current level of physical activity and fitness for each of the five health-related fitness components. The results of the assessment tests will help you set specific fitness goals and plan your fitness program. Lab 2.2 gives you the opportunity to assess your current overall level of activity and determine if it is appropriate. Assessment tests in Chapters 3–6 will help you evaluate your cardiorespiratory endurance, muscular strength, muscular endurance, flexibility, and body composition.

Setting Goals

The ultimate general goal of every health-related fitness program is the same—wellness that lasts a lifetime. Whatever your specific goals, they must be important enough to you to keep you motivated. Most sports psychologists believe that setting and achieving goals is the most effective way to stay motivated about exercise. (Refer to Chapter 1 for more on goal setting, as well as Common Questions Answered at the end of this chapter.) After you complete the assessment tests in Chapters 3–6, you will be able to set goals directly related to each fitness component, such as working toward a 3-mile jog or doing 20 push-ups. First, though, think carefully about your overall goals, and be clear about why you are starting a program.

Choosing Activities for a Balanced Program

An ideal fitness program combines a physically active lifestyle with a systematic exercise program to develop and maintain physical fitness. This overall program is shown in the physical activity pyramid in Figure 2.3. If you are currently sedentary, your goal should be to focus on activities at the bottom of the pyramid and gradually increase the amount of moderate-intensity physical activity in your daily life. Appropriate activities include

exercise stress test   A test usually administered on a treadmill or cycle ergometer that involves analysis of the changes in electrical activity in the heart from an electrocardiogram (EKG or ECG) taken during exercise; used to determine if any heart disease is present and to assess current fitness level.

graded exercise test (GXT)   An exercise test that starts at an easy intensity and progresses to maximum capacity.

WEB

TERMS

Is Exercise Safe?

Participating in exercise and sports is usually a wonderful experience that improves wellness in both the short and long term. In rare instances, however, vigorous exertion is associated with sudden death. It may seem difficult to understand that although regular exercise protects people from heart disease, it also increases the risk of sudden death.

Congenital heart defects (heart abnormalities present at birth) are the most common cause of exercise-related sudden death in people under 35. In nearly all other cases, coronary artery disease is responsible. In this condition, fat and other substances build up in the arteries that supply blood to the heart. Death can result if an artery becomes blocked or if the heart's rhythm and pumping action are disrupted. Exercise, particularly intense exercise, may trigger a heart attack in someone with underlying heart disease.

A study of jogging deaths in Rhode Island found that there was one death per 396,000 hours of jogging, or about one death per 7620 joggers per year—an extremely low risk for each individual jogger. Another study of men involved in a variety of physical activities found one death per 1.51 million hours of exercise. This 12-year study of more than 21,000 men found that those who didn't exercise vigorously were 74 times more likely to die suddenly from cardiac arrest during or shortly after exercise. It is also important to note that people are much safer exercising than engaging in many other common activities, including driving a car.

Although quite small, the risk does exist and may lead some people to wonder why exercise is considered such an important part of a wellness lifestyle. Exercise causes many positive changes in the body—in healthy people as well as those with heart disease—that more than make up for the slightly increased short-term risk of sudden death. Training slows or reverses the fatty buildup in arteries and helps protect people from deadly heart rhythm abnormalities.

People who exercise regularly have an overall risk of sudden death only about two-thirds that of nonexercisers. Active people who stop exercising can expect their heart attack risk to increase by 300%.

Obviously, someone with underlying coronary artery disease is at greater risk than someone who is free from the condition. However, many cases of heart disease go undiagnosed. The riskiest scenario may involve the middle-aged or older individual who suddenly begins participating in a vigorous sport or activity after being sedentary for a long time. This finding provides strong evidence for the recommendation that people increase their level of physical activity gradually and engage in regular, rather than sporadic, activity.

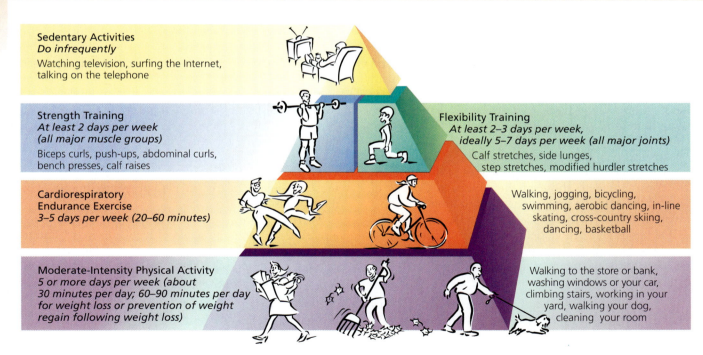

SOURCES: Thompson, P. D. 2001. Cardiovascular risks of exercise. *Physician and Sportsmedicine* 29(4). Albert, C. M., et al. 2000. Trigger of sudden death from cardiac causes by vigorous exertion. *New England Journal of Medicine* 343(19): 1355–1361.

Sedentary Activities
Do infrequently
Watching television, surfing the Internet, talking on the telephone

Strength Training
At least 2 days per week (all major muscle groups)
Biceps curls, push-ups, abdominal curls, bench presses, calf raises

Flexibility Training
At least 2–3 days per week, ideally 5–7 days per week (all major joints)
Calf stretches, side lunges, step stretches, modified hurdler stretches

Cardiorespiratory Endurance Exercise
3–5 days per week (20–60 minutes)
Walking, jogging, bicycling, swimming, aerobic dancing, in-line skating, cross-country skiing, dancing, basketball

Moderate-Intensity Physical Activity
5 or more days per week (about 30 minutes per day; 60–90 minutes per day for weight loss or prevention of weight regain following weight loss)
Walking to the store or bank, washing windows or your car, climbing stairs, working in your yard, walking your dog, cleaning your room

FIGURE 2.3   Physical activity pyramid. This physical activity pyramid shows the components of a balanced fitness program and emphasizes the importance of daily moderate-intensity physical activity. If you are currently sedentary, gradually increase the amount of moderate-intensity physical activity in your life. If you are already moderately active, begin a formal exercise program that includes cardiorespiratory endurance exercise, flexibility training, and strength training to help you develop all the health-related components of fitness.

Table 2.2	ACSM Exercise Recommendations for Fitness Development in Healthy Adults

Exercise to Develop and Maintain Cardiorespiratory Endurance and Body Composition

Frequency of training	3–5 days per week.
Intensity of training	55/65–90% of maximum heart rate or 40/50–85% of heart rate reserve or maximum oxygen uptake reserve.* The lower intensity values (55–64% of maximum heart rate and 40–49% of heart rate reserve) are most applicable to individuals who are quite unfit. For average individuals, intensities of 70–85% of maximum heart rate or 60–80% of heart rate reserve are appropriate.
Time (duration) of training	20–60 total minutes of continuous or intermittent (in sessions lasting 10 or more minutes) aerobic activity. Duration is dependent on the intensity of activity; thus, low-intensity activity should be conducted over a longer period of time (30 minutes or more). Low-to-moderate-intensity activity of longer duration is recommended for nonathletic adults.
Type (mode) of activity	Any activity that uses large-muscle groups, can be maintained continuously, and is rhythmic and aerobic in nature—for example, walking-hiking, running-jogging, cycling-bicycling, cross-country skiing, aerobic dancing and other forms of group exercise, rope skipping, rowing, stair climbing, swimming, skating, and endurance game activities.

Exercise to Develop and Maintain Muscular Strength and Endurance, Flexibility, and Body Composition

Resistance training	One set of 8–10 exercises that condition the major muscle groups, performed at least 2 days per week. Most people should complete 8–12 repetitions of each exercise to the point of fatigue; practicing other repetition ranges (for example, 3–5 or 12–15) also builds strength and endurance; for older and frailer people (approximately 50–60 and older), 10–15 repetitions with a lighter weight may be more appropriate. Multiple-set regimens will provide greater benefits if time allows. Any mode of exercise that is comfortable throughout the full range of motion is appropriate (for example, free weights, bands, or machines).
Flexibility training	Static stretches, performed for the major muscle groups at least 2–3 days per week, ideally 5–7 days per week. Stretch to the point of tightness, holding each stretch for 15–30 seconds; perform 2–4 repetitions of each stretch.

*Instructions for calculating target heart rate intensity for cardiorespiratory endurance exercise are presented in Chapter 3.

SOURCE: Adapted from American College of Sports Medicine. 2006. *ACSM's Guidelines for Exercise Testing and Prescription*, 7th ed. Philadelphia: Lippincott Williams and Wilkins.

walking briskly, climbing stairs, doing yard work, and washing your car. You don't have to exercise vigorously, but you should experience a moderate increase in your heart and breathing rates. As described earlier, your activity time can be broken up into small blocks over the course of a day.

The next two levels of the pyramid illustrate parts of a formal exercise program. The principles of this program are consistent with those of the American College of Sports Medicine, the professional organization for people involved in sports medicine and exercise science. The ACSM has established guidelines for creating an exercise program that will develop physical fitness (Table 2.2). A balanced program includes activities to develop all the health-related components of fitness:

• *Cardiorespiratory endurance* is developed by continuous rhythmic movements of large-muscle groups in activities such as walking, jogging, cycling, swimming, and aerobic dance and other forms of group exercise. Choose activities that you enjoy and that are convenient. Other popular choices are in-line skating, dancing, and backpacking. Start-and-stop activities such as tennis, racquetball, and soccer can also develop endurance if your skill level is sufficient to enable periods of continuous

play. Training for cardiorespiratory endurance is discussed in Chapter 3.

• *Muscular strength and endurance* can be developed through resistance training—training with weights or performing calisthenic exercises such as push-ups and curl-ups. Training for muscular strength and endurance is discussed in Chapter 4.

• *Flexibility* is developed by stretching the major muscle groups regularly and with proper technique. Flexibility is discussed in Chapter 5.

• *Healthy body composition* can be developed through a sensible diet and a program of regular exercise. Endurance exercise is best for reducing body fat; resistance training builds muscle mass, which, to a small extent, helps increase metabolism. Body composition is discussed in Chapter 6.

Chapter 7 contains guidelines to help you choose activities and put together a complete exercise program that will suit your goals and preferences. (Refer to Figure 2.4 for a summary of the health and fitness benefits of different levels of physical activity.)

What about the tip of the activity pyramid? Although sedentary activities are often unavoidable—attending class, studying, working in an office, and so on—many

	Lifestyle physical activity	Moderate exercise program	Vigorous exercise program
Description	Moderate physical activity—an amount of activity that uses about 150 calories per day	Cardiorespiratory endurance exercise (20–60 minutes, 3–5 days per week); strength training (at least 2 days per week) and stretching exercises (2 or more days per week)	Cardiorespiratory endurance exercise (20–60 minutes, 3–5 days per week); interval training; strength training (3–4 nonconsecutive days per week); and stretching exercises (5–7 days per week)
Sample activities or program	*One of the following:* • Walking to and from work, 15 minutes each way • Cycling to and from class, 10 minutes each way • Doing yard work for 30 minutes • Dancing (fast) for 30 minutes • Playing basketball for 20 minutes	• Jogging for 30 minutes, 3 days per week • Weight training, 1 set of 8 exercises, 2 days per week • Stretching exercises, 3 days per week	• Running for 45 minutes, 3 days per week • Intervals: running 400 m at high effort, 4 sets, 2 days per week • Weight training, 3 sets of 10 exercises, 3 days per week • Stretching exercises, 6 days per week
Health and fitness benefits	Better blood cholesterol levels, reduced body fat, better control of blood pressure, improved metabolic health, and enhanced glucose metabolism; improved quality of life; reduced risk of some chronic diseases Greater amounts of activity can help prevent weight gain and promote weight loss	All the benefits of lifestyle physical activity, plus improved physical fitness (increased cardiorespiratory endurance, muscular strength and endurance, and flexibility) and even greater improvements in health and quality of life and reductions in chronic disease risk	All the benefits of lifestyle physical activity and a moderate exercise program, with greater increases in fitness and somewhat greater reductions in chronic disease risk Participating in a vigorous exercise program may increase risk of injury and overtraining

FIGURE 2.4   Health and fitness benefits of different amounts of physical activity and exercise.

people choose inactivity over activity during their leisure time. Change sedentary patterns by becoming more active whenever you can. Move more and sit less.

MOTIVATION BOOSTER

Locate resources. Your school and community may present challenges to making healthy lifestyle choices, but they also have resources that can help you. Find out what local resources are available and will support your efforts at change. For example, go to your school's physical education office and ask for a comprehensive listing of all the exercise and fitness facilities and courses available on your campus. Obtain the same information about facilities and classes in your neighborhood, including those offered by the city or county recreation department. What fitness facilities and/or courses fit your goals, schedule, preferences, and budget? If you can't find a local program or facility to fit your needs, check out the programs available through the President's Challenge (http://www.presidentschallenge.org).

Guidelines for Training

The following guidelines will make your exercise program more effective and successful.

Train the Way You Want Your Body to Change   Stress your body so it adapts in the desired manner. To have a more muscular build, lift weights. To be more flexible, do stretching exercises. To improve performance in a particular sport, practice that sport or its movements.

Train Regularly   Consistency is the key to improving fitness. Fitness improvements are lost if too much time passes between exercise sessions.

Start Slowly, and Get in Shape Gradually   As Figure 2.5 (p. 42) shows, an exercise program can be divided into three phases:

* *Beginning phase.* The body adjusts to the new type and level of activity.
* *Progress phase.* Fitness increases.
* *Maintenance phase.* The targeted level of fitness is sustained over the long term.

FIGURE 2.5 Progression of an exercise program. This figure shows how the amount of overload is increased gradually over time in a sample walking program. Regardless of the activity chosen, it is important that an exercise program begin slowly and progress gradually. Once you achieve the desired level of fitness, you can maintain it by exercising 3–5 days a week.

SOURCE: Progression data from American College of Sports Medicine. 2006. *ACSM's Guidelines for Exercise Testing and Prescription*, 7th ed. Philadelphia: Lippincott Williams and Wilkins.

When beginning a program, start slowly to give your body time to adapt to the stress of exercise. Choose activities carefully according to your fitness status; if you have been sedentary or are overweight, try an activity such as walking or swimming that won't jar the body or strain the joints.

As you progress, increase duration and frequency before increasing intensity. If you train too much or too intensely, you are more likely to suffer injuries or become **overtrained**, a condition characterized by lack of energy, aching muscles and joints, and decreased physical performance. Injuries and overtraining slow down an exercise program and impede motivation. The goal is not to get in shape as quickly as possible but to gradually become and then remain physically fit.

Warm Up Before Exercise   Warming up can decrease your chances of injury by helping your body gradually progress from rest to activity. A good warm-up can increase muscle temperature, reduce joint stiffness, bathe the joint surfaces in lubricating fluid, and increase blood flow to the muscles, including the heart. Some studies

suggest that warming up may also enhance muscle metabolism and mentally prepare you for a workout.

A warm-up should include low-intensity, whole-body movements similar to those used in the activity that will follow. For example, runners may walk and jog slowly prior to running at full speed. A tennis player might hit forehands and backhands at a low intensity before playing a vigorous set of tennis. It is important to note that a warm-up is not the same thing as a stretching workout. For safety and effectiveness, it is best to stretch *after* an endurance or strength training workout, when muscles are warm—and not as part of a warm-up. (Appropriate and effective warm-ups are discussed in greater detail in Chapters 3–5.)

Cool Down After Exercise   During exercise, as much as 90% of circulating blood is directed to the muscles and skin, up from as little as 20% during rest. If you suddenly stop moving after exercise, the amount of blood returning to your heart and brain may be insufficient, and you may experience dizziness, a drop in blood pressure, or other problems. Cooling down at the end of a workout helps safely restore circulation to its normal resting condition. So don't sit or lie down or jump into the shower after exercise without cooling down first. Cool down by continuing to move at a slow pace—walking, for example—for 5–10 minutes, as your heart and breathing rate slowly return to normal. At the end of the cool-down period, do stretching exercises while your muscles are still warm. Cool down longer after intense exercise sessions.

Exercise Safely   Physical activity can cause injury or even death if you don't consider safety. For example, you should always:

- Wear a helmet when biking, skiing, or rock climbing.
- Wear eye protection when playing racquetball or squash.
- Wear bright clothing when exercising on a public street.
- Walk or run with a partner in a park or on a deserted track.
- Give vehicles plenty of leeway, even when you have the right of way.

Train within your capacity because overloading your muscles and joints can lead to serious injury. Use high-quality equipment and keep it in good repair. Report broken gym equipment to the health club manager. (See Appendix A for more information on personal safety.)

Listen to Your Body and Get Adequate Rest   Rest can be as important as exercise for improving fitness. Fitness reflects an adaptation to the stress of exercise. Building fitness involves a series of exercise stresses, recuperation, and adaptation leading to improved fitness, followed by further stresses. Build rest into your training

TERMS

overtraining   A condition caused by training too much or too intensely, characterized by lack of energy, decreased physical performance, fatigue, depression, aching muscles and joints, and susceptibility to injury.

Vary Your Activities

Do you have a hard time thinking of new activities to try? Check the boxes next to the activities listed here that interest you. Then look for resources and facilities on your campus or in your community.

Outdoor Exercises

- ☐ Walking
- ☐ Inline skating
- ☐ Hiking
- ☐ Running
- ☐ Skateboarding
- ☐ Backpacking
- ☐ Cycling
- ☐ Rowing
- ☐ Ice skating
- ☐ Swimming
- ☐ Horseback riding
- ☐ Fly fishing

Sports and Games

- ☐ Basketball
- ☐ Softball
- ☐ Bowling
- ☐ Tennis
- ☐ Water skiing
- ☐ Surfing
- ☐ Volleyball
- ☐ Windsurfing
- ☐ Dancing
- ☐ Golf
- ☐ Badminton
- ☐ Snow skiing
- ☐ Soccer
- ☐ Ultimate Frisbee
- ☐ Gymnastics

Exercises You Can Do at Home and Work

- ☐ Desk exercises
- ☐ Yard work
- ☐ Painting the walls
- ☐ Calisthenics
- ☐ Sweeping the walkway
- ☐ Walking the dog
- ☐ Gardening
- ☐ Exploring on foot
- ☐ Shopping
- ☐ Housework
- ☐ Entering a walk-a-thon
- ☐ Running errands

Health Club Exercises

- ☐ Weight training
- ☐ Ski machine
- ☐ Elliptical trainer
- ☐ Circuit training
- ☐ Supine bike
- ☐ Medicine ball
- ☐ Group exercise
- ☐ Rowing machine
- ☐ Rope skipping
- ☐ Treadmill
- ☐ Plyometrics
- ☐ Punching bag
- ☐ Stationary bike
- ☐ Water aerobics
- ☐ Racquetball

program, and don't exercise if it doesn't feel right. Sometimes you need a few days of rest to recover enough to train with the intensity required for improving fitness. Getting enough sleep is an important part of the recovery process. On the other hand, you can't train sporadically, either. If you listen to your body and it always tells you to rest, you won't make any progress.

Cycle the Volume and Intensity of Your Workouts   To add enjoyment and variety to your program, and to further improve fitness, don't train at the same intensity during every workout. Train intensely on some days and train lightly on others. Proper management of the level of workout intensity is a key to improved physical fitness. Use cycle training, also known as periodization, to provide enough recovery for intense training: Because you trained lightly one workout, you can train harder the next. However, take care to increase the volume and intensity of your program gradually—never more than 10% per week.

Vary Your Activities   Change your exercise program from time to time to keep things fresh and help develop a higher degree of fitness. The body adapts quickly to an exercise stress, such as walking, cycling, or swimming. Gains in fitness in a particular activity become more difficult with time. Varying the kinds of exercises in your program allows you to adapt to many types of exercise and develops fitness in a variety of activities. (see the box "Vary Your Activities"). Changing activities may also help reduce your risk of injury.

Try varying the type of training you do during different times of the year. During the summer, you might emphasize conditioning by jogging, playing basketball, and doing high-volume strength training exercises. During the fall, you might emphasize resistance training using more weights and fewer repetitions, gradually introducing more cardiovascular exercise into your program. In the spring, you might try a variety of activities, continue weight training, and get in great shape for the summer.

Train with a Partner   Training partners can motivate and encourage each other through rough spots and help each other develop proper exercise techniques. Training with a partner can make exercising seem easier and more fun. It can also help you keep motivated and on track. For example, you may find it easy to hit the snooze button and skip a planned solo 20-minute morning walk. But would you stay in bed if you knew a friend was waiting for you? A commitment to a friend is a powerful motivator.

Train Your Mind   Becoming fit requires commitment, discipline, and patience. These qualities come from understanding the importance of exercise and having clear and reachable goals. Use the lifestyle management techniques discussed in Chapter 1 to keep your program on track.

Fuel Your Activity Appropriately   Good nutrition, including rehydration and resynthesis of liver and muscle carbohydrate stores, is part of optimal recuperation from exercise. Consume enough calories to support your exercise program without gaining body fat. Many studies show that consuming carbohydrates and protein before or after exercise promotes restoration of stored fuels so that you can exercise intensely again shortly. Nutrition for exercise is discussed in greater detail in Chapters 3 and 8.

Have Fun   You are more likely to stick with an exercise program if it's fun. Choose a variety of activities that you enjoy. Some people like to play competitive sports, such as tennis, golf, or volleyball. Competition can boost motivation, but remember: Sports are competitive, whereas

QUESTIONS FOR CRITICAL THINKING AND REFLECTION

What kind of physical activity or exercise program would be most appropriate for you at this point in your life? If you were to start planning a program, what would be your three most important long-term goals? What would you set as short-term goals? What rewards would be meaningful to you?

training for fitness is not. Other people like more solitary activities, such as jogging, walking, or swimming. Still others like high-skill individual sports, such as skiing, surfing, or skateboarding. Many activities can help you get fit, so choose the ones you enjoy. You can also boost your enjoyment and build your social support network by exercising with friends and family.

Track Your Progress   Monitoring the progress of your program can help keep you motivated and on track. Depending on the activities you've included in your program, you may track different measures of your program—minutes of jogging, miles of cycling, laps of swimming, number of push-ups, amount of weight lifted, and so on. If your program is focused on increasing daily physical activity, consider using an inexpen-

TIPS FOR TODAY AND THE FUTURE

Physical activity and exercise offer benefits in nearly every area of wellness. Even a low-to-moderate level of activity provides valuable health benefits. The important thing is to get moving!

RIGHT NOW YOU CAN

■ Go outside and take a brisk 15-minute walk.
■ Look at your calendar for the rest of the week and write in some physical activity—such as walking, running, biking, skating, swimming, hiking, or playing Frisbee—on as many days as you can. Schedule the activity for a specific time and stick to it.
■ Call a friend and invite her or him to start planning a regular exercise program with you.

IN THE FUTURE YOU CAN

■ Schedule a session with a qualified personal trainer who can evaluate your current fitness level and help you set personalized fitness goals.
■ Create seasonal workout programs for the summer, spring, fall, and winter. Develop programs that are varied but consistent with your overall fitness goals.

sive pedometer to monitor the number of steps you take each day (see Lab 2.3 for more information on setting goals and monitoring activity with a pedometer). Specific examples of program monitoring can be found in the labs for Chapters 3–5 and in the Daily Fitness and Nutrition Journal.

Keep Your Exercise Program in Perspective   As important as physical fitness is, it is only part of a well-rounded life. You have to have time for work and school, family and friends, relaxation and hobbies. Some people become overinvolved in exercise and neglect other parts of their lives. They think of themselves as runners, dancers, swimmers, or triathletes rather than as people who participate in those activities. Balance and moderation are the key ingredients of a fit and well life.

SUMMARY

• Moderate daily exercise contributes substantially to good health. Even without a formal, vigorous exercise program, you can get many of the same health benefits by becoming more physically active.

• If you are already active, you benefit even more by increasing the intensity or duration of your activities.

• The five components of physical fitness most important for health are cardiorespiratory endurance, muscular strength, muscular endurance, flexibility, and body composition.

• Physical training is the process of producing long-term improvements in the body's functioning through exercise. All training is based on the fact that the body adapts to physical stress.

• According to the principle of specificity, bodies change specifically in response to the type of training received.

• Bodies also adapt to progressive overload. When you progressively increase the frequency, intensity, and time (duration) of the right type of exercise, you become increasingly fit.

• Bodies adjust to lower levels of activity by losing fitness, a principle known as reversibility. To counter the effects of reversibility, it's important to keep training at the same intensity, even if you have to reduce the number or length of sessions.

• According to the principle of individual differences, people vary in the maximum level of fitness they can achieve.

• When designing an exercise program, determine if medical clearance is needed, assess your current level of fitness, set realistic goals, and choose activities that develop all the components of fitness.

• Train regularly, get in shape gradually, warm up and cool down, maintain a structured but flexible program, exercise safely, consider training with a partner, train your mind, have fun, and keep exercise in perspective.

Q Where can I work out?

A Identify accessible and pleasant places to work out. For running, find a field or park with a soft surface. For swimming, find a pool that's open at times convenient for you. For cycling, find an area with minimal traffic and air pollution. Make sure the location is safe and convenient. If you join a health club or fitness center, follow the guidelines in the box "Choosing a Fitness Center," on p. 46.

Q What should my fitness goals be?

A Begin by thinking about your general overall goals—the benefits you want to obtain by increasing your activity level and/or beginning a formal exercise program. Examples of long-term goals include reducing your risk of chronic diseases, increasing your energy level, and maintaining a healthy body weight.

To help shape your fitness program, you need to also set specific, short-term goals based on measurable factors. These specific goals should be an extension of your overall goals—the specific changes to your current activity and exercise habits needed to achieve your general goals. In setting short-term goals, be sure to use the SMART criteria described in Chapter 1 (p. 16–17). As noted there, your goals should be **S**pecific, **M**easurable, **A**ttainable, **R**ealistic, and **T**ime frame–specific (SMART).

You need information about your current levels of physical activity and physical fitness in order to set appropriate goals. The labs in this chapter will help you determine your physical activity level—for example, how many minutes per day you engage in moderate or vigorous activity or how many daily steps you take. Using this information, you can set goals for lifestyle physical activity to help you meet your overall goals. For example, if your general long-term goals are to reduce the risk of chronic disease and prevent weight gain, the Dietary Guidelines recommend 60 minutes of moderate physical activity daily. If you currently engage in 30 minutes of moderate activity daily, then your behavior change goal would be to add 30 additional minutes of daily physical activity (or an equivalent number of additional daily steps— about 3500–4000); your time frame for the change might be 8–12 weeks.

Labs in Chapters 3–6 provide opportunities to specifically assess your fitness status for all the health-related components of fitness. The results of these assessments can guide you in setting specific fitness goals. For instance, if the labs in Chapter 4 indicate that you have good muscular strength and endurance in your lower body but poor strength and endurance in your upper body, then setting a specific goal for improving upper-body muscle fitness would be an appropriate goal—increasing the number of push-ups you can do from 22 to 30, for example. Chapters 3–6 include additional advice for setting appropriate goals.

Once you start your behavior change program, you may discover that your goals aren't quite appropriate—perhaps you were overly optimistic, or maybe you set the bar too low. There are limits to the amount of fitness you can achieve, but within the limits of your genes and health status, you can make significant improvements in fitness. Adjust your goals as needed.

Q How can I fit a workout into my day?

A Good time management is an important skill in creating and maintaining an exercise program. Choose a regular time to exercise, preferably the same time every day. Don't tell yourself you'll exercise "sometime during the day" when you have free time—that free time may never come. Schedule your workout, and make it a priority. Include alternative plans in your program to account for circumstances like bad weather or vacations. (You'll have the chance to develop strategies for successful time management in the Behavior Change Workbook at the end of the text.)

Q Where can I get help and advice about exercise?

A One of the best places to get help is an exercise class. There, expert instructors can help you learn the basics of training and answer your questions. Make sure the instructor is certified by a recognized professional organization and/or has formal training in exercise physiology. Read articles by credible experts in fitness magazines. Many of these magazines include articles by leading experts in exercise science written at a layperson's level.

A qualified personal trainer can also help you get started in an exercise program or a new form of training. Make sure this person has proper qualifications, such as a college degree in exercise physiology or physical education or ACSM, National Strength and Conditioning Association (NSCA), or American Council on Exercise (ACE) certification. Don't seek out a person for advice simply because he or she looks fit. UCLA researchers found that 60% of the personal trainers in their study couldn't pass a basic exam on training methods, exercise physiology, or biomechanics. Trainers who performed best had college degrees in exercise physiology, physical education, or physical therapy. So choose your trainer carefully and don't get caught up with fads.

Q Should I follow my exercise program if I'm sick?

A If you have a mild head cold or feel one coming on, it is probably OK to exercise moderately. Just begin slowly and see how you feel. However, if you have symptoms of a more serious illness—fever, swollen glands, nausea, extreme tiredness, muscle aches—wait until you have fully recovered before resuming your exercise program. Continuing to exercise while suffering from an illness more serious than a cold can compromise your recovery and may even be dangerous.

For more Common Questions Answered about fitness, visit the Online Learning Center.

Choosing a Fitness Center

Fitness centers can provide you with many benefits—motivation and companionship are among the most important. A fitness center may also offer expert instruction and supervision as well as access to better equipment than you could afford on your own. There are an estimated 17,000 health clubs in the United States, serving more than 30 million members. All fitness centers, however, are not of the same overall quality. Many health facilities cater to people with very specific exercise or fitness goals. In other words, every fitness center is not for every person. If you're thinking of joining a fitness center, here are some guidelines to help you choose a club that's right for you.

Convenience

- Look for an established facility that's within 10–15 minutes of your home or work. If it's farther away, your chances of sticking to an exercise regimen start to diminish.
- Check out the facility's hours, then visit it at the time you would normally exercise. Is there adequate parking? Will you have easy access to the equipment and exercise classes you want at that time?
- If needed, ask about child-care or youth programs. What services are available, and how are they supervised?

Atmosphere

- Look around to see if there are other members who are your age and at about your fitness level. Some clubs cater to a certain age group or lifestyle, such as hard-core body-builders.
- If you like to exercise to music, make sure you like the music played there, both its type and volume.
- Observe how the members dress. Will you fit in, or will you be uncomfortable?
- Observe the staff. Are they easy to identify? Are they friendly and helpful?
- Check to see that the facility is clean, including showers and lockers. Make sure the facility is climate controlled, well ventilated, and well lit.

Safety

- Find out if the facility offers some type of preactivity screening as well as basic fitness testing that includes cardiovascular screening.
- Determine if personnel are trained in CPR and if there is emergency equipment such as automated external defibrillators (AEDs) on the premises. An AED can help someone with cardiac arrest.
- Ask if at least one staff member on each shift is trained in first aid.
- Find out if the club has an emergency plan in case a member has a heart attack or serious injury (many clubs do not). The facility should also have an evacuation plan, as well as established procedures for responding to other types of emergencies. All personnel should be trained in carrying out these plans.

Trained Personnel

- Determine if the personal trainers and fitness instructors are certified by a recognized professional association such as the American College of Sports Medicine (ACSM), Aerobics and Fitness Association of America (AFAA), National Strength and Conditioning Association (NSCA), or American Council on Exercise (ACE). All personal trainers are not equal; more than 100 organizations certify trainers, and few of these require much formal training. Trainers with college degrees in exercise physiology or physical education are usually the most knowledgeable.
- Find out if the club has a trained exercise physiologist on staff, such as someone with a degree in exercise physiology, kinesiology, or exercise science. If the facility offers nutritional counseling, it should employ someone who is a registered dietitian (RD) or has similar formal training.
- Ask how much experience the instructors have. Clubs may employ people because they were good athletes or look fit; by themselves, these are not good reasons to hire someone. Ideally, trainers should have both academic preparation and practical experience.

Cost

- Buy only what you need and can afford. If you want to use only workout equipment, you may not need a club that has racquetball courts and saunas.
- Check the contract. Choose the one that covers the shortest period of time possible, especially if it's your first fitness club experience. Don't feel pressured to sign a long-term contract.
- Make sure the contract permits you to extend your membership if you have a prolonged illness or go on vacation.
- Try out the club. Ask for a free trial workout, or a 1-day pass, or an inexpensive 1- or 2-week trial membership.
- Find out whether there is an extra charge for the particular services you want. Get any special offers in writing.

Effectiveness

- Tour the facility. Does it offer what the brochure says it does? Does it offer the activities and equipment you want?
- Check the equipment. A good club will have treadmills, bikes, stair-climbers, resistance machines, and weights. Make sure these machines are up-to-date and well maintained.
- Find out if new members get a formal orientation and instruction on how to safely use the equipment. Will a staff member help you develop a program that is appropriate for your current fitness level and goals?
- Make sure the facility is certified. Look for the displayed names American College of Sports Medicine (ACSM), American Council on Exercise (ACE), Aerobics and Fitness Association of America (AFAA), or International Health, Racquet, and Sportsclub Association (IHRSA).
- Don't get cheated. Check with your Better Business Bureau or Consumer Affairs office to see if others have complained about the facility.

BOOKS

American College of Sports Medicine. 2003. *ACSM Fitness Book,* 3rd ed. Champaign, Ill.: Human Kinetics. *Provides a step-by-step approach to becoming more active and developing a fitness program.*

American College of Sports Medicine. 2006. *ACSM's Guidelines for Exercise Testing and Prescription,* 7th ed. Philadelphia: Lippincott Williams and Wilkins. *Includes the ACSM guidelines for safety of exercising, a basic discussion of exercise physiology, and information about fitness testing and prescription.*

Earle, R. W., and T. R. Baechle, eds. 2004. *NSCA's Essentials of Personal Training.* Champaign, Ill.: Human Kinetics. *Comprehensive discussions of fitness testing, exercise and disease, nutrition and physical performance, and exercise prescription.*

Mayo Clinic. 2005. *Mayo Clinic Fitness for Everybody.* Rochester, Minn.: Mayo Clinic. *An illustrated guide to designing and maintaining a personalized fitness program, with hundreds of fully illustrated exercises.*

JOURNALS

ACSM Health and Fitness Journal (401 West Michigan Street, Indianapolis, IN 46202; http://www.acsm-healthfitness.org)

Physician and Sportsmedicine (4530 W. 77th Street, Minneapolis, MN 55435; many of the journal's articles are also available online at http://ww.postgradmed.com/journal.htm)

ORGANIZATIONS, HOTLINES, AND WEB SITES

American Alliance for Health, Physical Education, Recreation, and Dance (AAHPERD). A professional organization dedicated to promoting quality health and physical education programs.
> 800-213-7193
> http://www.aahperd.org

American College of Sports Medicine (ACSM). The principal professional organization for sports medicine and exercise science. Provides brochures, publications, and audio- and videotapes.
> 317-637-9200
> http://www.acsm.org

American Council on Exercise (ACE). Promotes exercise and fitness; the Web site features fact sheets on many consumer topics, including choosing shoes, cross-training, and steroids.
> 888-825-3636
> http://www.acefitness.org

American Heart Association: Start! Provides practical advice for people of all fitness levels plus an online fitness diary.
> http://www.heart.org/presenter.jhtml?identifier=3040778

CDC Physical Activity Information. Provides information on the benefits of physical activity and suggestions for incorporating moderate physical activity into daily life.
> http://www.cdc.gov/nccdphp/dnpa/

Disabled Sports USA. Provides sports and recreation services to people with physical or mobility disorders.
> http://www.dsusa.org

Health Canada's Physical Activity Guide. Offers many suggestions for incorporating physical activity into everyday life.
> http://www.hc-sc.gc.ca/hl-vs/physactiv/index_e.html

International Health, Racquet, and Sportsclub Association (IHRSA): Health Clubs. Provides guidelines for choosing a health or fitness facility and links to clubs that belong to IHRSA.
> http://www.healthclubs.com

MedlinePlus: Exercise and Physical Fitness. Provides links to news and reliable information about fitness and exercise from government agencies and professional associations.
> http://www.nlm.nih.gov/medlineplus/exercisephysicalfitness.html

President's Council on Physical Fitness and Sports (PCPFS). Provides information on PCPFS programs and publications, including fitness guides and fact sheets.
> http://www.fitness.gov
> http://www.presidentschallenge.org

Shape Up America! A nonprofit organization that provides information and resources on exercise, nutrition, and weight loss.
> http://www.shapeup.org

SmallStep.Gov. Provides resources for increasing activity and improving diet through small changes in daily habits.
> http://www.smallstep.gov

The following provide links to sites with information on a wide variety of activities and fitness issues; evaluate commercial sites carefully.

Fitness Jumpsite: http://www.primusweb.com/fitnesspartner
NetSweat: The Internet's Fitness Resource: http://www.netsweat.com
Yahoo!Fitness: http://dir.yahoo.com/Health/Fitness

SELECTED BIBLIOGRAPHY

American College of Sports Medicine. 2007. *ACSM's Health/Fitness Facility Standards and Guidelines,* 3rd ed. Champaign, Ill.: Human Kinetics.

American College of Sports Medicine. 2006. *ACSM's Guidelines for Exercise Testing and Prescription.* Philadelphia: Lippincott Williams and Wilkins.

American College of Sports Medicine. 2006. *ACSM's Resource Manual for Guidelines for Exercise Testing and Prescription,* 5th ed. Philadelphia: Lippincott Williams and Wilkins.

American College of Sports Medicine. 1998. The recommended quantity and quality of exercise for developing and maintaining cardiorespiratory and muscular fitness, and flexibility in healthy adults. ACSM position paper. *Medicine and Science in Sports and Exercise* 30(6): 975–991.

American College of Obstetrics and Gynecology Committee on Obstetric Practice. 2002. Exercise during pregnancy and the postpartum period. Committee Opinion No. 267. *International Journal of Gynaecology and Obstetrics* 77:79–81.

American Heart Association. 2007. Resistance exercise in individuals with and without cardiovascular disease, 2007 update: A scientific statement from the American Heart Association Council on Clinical Cardiology and Council on Nutrition, Physical Activity, and Metabolism. *Circulation* 116: 572–584.

Bouchard, C., et al. 2007. *Physical Activity and Health.* Champaign, Ill.: Human Kinetics.

Centers for Disease Control and Prevention. 2005. Trends in leisure-time physical inactivity by age, sex, and race/ethnicity—United States, 1994–2004. *Morbidity and Mortality Weekly Report* 54(39): 991–994.

Centers for Disease Control and Prevention. 2007. Prevalence of regular physical activity among adults-United States, 2001 and 2005. *Morbidity and Mortality Weekly Report* 56(46): 12-9-1212

Colcombe, S. J., et al. 2006. Aerobic exercise training increases brain volume in aging humans. *The Journals of Gerontology: Series A, Biological Sciences and Medical Sciences* 61(11): 1166–1170.

Department of Health and Human Services. 1996. *Physical Activity and Health: A Report of the Surgeon General*. Atlanta: DHHS.

Dong, L., G. Block, and S. Mandel. 2004. Activities contributing to total energy expenditure in the United States: Results from the NHAPS Study. *International Journal of Behavioral Nutrition and Physical Activity* 1(4).

Ekelund, U., et al. 2007. Physical activity and metabolic risk in individuals with a family history of type 2 diabetes. *Diabetes Care* 30(2): 337–342.

Exercise for health: How much exercise is enough? ACSM works with others to avoid misunderstanding. 2003. *ACSM Fit Society Page,* Winter.

Garman, J. F., et al. 2004. Occurrence of exercise dependence in a college-aged population. *Journal of American College Health* 52(5): 221–228.

Greaney, M. L., et al. 2004. What older adults find useful for maintaining healthy eating and exercise habits. *Journal of Nutrition for the Elderly* 24: 19–35.

Haskell, W. L., et al. 2007. Physical activity and public health: Updated recommendation for adults from the American College of Sports Medicine and the American Heart Association. *Medicine & Science in Sports & Exercise* 39: 1423–1434.

Haskell, W. L., et al. 2007. Physical activity and public health in older adults: Recommendation from the American College of Sports Medicine and the American Heart Association. *Medicine & Science in Sports & Exercise* 39: 1435–1445.

Hu, F. B. 2003. Sedentary lifestyle and risk of obesity and type 2 diabetes. *Lipids* 38(2): 103–108.

Institutes of Medicine, National Academies. 2002. *Dietary Reference Intakes for Energy, Carbohydrate, Fiber, Fat, Fatty Acids, Cholesterol, Protein, and Amino Acids*. Washington, D.C.: National Academy Press.

Is easy-does-it exercise enough? 2004. *Consumer Reports on Health,* February.

Jonker, J. T., et al. 2006. Physical activity and life expectancy with and without diabetes. *Diabetes Care* 29: 38–43.

Kushi, L. H., et al. 2006. American Cancer Society guidelines on nutrition and physical activity for cancer prevention: Reducing the risk of cancer with healthy food choices and physical activity. *CA: A Cancer Journal for Clinicians* 56: 254–281.

Kruger, J., et al. 2005. Physical activity profiles of U.S. adults trying to lose weight: NHIS 1998. *Medicine and Science in Sports and Exercise* 37: 364–368.

Le Masurier, G. 2005. Walkee talkee: Answers to pedometer FAQs. *ACSM Fit Society Page,* Spring.

Lucas, J. W., J. S. Schiller, and V. Benson. 2004. Summary health statistics for U.S. adults: National Health Interview Survey, 2001. *Vital Health Statistics* 10: 1–134.

Lustyk, M. K., et al. 2004. Physical activity and quality of life: Assessing the influence of activity frequency, intensity, volume, and motives. *Behavioral Medicine* 30: 124–131.

Macfarlane, D. J., et al. 2006. Very short intermittent versus continuous bouts of activity in sedentary adults. *Preventive Medicine* 43(4): 332–336.

Malek, M. H., et al. 2002. Importance of health science education for personal fitness trainers. *Journal of Strength and Conditioning Research* 16: 19–24.

Marks, B. L., et al. Role of aerobic fitness and aging on cerebral white matter integrity. *Annals of the New York Academy of Sciences* 1097: 171–174.

Pate, R. R., et al. 1995. Physical activity and public health: A recommendation from the Centers for Disease Control and Prevention and the American College of Sports Medicine. *Journal of the American Medical Association* 273: 402–407.

President's Council on Physical Fitness and Sports. 2000. Definitions: Health, fitness, and physical activity. *Research Digest* 3(9).

Rosenbloom, C., and M. Bahns. 2006. What can we learn about diet and physical activity from master athletes? *Holistic Nursing Practice* 20(4): 161–166.

Sorensen, J. B., et al. 2007. Exercise on prescription: Trial protocol and evaluation of outcomes. *BMC Health Services Research* 7: 36.

Swain, D. P. 2005. Moderate or vigorous intensity exercise: Which is better for improving aerobic fitness? *Preventive Cardiology* 8: 55–58.

Vanhees, L., et al. 2005. How to assess physical activity? How to assess physical fitness? *European Journal of Cardiovascular Prevention and Rehabilitation* 12: 102–114.

U.S. Department of Health and Human Services and U.S. Department of Agriculture. 2005. *Dietary Guidelines for Americans, 2005,* 6th ed. Washington, D.C.: U.S. Government Printing Office.

World Health Organization/FAO Expert Consultation. 2003. *Diet, Nutrition and the Prevention of Chronic Diseases*. WHO Technical Report Series 916. Geneva: World Health Organization.

LAB 2.1 Safety of Exercise Participation

Physical Activity Readiness
Questionnaire - PAR-Q
(revised 2002)

PAR-Q & YOU

(A Questionnaire for People Aged 15 to 69)

Regular physical activity is fun and healthy, and increasingly more people are starting to become more active every day. Being more active is very safe for most people. However, some people should check with their doctor before they start becoming much more physically active.

If you are planning to become much more physically active than you are now, start by answering the seven questions in the box below. If you are between the ages of 15 and 69, the PAR-Q will tell you if you should check with your doctor before you start. If you are over 69 years of age, and you are not used to being very active, check with your doctor.

Common sense is your best guide when you answer these questions. Please read the questions carefully and answer each one honestly: check YES or NO.

YES	NO		
☐	☐	1.	**Has your doctor ever said that you have a heart condition <u>and</u> that you should only do physical activity recommended by a doctor?**
☐	☐	2.	**Do you feel pain in your chest when you do physical activity?**
☐	☐	3.	**In the past month, have you had chest pain when you were not doing physical activity?**
☐	☐	4.	**Do you lose your balance because of dizziness or do you ever lose consciousness?**
☐	☐	5.	**Do you have a bone or joint problem (for example, back, knee or hip) that could be made worse by a change in your physical activity?**
☐	☐	6.	**Is your doctor currently prescribing drugs (for example, water pills) for your blood pressure or heart condition?**
☐	☐	7.	**Do you know of <u>any other reason</u> why you should not do physical activity?**

If

you

answered

YES to one or more questions

Talk with your doctor by phone or in person BEFORE you start becoming much more physically active or BEFORE you have a fitness appraisal. Tell your doctor about the PAR-Q and which questions you answered YES.

- You may be able to do any activity you want — as long as you start slowly and build up gradually. Or, you may need to restrict your activities to those which are safe for you. Talk with your doctor about the kinds of activities you wish to participate in and follow his/her advice.
- Find out which community programs are safe and helpful for you.

NO to all questions

If you answered NO honestly to <u>all</u> PAR-Q questions, you can be reasonably sure that you can:
- start becoming much more physically active — begin slowly and build up gradually. This is the safest and easiest way to go.
- take part in a fitness appraisal – this is an excellent way to determine your basic fitness so that you can plan the best way for you to live actively. It is also highly recommended that you have your blood pressure evaluated. If your reading is over 144/94, talk with your doctor before you start becoming much more physically active.

→

DELAY BECOMING MUCH MORE ACTIVE:
- if you are not feeling well because of a temporary illness such as a cold or a fever — wait until you feel better; or
- if you are or may be pregnant — talk to your doctor before you start becoming more active.

PLEASE NOTE: If your health changes so that you then answer YES to any of the above questions, tell your fitness or health professional. Ask whether you should change your physical activity plan.

<u>Informed Use of the PAR-Q</u>: The Canadian Society for Exercise Physiology, Health Canada, and their agents assume no liability for persons who undertake physical activity, and if in doubt after completing this questionnaire, consult your doctor prior to physical activity.

No changes permitted. You are encouraged to photocopy the PAR-Q but only if you use the entire form.

NOTE: If the PAR-Q is being given to a person before he or she participates in a physical activity program or a fitness appraisal, this section may be used for legal or administrative purposes.

"I have read, understood and completed this questionnaire. Any questions I had were answered to my full satisfaction."

NAME _____

SIGNATURE _____

SIGNATURE OF PARENT _____
or GUARDIAN (for participants under the age of majority)

DATE _____

WITNESS _____

Note: This physical activity clearance is valid for a maximum of 12 months from the date it is completed and becomes invalid if your condition changes so that you would answer YES to any of the seven questions.

© Canadian Society for Exercise Physiology

Supported by: Health Santé
Canada Canada

General Health Profile

To help further assess the safety of exercise for you, complete as much of this health profile as possible.

General Information

Age: _____

Height: _____

Weight: _____

Total cholesterol: _____

HDL: _____

LDL: _____

Blood pressure: _____ / _____

Triglycerides: _____

Blood glucose level: _____

Are you currently trying to _____ gain or _____ lose weight? (check one if appropriate)

Medical Conditions/Treatments

Check any of the following that apply to you, and add any other conditions that might affect your ability to exercise safely.

_____ heart disease

_____ lung disease

_____ diabetes

_____ allergies

_____ asthma

_____ depression, anxiety, or other psychological disorder

_____ eating disorder

_____ back pain

_____ arthritis

_____ other injury or joint problem: _____

_____ substance abuse problem

_____ other: _____

_____ other: _____

_____ other: _____

_____ Do you have a family history of cardiovascular disease (CVD) (a parent, sibling, or child who had a heart attack or stroke before age 55 for men or 65 for women)?

List any medications or supplements you are taking or any medical treatments you are undergoing. Include the name of the substance or treatment and its purpose. Include both prescription and over-the-counter drugs and supplements.

_____   _____

_____   _____

Lifestyle Information

Check any of the following that is true for you, and fill in the requested information.

_____ I usually eat high-fat foods (fatty meats, cheese, fried foods, butter, full-fat dairy products) every day.

_____ I consume fewer than 5 servings of fruits and vegetables on most days.

_____ I smoke cigarettes or use other tobacco products. If true, describe your use of tobacco (type and frequency): _____

_____ I regularly drink alcohol. If true, describe your typical weekly consumption pattern: _____

_____ I often feel as if I need more sleep. (I need about _____ hours per day; I get about _____ hours per day.)

_____ I feel as though stress has adversely affected my level of wellness during the past year.

Describe your current activity pattern. What types of moderate physical activity do you engage in on a daily basis? Are you involved in a formal exercise program, or do you regularly participate in sports or recreational activities?

_____

_____

Using Your Results

How did you score? Did the PAR-Q indicate that exercise is likely to be safe for you? Is there anything in your health profile that you think may affect your ability to exercise safely? Have you had any problems with exercise in the past?

What should you do next? If the assessments in this lab indicate that you should see your physician before beginning an exercise program, or if you have any questions about the safety of exercise for you, make an appointment to talk with your health care provider to address your concerns.

LAB 2.2 Overcoming Barriers to Being Active

Barriers to Being Active Quiz

Directions: Listed below are reasons that people give to describe why they do not get as much physical activity as they think they should. Please read each statement and indicate how likely you are to say each of the following statements.

How likely are you to say this?	Very likely	Somewhat likely	Somewhat unlikely	Very unlikely
1. My day is so busy now, I just don't think I can make the time to include physical activity in my regular schedule.	3	2	1	0
2. None of my family members or friends like to do anything active, so I don't have a chance to exercise.	3	2	1	0
3. I'm just too tired after work to get any exercise.	3	2	1	0
4. I've been thinking about getting more exercise, but I just can't seem to get started.	3	2	1	0
5. I'm getting older so exercise can be risky.	3	2	1	0
6. I don't get enough exercise because I have never learned the skills for any sport.	3	2	1	0
7. I don't have access to jogging trails, swimming pools, bike paths, etc.	3	2	1	0
8. Physical activity takes too much time away from other commitments—like work, family, etc.	3	2	1	0
9. I'm embarrassed about how I will look when I exercise with others.	3	2	1	0
10. I don't get enough sleep as it is. I just couldn't get up early or stay up late to get some exercise.	3	2	1	0
11. It's easier for me to find excuses not to exercise than to go out and do something.	3	2	1	0
12. I know of too many people who have hurt themselves by overdoing it with exercise.	3	2	1	0
13. I really can't see learning a new sport at my age.	3	2	1	0
14. It's just too expensive. You have to take a class or join a club or buy the right equipment.	3	2	1	0
15. My free times during the day are too short to include exercise.	3	2	1	0
16. My usual social activities with family or friends do not include physical activity.	3	2	1	0
17. I'm too tired during the week and I need the weekend to catch up on my rest.	3	2	1	0

How likely are you to say this?	Very likely	Somewhat likely	Somewhat unlikely	Very unlikely
18. I want to get more exercise, but I just can't seem to make myself stick to anything.	3	2	1	0
19. I'm afraid I might injure myself or have a heart attack.	3	2	1	0
20. I'm not good enough at any physical activity to make it fun.	3	2	1	0
21. If we had exercise facilities and showers at work, then I would be more likely to exercise.	3	2	1	0

Scoring

- Enter the circled numbers in the spaces provided, putting the number for statement 1 on line 1, statement 2 on line 2, and so on.

- Add the three scores on each line. Your barriers to physical activity fall into one or more of seven categories: lack of time, social influence, lack of energy, lack of willpower, fear of injury, lack of skill, and lack of resources. A score of 5 or above in any category shows that this is an important barrier for you to overcome.

```
____  +  ____  +  ____  =  _____
  1         8        15         Lack of time

____  +  ____  +  ____  =  _____
  2         9        16         Social influence

____  +  ____  +  ____  =  _____
  3        10        17         Lack of energy

____  +  ____  +  ____  =  _____
  4        11        18         Lack of willpower

____  +  ____  +  ____  =  _____
  5        12        19         Fear of injury

____  +  ____  +  ____  =  _____
  6        13        20         Lack of skill

____  +  ____  +  ____  =  _____
  7        14        21         Lack of resources
```

Using Your Results

How did you score? How many key barriers did you identify? Are they what you expected?

What should you do next? For your key barriers, try the strategies listed on the following pages and/or develop additional strategies that work for you. Check off any strategy that you try.

Suggestions for Overcoming Physical Activity Barriers

Lack of time

_____ Identify available time slots. Monitor your daily activities for 1 week. Identify at least three 30-minute time slots you could use for physical activity.

_____ Add physical activity to your daily routine. For example, walk or ride your bike to work or shopping, organize social activities around physical activity, walk the dog, exercise while you watch TV, park farther from your destination, etc.

_____ Make time for physical activity. For example, walk, jog, or swim during your lunch hour, or take fitness breaks instead of coffee breaks.

_____ Select activities requiring minimal time, such as walking, jogging, or stair climbing.

_____ Other: _____

Social influence

_____ Explain your interest in physical activity to friends and family. Ask them to support your efforts.

_____ Invite friends and family members to exercise with you. Plan social activities involving exercise.

_____ Develop new friendships with physically active people. Join a group, such as the YMCA or a hiking club.

_____ Other: _____

Lack of energy

_____ Schedule physical activity for times in the day or week when you feel energetic.

_____ Convince yourself that if you give it a chance, exercise will increase your energy level; then, try it.

_____ Other: _____

Lack of willpower

_____ Plan ahead. Make physical activity a regular part of your daily or weekly schedule and write it on your calendar.

_____ Invite a friend to exercise with you on a regular basis and write it on _both_ your calendars.

_____ Join an exercise group or class.

_____ Other: _____

Fear of injury

_____ Learn how to warm up and cool down to prevent injury.

_____ Learn how to exercise appropriately considering your age, fitness level, skill level, and health status.

_____ Choose activities involving minimal risk.

_____ Other: _____

Lack of skill

_____ Select activities requiring no new skills, such as walking, jogging, or stair climbing.

_____ Exercise with friends who are at the same skill level as you are.

_____ Find a friend who is willing to teach you some new skills.

_____ Take a class to develop new skills.

_____ Other: _____

Lack of resources

_____ Select activities that require minimal facilities or equipment, such as walking, jogging, jumping rope, or calisthenics.

_____ Identify inexpensive, convenient resources available in your community (community education programs, park and recreation programs, worksite programs, etc.).

_____ Other: _____

Are any of the following additional barriers important for you? If so, try some of the strategies listed here or invent your own.

Weather conditions

_____ Develop a set of regular activities that are always available regardless of weather (indoor cycling, aerobic dance, indoor swimming, calisthenics, stair climbing, rope skipping, mall walking, dancing, gymnasium games, etc.).

_____ Look on outdoor activities that depend on weather conditions (cross-country skiing, outdoor swimming, outdoor tennis, etc.) as "bonuses"—extra activities possible when weather and circumstances permit.

_____ Other: _____

Travel

_____ Put a jump rope in your suitcase and jump rope.

_____ Walk the halls and climb the stairs in hotels.

_____ Stay in places with swimming pools or exercise facilities.

_____ Join the YMCA or YWCA (ask about reciprocal membership agreements).

_____ Visit the local shopping mall and walk for half an hour or more.

_____ Bring a small tape recorder and your favorite aerobic exercise tape.

_____ Other: _____

Family obligations

_____ Trade babysitting time with a friend, neighbor, or family member who also has small children.

_____ Exercise _with_ the kids—go for a walk together, play tag or other running games, or get an aerobic dance or exercise tape for kids (there are several on the market) and exercise together. You can spend time together and still get your exercise.

_____ Hire a babysitter and look at the cost as a worthwhile investment in your physical and mental health.

_____ Jump rope, do calisthenics, ride a stationary bicycle, or use other home gymnasium equipment while the kids watch TV or when they are sleeping.

_____ Try to exercise when the kids are not around (e.g., during school hours or their nap time).

_____ Other: _____

Retirement years

_____ Look on your retirement as an opportunity to become more active instead of less. Spend more time gardening, walking the dog, and playing with your grandchildren. Children with short legs and grandparents with slower gaits are often great walking partners.

_____ Learn a new skill you've always been interested in, such as ballroom dancing, square dancing, or swimming.

_____ Now that you have the time, make regular physical activity a part of every day. Go for a walk every morning or every evening before dinner. Treat yourself to an exercycle and ride every day during a favorite TV show.

_____ Other: _____

SOURCE: CDC Division of Nutrition and Physical Activity. 1999. _Promoting Physical Activity: A Guide for Community Action._ Champaign, Ill.: Human Kinetics.

LAB 2.3 Using a Pedometer to Track Physical Activity

How physically active are you? Would you be more motivated to increase daily physical activity if you had an easy way to monitor your level of activity? If so, consider wearing a pedometer to track the number of steps you take each day—a rough but easily obtainable reflection of daily physical activity.

Determine Your Baseline

Wear the pedometer for a week to obtain a baseline average daily number of steps.

	M	T	W	Th	F	Sa	Su	Average
Steps								

Set Goals

Set an appropriate goal for increasing steps. The goal of 10,000 steps per day is widely recommended, but your personal goal should reflect your baseline level of steps. For example, if your current daily steps are far below 10,000, a goal of walking 2000 additional steps each day might be appropriate. If you are already close to 10,000 steps per day, choose a higher goal. Also consider the physical activity goals in the 2005 Dietary Guidelines:

- To reduce the risk of chronic disease, aim to accumulate at least 30 minutes of moderate physical activity per day.
- To help manage body weight and prevent gradual, unhealthy weight gain, engage in 60 minutes of moderate-to-vigorous-intensity activity on most days of the week.
- To sustain weight loss, engage daily in at least 60–90 minutes of moderate-intensity physical activity.

To help gauge how close you are to meeting these time-based physical activity goals, you might walk for 10–15 minutes while wearing your pedometer to determine how many steps correspond with the time-based goals from the Dietary Guidelines.

Once you have set your overall goal, break it down into several steps. For example, if your goal is to increase daily steps by 2000, set mini-goals of increasing daily steps by 500, allowing 2 weeks to reach each mini-goal. Smaller goals are easier to achieve and can help keep you motivated and on track. Having several interim goals also gives you the opportunity to reward yourself more frequently. Note your goals below:

Mini-goal 1: _____ Target date: _____ Reward: _____

Mini-goal 2: _____ Target date: _____ Reward: _____

Mini-goal 3: _____ Target date: _____ Reward: _____

Overall goal: _____ Target date: _____ Reward: _____

Develop Strategies for Increasing Steps

What can you do to become more active? Your text includes a variety of suggestions, including walking when you do errands, getting off one stop from your destination on public transportation, parking an extra block or two away from your destination, and doing at least one chore every day that requires physical activity. If weather or neighborhood safety is an issue, look for alternative locations to walk. For example, find an indoor gym or shopping mall or even a long hallway. Check out locations that are near or on the way to your campus, workplace, or residence. If you think walking indoors will be dull, walk with friends or family members or wear headphones (if safe) and listen to music or books on tape.

Are there any days of the week for which your baseline steps are particularly low and/or it will be especially difficult because of your schedule to increase your number of steps? Be sure to develop specific strategies for difficult situations.

Below, list at least five strategies for increasing daily steps:

_____   _____

_____   _____

_____   _____

Track Your Progress

Based on the goals you set, fill in your goal portion of the progress chart with your target average daily steps for each week. Then wear your pedometer every day and note your total daily steps. Track your progress toward each mini-goal and your final goal. Every few weeks, stop and evaluate your progress. If needed, adjust your plan and develop additional strategies for increasing steps. In addition to the chart in this worksheet, you might also want to graph your daily steps to provide a visual reminder of how you are progressing toward your goals. Make as many copies of this chart as you need.

Week	Goal	M	Tu	W	Th	F	Sa	Su	Average
1									
2									
3									
4									

Progress Checkup

How close are you to meeting your goal? How do you feel about your program and your progress?

If needed, describe changes to your plan and additional strategies for increasing steps:

Week	Goal	M	Tu	W	Th	F	Sa	Su	Average
5									
6									
7									
8									

Progress Checkup

How close are you to meeting your goal? How do you feel about your program and your progress?

If needed, describe changes to your plan and additional strategies for increasing steps:

Week	Goal	M	Tu	W	Th	F	Sa	Su	Average
9									
10									
11									
12									

Progress Checkup

How close are you to meeting your goal? How do you feel about your program and your progress?

If needed, describe changes to your plan and additional strategies for increasing steps:

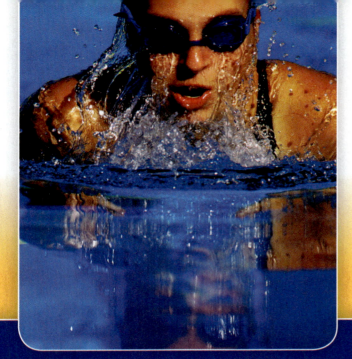

LOOKING AHEAD>>>>>

AFTER READING THIS CHAPTER, YOU SHOULD BE ABLE TO:

- Describe how the body produces the energy it needs for exercise
- List the major effects and benefits of cardiorespiratory endurance exercise
- Explain how cardiorespiratory endurance is measured and assessed
- Describe how frequency, intensity, time (duration), and type of exercise affect the development of cardiorespiratory endurance
- Explain the best ways to prevent and treat common exercise injuries

CARDIORESPIRATORY ENDURANCE

3

TEST YOUR KNOWLEDGE

1. **Compared to sedentary people, those who engage in regular moderate endurance exercise are likely to**
   a. have fewer colds.
   b. be less anxious and depressed.
   c. fall asleep more quickly and sleep better.
   d. be more alert and creative.

2. **About how much blood does the heart pump each minute during aerobic exercise?**
   a. 5 quarts
   b. 10 quarts
   c. 20 quarts

3. **During an effective 30-minute cardiorespiratory endurance workout, you should lose 1–2 pounds.**

   True or false?

ANSWERS

1. **ALL FOUR.** Endurance exercise has many immediate benefits that affect all the dimensions of wellness and improve overall quality of life.

2. **c.** During exercise, cardiac output increases to 20 or more quarts per minute, compared to about 5 quarts per minute at rest.

3. **FALSE.** Any weight loss during an exercise session is due to fluid loss that needs to be replaced to prevent dehydration and enhance performance. It is best to drink enough during exercise to match fluid loss in sweat (usually about 6–12 ounces every 15–20 minutes of exercise); weigh yourself before and after a workout to make sure that you are drinking enough.

FIT AND WELL ONLINE LEARNING CENTER www.mhhe.com/fahey

Visit the *Fit and Well* Online Learning Center for resources that will help you get the most out of your course!

- Study and review aids include practice quizzes, glossary flashcards, chapter summaries, learning objectives, PowerPoint presentations, Common Questions Answered, student handouts, crossword puzzles, Internet activities, and links to wellness Web sites.
- Behavior change tools include a daily fitness and nutrition journal, a behavior change workbook, sample behavior change plans, and blank behavior change logs to print and use.
- Chapter 3 resources also include three "custom chapters" that provide more in-depth information on topics of special interest—"Developing Sport and Movement Skills," "Prevention and Care of Athletic Injuries," and "The Environment and Exercise."

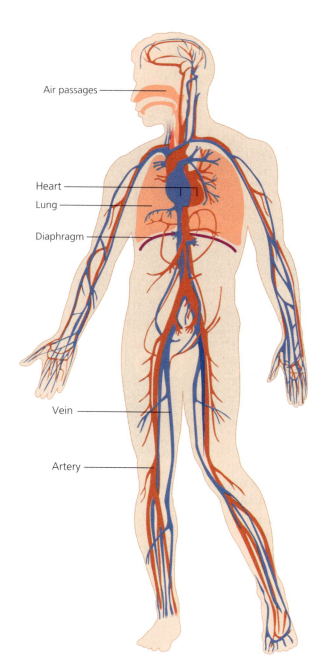

Cardiorespiratory endurance—the ability of the body to perform prolonged, large-muscle, dynamic exercise at moderate-to-high levels of intensity—is a key health-related component of fitness. As explained in Chapter 2, a healthy cardiorespiratory system is essential to high levels of fitness and wellness.

This chapter reviews the short- and long-term effects and benefits of cardiorespiratory endurance exercise. It then describes several tests that are commonly used to assess cardiorespiratory fitness. Finally, it provides guidelines for creating your own cardiorespiratory endurance program, one that is geared to your current level of fitness and built around activities you enjoy.

BASIC PHYSIOLOGY OF CARDIORESPIRATORY ENDURANCE EXERCISE

A basic understanding of the body processes involved in cardiorespiratory endurance exercise can help you design a safe and effective fitness program.

TERMS

cardiorespiratory system   The system that circulates blood through the body; consists of the heart, blood vessels, and respiratory system.

pulmonary circulation   The part of the circulatory system that moves blood between the heart and the lungs; controlled by the right side of the heart.

systemic circulation   The part of the circulatory system that moves blood between the heart and the rest of the body; controlled by the left side of the heart.

venae cavae   The large veins through which blood is returned to the right atrium of the heart.

atria   The two upper chambers of the heart in which blood collects before passing to the ventricles; also called *auricles*.

ventricles   The two lower chambers of the heart from which blood flows through arteries to the lungs and other parts of the body.

aorta   The large artery that receives blood from the left ventricle and distributes it to the body.

systole   Contraction of the heart.

diastole   Relaxation of the heart.

blood pressure   The force exerted by the blood on the walls of the blood vessels; created by the pumping action of the heart.

veins   Vessels that carry blood to the heart.

arteries   Vessels that carry blood away from the heart.

Air passages

Heart

Lung

Diaphragm

Vein

Artery

FIGURE 3.1   The cardiorespiratory system.

The Cardiorespiratory System

The **cardiorespiratory system** consists of the heart, the blood vessels, and the respiratory system (Figure 3.1). The cardiorespiratory system transports oxygen, nutrients, and other key substances to the organs and tissues that need them; it also carries waste products to where they can be used or expelled.

The Heart   The heart is a four-chambered, fist-sized muscle located just beneath the sternum (breastbone). It pumps oxygen-poor blood to the lungs and oxygenated (oxygen-rich) blood to the rest of the body. Blood

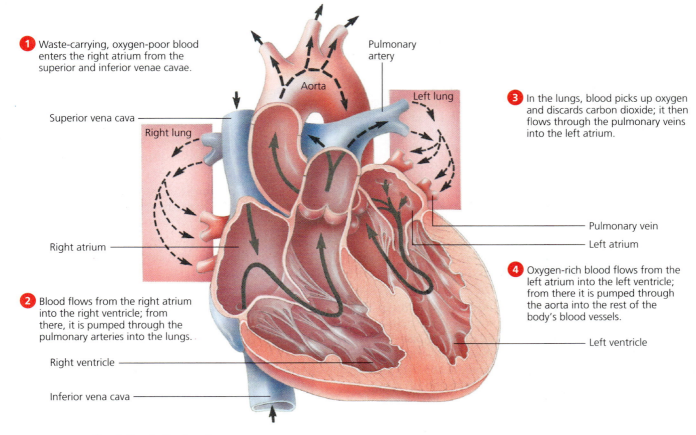

1 Waste-carrying, oxygen-poor blood enters the right atrium from the superior and inferior venae cavae.

Pulmonary artery

Aorta

Superior vena cava

Right lung

Left lung

3 In the lungs, blood picks up oxygen and discards carbon dioxide; it then flows through the pulmonary veins into the left atrium.

Right atrium

Pulmonary vein

Left atrium

2 Blood flows from the right atrium into the right ventricle; from there, it is pumped through the pulmonary arteries into the lungs.

4 Oxygen-rich blood flows from the left atrium into the left ventricle; from there it is pumped through the aorta into the rest of the body's blood vessels.

Right ventricle

Left ventricle

Inferior vena cava

FIGURE 3.2   Circulation in the heart.

actually travels through two separate circulatory systems: The right side of the heart pumps blood to the lungs in what is called **pulmonary circulation**, and the left side pumps blood through the rest of the body in **systemic circulation.**

The following steps describe the path blood follows as it travels through the cardiorespiratory system (Figure 3.2):

1. Waste-laden, oxygen-poor blood travels through large vessels, called **venae cavae**, into the heart's right upper chamber, or **atrium.**

2. After the right atrium fills, it contracts and pumps blood into the heart's right lower chamber, or **ventricle.**

3. When the right ventricle is full, it contracts and pumps blood through the pulmonary artery into the lungs.

4. In the lungs, blood picks up oxygen and discards carbon dioxide.

5. The cleaned, oxygenated blood flows from the lungs through the pulmonary veins into the heart's left atrium.

6. After the left atrium fills, it contracts and pumps blood into the left ventricle.

7. When the left ventricle is full, it pumps blood through the **aorta**—the body's largest artery—for distribution to the rest of the body's blood vessels.

The period of the heart's contraction is called **systole;** the period of relaxation is called **diastole**. During systole, the atria contract first, pumping blood into the ventricles. A fraction of a second later, the ventricles contract, pumping blood to the lungs and the body. During diastole, blood flows into the heart.

Blood pressure, the force exerted by blood on the walls of the blood vessels, is created by the pumping action of the heart; blood pressure is greater during systole than during diastole. A person weighing 150 pounds has about 5 quarts of blood, which are circulated about once every minute.

The heartbeat—the split-second sequence of contractions of the heart's four chambers—is controlled by nerve impulses. These signals originate in a bundle of specialized cells in the right atrium called the pacemaker or sinoatrial (SA) node. Unless it is speeded up or slowed down by the brain in response to such stimuli as danger or the tissues' need for more oxygen, the heart produces nerve impulses at a steady rate.

The Blood Vessels   Blood vessels are classified by size and function. **Veins** carry blood to the heart; **arteries**

carry it away from the heart. Veins have thin walls, but arteries have thick elastic walls that enable them to expand and relax with the volume of blood being pumped through them.

After leaving the heart, the aorta branches into smaller and smaller vessels. The smallest arteries branch still further into **capillaries,** tiny vessels only one cell thick. The capillaries deliver oxygen and nutrient-rich blood to the tissues and pass on oxygen-poor, waste-laden blood. From the capillaries, this blood empties into small veins (*venules*) and then into larger veins that return it to the heart to repeat the cycle.

Blood pumped through the heart doesn't reach the cells of the heart, so the organ has its own network of arteries, veins, and capillaries. Two large vessels, the right and left coronary arteries, branch off the aorta and supply the heart muscle with oxygenated blood. Blockage of a coronary artery is a leading cause of heart attacks (see Chapter 11).

The Respiratory System

The **respiratory system** supplies oxygen to the body, carries off carbon dioxide—a waste product of body processes—and helps regulate acid produced during metabolism. Air passes in and out of the lungs as a result of pressure changes brought about by the contraction and relaxation of the diaphragm and rib muscles; the lungs expand and contract about 12–20 times per minute. As air is inhaled, it passes through the nasal passages, the throat, larynx, trachea (windpipe), and bronchi into the lungs. The lungs consist of many branching tubes that end in tiny, thin-walled air sacs called **alveoli.**

Carbon dioxide and oxygen are exchanged between alveoli and capillaries in the lungs. Carbon dioxide passes from blood cells into the alveoli, where it is carried up and out of the lungs (exhaled). Oxygen from inhaled air is passed from the alveoli into blood cells; these oxygen-rich blood cells then return to the heart and are pumped throughout the body. Oxygen is an important component of the body's energy-producing system, so the cardiorespiratory system's ability to pick up and deliver oxygen is critical for the functioning of the body.

The Cardiorespiratory System at Rest and During Exercise

At rest and during light activity, the cardiorespiratory system functions at a fairly steady pace. Your heart beats at a rate of about 50–90 beats per minute, and you take about 12–20 breaths per minute. A typical resting blood pressure in a healthy adult, measured in millimeters of mercury, is 120 systolic and 80 diastolic (120/80).

During exercise, the demands on the cardiorespiratory system increase. Body cells, particularly working muscles, need to obtain more oxygen and fuel and to eliminate more waste products. To meet these demands, your body makes the following changes:

- Heart rate increases, up to 170–210 beats per minute during intense exercise.

- The heart's **stroke volume** increases, meaning that the heart pumps out more blood with each beat.

- The heart pumps and circulates more blood per minute as a result of the faster heart rate and greater stroke volume. During exercise, this **cardiac output** increases to 20 or more quarts per minute, compared to about 5 quarts per minute at rest.

- Blood flow changes, so as much as 85–90% of the blood may be delivered to working muscles. At rest, about 15–20% of blood is distributed to the skeletal muscles.

- Systolic blood pressure increases, while diastolic blood pressure holds steady or declines slightly. A typical exercise blood pressure might be 175/65.

- To oxygenate this increased blood flow, you take deeper breaths and breathe faster, up to 40–60 breaths per minute.

All of these changes are controlled and coordinated by special centers in the brain, which use the nervous system and chemical messengers to control the process.

Energy Production

Metabolism is the sum of all the chemical processes necessary to maintain the body. Energy is required to fuel vital body functions—to build and break down tissue, contract muscles, conduct nerve impulses, regulate body temperature, and so on.

The rate at which your body uses energy—its **metabolic rate**—depends on your level of activity. At rest, you have a low metabolic rate; if you begin to walk, your metabolic rate increases. If you jog, your metabolic rate may increase more than 800% above its resting level. Olympic-caliber distance runners can increase their metabolic rate by 2000% or more.

Energy from Food

The body converts chemical energy from food into substances that cells can use as fuel. These fuels can be used immediately or stored for later use. The body's ability to store fuel is critical, because if all the energy from food were released immediately, much of it would be wasted.

The three classes of energy-containing nutrients in food are carbohydrates, fats, and proteins. During digestion, most carbohydrates are broken down into the simple sugar **glucose.** Some glucose remains circulating in the blood ("blood sugar"), where it can be used as a quick source of fuel to produce energy. Glucose may also be converted to **glycogen** and stored in the liver, muscles, and kidneys. If glycogen stores are full and the body's immediate need for energy is met, the remaining glucose is converted to fat and stored in the body's fatty tissues. Excess energy from dietary fat is also stored as body fat. Protein in the diet is used primarily to build new tissue, but it can be broken down

Table 3.1 Characteristics of the Body's Energy Systems

	Energy System*		
	Immediate	**Nonoxidative**	**Oxidative**
Duration of Activity for Which System Predominates	0–10 seconds	10 seconds–2 minutes	>2 minutes
Intensity of Activity for Which System Predominates	High	High	Low to moderately high
Rate of ATP Production	Immediate, very rapid	Rapid	Slower, but prolonged
Fuel	Adenosine triphosphate (ATP), creatine phosphate (CP)	Muscle stores of glycogen and glucose	Body stores of glycogen, glucose, fat, and protein
Oxygen Used?	No	No	Yes
Sample Activities	Weight lifting, picking up a bag of groceries	400-meter run, running up several flights of stairs	1500-meter run, 30-minute walk, standing in line for a long time

*For most activities, all three systems contribute to energy production; the duration and intensity of the activity determine which system predominates.

SOURCE: Adapted from Brooks, G. A., et. al. 2005. *Exercise Physiology: Human Bioenergetics and its Applications,* 4th ed. New York: McGraw-Hill. Copyright © 2005 The McGraw-Hill Companies. Reproduced with permission of The McGraw-Hill Companies.

for energy or incorporated into fat stores. Glucose, glycogen, and fat are important fuels for the production of energy in the cells; protein is a significant energy source only when other fuels are lacking. (See Chapter 8 for more on the roles of carbohydrate, fat, and protein in the body.)

ATP: The Energy "Currency" of Cells

The basic form of energy used by cells is **adenosine triphosphate,** or **ATP.** When a cell needs energy, it breaks down ATP, a process that releases energy in the only form the cell can use directly. Cells store a small amount of ATP; when they need more, they create it through chemical reactions that utilize the body's stored fuels—glucose, glycogen, and fat. When you exercise, your cells need to produce more energy. Consequently, your body mobilizes its stores of fuel to increase ATP production.

Exercise and the Three Energy Systems

The muscles in your body use three energy systems to create ATP and fuel cellular activity. These systems use different fuels and chemical processes and perform different, specific functions during exercise (Table 3.1).

The Immediate Energy System

The **immediate ("explosive") energy system** provides energy rapidly but for only a short period of time. It is used to fuel activities that last for about 10 or fewer seconds—examples in sports include weight lifting and shot-putting; examples in daily life include rising from a chair or picking up a bag of groceries. The components of this energy system include existing cellular ATP stores and creatine phosphate (CP), a chemical that cells can use to make

ATP. CP levels are depleted rapidly during exercise, so the maximum capacity of this energy system is reached within a few seconds. Cells must then switch to the other energy systems to restore levels of ATP and CP. (Without adequate ATP, muscles will stiffen and become unusable.)

capillaries   Very small blood vessels that distribute blood to all parts of the body.

respiratory system   The lungs, air passages, and breathing muscles; supplies oxygen to the body and carries off carbon dioxide.

alveoli   Tiny air sacs in the lungs through whose walls gases such as oxygen and carbon dioxide diffuse in and out of blood.

stroke volume   The amount of blood the heart circulates with each beat.

cardiac output   The amount of blood pumped by the heart each minute; a function of heart rate and stroke volume (the amount of blood pumped during each beat).

metabolic rate   The rate at which the body uses energy.

glucose   A simple sugar that circulates in the blood and can be used by cells to fuel adenosine triphosphate (ATP) production.

glycogen   A complex carbohydrate stored principally in the liver and skeletal muscles; the major fuel source during most forms of intense exercise. Glycogen is the storage form of glucose.

adenosine triphosphate (ATP)   The energy source for cellular processes.

immediate ("explosive") energy system   The system that supplies energy to muscle cells through the breakdown of cellular stores of ATP and creatine phosphate (CP).

The Nonoxidative Energy System The **nonoxidative (anaerobic) energy system** is used at the start of an exercise session and for high-intensity activities lasting for about 10 seconds to 2 minutes, such as the 400-meter run. During daily activities, this system may be called on to help you run to catch a bus or dash up several flights of stairs. The nonoxidative energy system creates ATP by breaking down glucose and glycogen. This system doesn't require oxygen, which is why it is sometimes referred to as the **anaerobic** system. The capacity of this system to produce energy is limited, but it can generate a great deal of ATP in a short period of time. For this reason, it is the most important energy system for very intense exercise.

There are two key limiting factors for the nonoxidative energy system. First, the body's supply of glucose and glycogen is limited. If these are depleted, a person may experience fatigue and dizziness, and judgment may be impaired. (The brain and nervous system rely on carbohydrates as fuel.) Second, the nonoxidative system releases substances called **hydrogen ions** that are thought to interfere with metabolism and muscle contraction, thereby causing fatigue. During heavy exercise, such as sprinting, the body produces large amounts of hydrogen ions and muscles fatigue rapidly. The anaerobic energy system also creates metabolic acids. Fortunately, exercise training increases the body's ability to cope with metabolic acid. One of these acids, called **lactic acid,** is often linked to fatigue during intense exercise. However, it is an important fuel at rest and during exercise and may actually prevent fatigue.

TERMS

nonoxidative (anaerobic) energy system The system that supplies energy to muscle cells through the breakdown of muscle stores of glucose and glycogen; also called the *anaerobic system* or the *lactic acid system* because chemical reactions take place without oxygen and produce lactic acid.

anaerobic Occurring in the absence of oxygen.

hydrogen ion A positively charged atom of hydrogen; high concentrations during exercise slow metabolism and contribute to fatigue.

lactic acid A metabolic acid resulting from the metabolism of glucose and glycogen.

oxidative (aerobic) energy system The system that supplies energy to cells through the breakdown of glucose, glycogen, fats, and amino acids; also called the *aerobic system* because chemical reactions require oxygen.

aerobic Dependent on the presence of oxygen.

mitochondria Intracellular structures containing enzymes used in the chemical reactions that convert the energy in food to a form the body can use.

maximal oxygen consumption ($\dot{V}O_{2max}$) The highest rate of oxygen consumption an individual is capable of during maximum physical effort, reflecting the body's ability to transport and use oxygen; measured in milliliters used per minute per kilogram of body weight.

The Oxidative Energy System The **oxidative (aerobic) energy system** is used during any physical activity that lasts longer than about 2 minutes, such as distance running, swimming, hiking, or even standing in line. The oxidative system requires oxygen to generate ATP, which is why it is considered an **aerobic** system. The oxidative system cannot produce energy as quickly as the other two systems, but it can supply energy for much longer periods of time. It provides energy during most daily activities.

In the oxidative energy system, ATP production takes place in cellular structures called **mitochondria.** Because mitochondria can use carbohydrates (glucose and glycogen) or fats to produce ATP, the body's stores of fuel for this system are much greater than those for the other two energy systems. The actual fuel used depends on the intensity and duration of exercise and on the fitness status of the individual. Carbohydrates are favored during more intense exercise (over 65% of maximum capacity); fats are used for mild, low-intensity activities. During a prolonged exercise session, carbohydrates are the predominant fuel at the start of the workout, but fat utilization increases over time. Fit individuals use a greater proportion of fat as fuel because increased fitness allows people to do activities at lower intensities. This is an important adaptation because glycogen depletion is one of the limiting factors for the oxidative energy system. Thus, by being able to use more fat as fuel, a fit individual can exercise for a longer time before glycogen is depleted and muscles become fatigued.

Oxygen is another limiting factor. The oxygen requirement of this energy system is proportional to the intensity of exercise—as intensity increases, so does oxygen consumption. There is a limit to the body's ability to increase the transport and use of oxygen; this limit is referred to as **maximal oxygen consumption,** or $\dot{V}O_{2max}$. $\dot{V}O_{2max}$ is influenced by genetics, fitness status (power-generating capacity and fatigue resistance), gender, and age. It depends on many factors, including the capacity of blood to carry oxygen, the rate at which oxygen is transported to the tissues, and the amount of oxygen that cells extract from the blood. $\dot{V}O_{2max}$ determines how intensely a person can perform endurance exercise and for how long, and it is considered the best overall measure of the capacity of the cardiorespiratory system. (The assessment tests described later in the chapter are designed to help you predict your $\dot{V}O_{2max}$.)

The Energy Systems in Combination Your body typically uses all three energy systems when you exercise. The intensity and duration of the activity determine which system predominates. For example, when you play tennis, you use the immediate energy system when hitting the ball, but you replenish cellular energy stores using the nonoxidative and oxidative systems. When cycling, the oxidative system predominates. However, if you must suddenly exercise intensely—ride up a steep hill, for example—the other systems become important because the oxidative system is unable to supply ATP fast enough to sustain high-intensity effort.

Physical Fitness and Energy Production Physically fit people can increase their metabolic rate substantially, generating the energy needed for powerful or sustained exercise. People who are not fit cannot respond to exercise in the same way. Their bodies are less capable of delivering oxygen and fuel to exercising muscles; they can't burn as many calories during or after exercise; and they are less able to cope with lactic acid and other substances produced during intense physical activity that contribute to fatigue. Because of this, they become fatigued more rapidly—their legs hurt and they breathe heavily walking up a flight of stairs, for example. Regular physical training can substantially improve the body's ability to produce energy and meet the challenges of increased physical activity.

In designing an exercise program, focus on the energy system most important to your goals. Because improving the functioning of the cardiorespiratory system is critical to overall wellness, endurance exercise that utilizes the oxidative energy system—activities performed at moderate-to-high intensities for a prolonged duration—is a key component of any health-related fitness program.

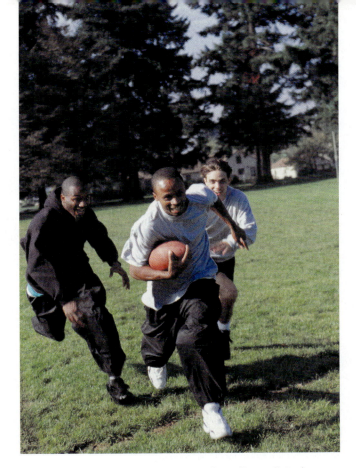

Exercise offers both long-term health benefits and immediate pleasures. Many popular sports and activities develop cardiorespiratory endurance.

QUESTIONS FOR CRITICAL THINKING AND REFLECTION
When you think about the types of physical activity you engage in during your typical day or week, which ones use the immediate energy system? The nonoxidative energy system? The oxidative energy system? How can you increase activities that use the oxidative energy system?

BENEFITS OF CARDIORESPIRATORY ENDURANCE EXERCISE

Cardiorespiratory endurance exercise helps the body become more efficient and better able to cope with physical challenges. It also lowers risk for many chronic diseases.

Improved Cardiorespiratory Functioning

Earlier in this chapter, we described some of the major changes that occur in the cardiorespiratory system when you exercise, such as increases in cardiac output and blood pressure, breathing rate, blood flow to the skeletal muscles, and sweating. In the short term, all these changes help the body respond to the challenge of exercise. When performed regularly, endurance exercise also leads to permanent adaptations in the cardiorespiratory system (Figure 3.3, p. 64). These improvements reduce the effort required to do everyday tasks and make the body better able to respond to physical challenges. This, in a nutshell, is what it means to be physically fit.

Endurance exercise enhances the heart's health by:

- Maintaining or increasing the heart's own blood and oxygen supply.
- Increasing the heart muscle's function, so it pumps more blood per beat. This improved function keeps the heart rate lower both at rest and during exercise. The resting heart rate of a fit person is often 10–20 beats per minute lower than that of an unfit person. This translates into as many as 10 million fewer beats in the course of a year.
- Strengthening the heart's contractions.
- Increasing the heart's cavity size (in young adults).
- Increasing blood volume so the heart pushes more blood into the circulatory system during each contraction.
- Reducing blood pressure.

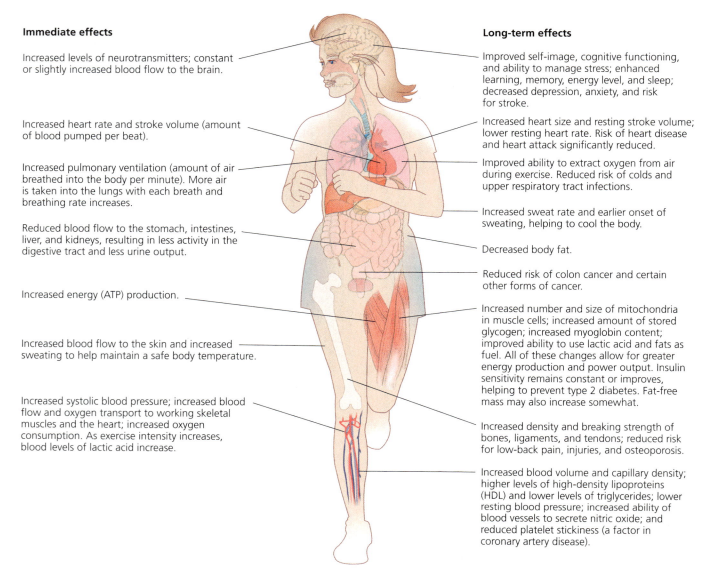

Immediate effects

Increased levels of neurotransmitters; constant or slightly increased blood flow to the brain.

Increased heart rate and stroke volume (amount of blood pumped per beat).

Increased pulmonary ventilation (amount of air breathed into the body per minute). More air is taken into the lungs with each breath and breathing rate increases.

Reduced blood flow to the stomach, intestines, liver, and kidneys, resulting in less activity in the digestive tract and less urine output.

Increased energy (ATP) production.

Increased blood flow to the skin and increased sweating to help maintain a safe body temperature.

Increased systolic blood pressure; increased blood flow and oxygen transport to working skeletal muscles and the heart; increased oxygen consumption. As exercise intensity increases, blood levels of lactic acid increase.

Long-term effects

Improved self-image, cognitive functioning, and ability to manage stress; enhanced learning, memory, energy level, and sleep; decreased depression, anxiety, and risk for stroke.

Increased heart size and resting stroke volume; lower resting heart rate. Risk of heart disease and heart attack significantly reduced.

Improved ability to extract oxygen from air during exercise. Reduced risk of colds and upper respiratory tract infections.

Increased sweat rate and earlier onset of sweating, helping to cool the body.

Decreased body fat.

Reduced risk of colon cancer and certain other forms of cancer.

Increased number and size of mitochondria in muscle cells; increased amount of stored glycogen; increased myoglobin content; improved ability to use lactic acid and fats as fuel. All of these changes allow for greater energy production and power output. Insulin sensitivity remains constant or improves, helping to prevent type 2 diabetes. Fat-free mass may also increase somewhat.

Increased density and breaking strength of bones, ligaments, and tendons; reduced risk for low-back pain, injuries, and osteoporosis.

Increased blood volume and capillary density; higher levels of high-density lipoproteins (HDL) and lower levels of triglycerides; lower resting blood pressure; increased ability of blood vessels to secrete nitric oxide; and reduced platelet stickiness (a factor in coronary artery disease).

FIGURE 3.3 Immediate and long-term effects of regular cardiorespiratory endurance exercise. When endurance exercise is performed regularly, short-term changes in the body develop into more permanent adaptations; these include improved ability to exercise, reduced risk of many chronic diseases, and improved psychological and emotional well-being.

Improved Cellular Metabolism

Regular endurance exercise improves the body's metabolism, down to the cellular level, enhancing your ability to produce and use energy efficiently. Cardiorespiratory training improves metabolism by doing the following:

- Increasing the number of capillaries in the muscles. Additional capillaries supply the muscles with more fuel and oxygen and more quickly eliminate waste products. Greater capillary density also helps heal injuries and reduce muscle aches.

- Training muscles to make the most of oxygen and fuel so they work more efficiently.

- Increasing the size of and number of mitochondria in muscle cells, increasing cells' energy capacity.

- Preventing glycogen depletion and increasing the muscles' ability to use lactic acid and fat as fuels.

Regular exercise may also help protect cells from chemical damage caused by agents called *free radicals*. (See Chapter 8 for details on free radicals and special enzymes the body uses to fight them.)

Fitness programs that best develop metabolic efficiency include both long-duration, moderately intense endurance exercise and brief periods of more intense effort. For example, climbing a small hill while jogging or cycling introduces the kind of intense exercise that leads to more efficient use of lactic acid and fats.

Benefits of Exercise for Older Adults

Research has shown that most aspects of physiological functioning peak when people are about 30 years old and then decline at a rate of about 0.5–1.0% per year. This decline in physical capacity is characterized by a decrease in maximal oxygen consumption, cardiac output, muscular strength, fat-free mass, joint mobility, and other factors. However, regular exercise can substantially alter the rate of decline in functional status, and it is associated with both longevity and improved quality of life.

Regular endurance exercise can improve maximal oxygen consumption in older people by up to 15–30%—the same degree of improvement seen in younger people. In fact, studies have shown that Masters athletes in their 70s have $\dot{V}O_{2max}$ values equivalent to those of sedentary 20-year-olds: At any age, endurance training can improve cardiorespiratory functioning, cellular

metabolism, body composition, and psychological and emotional well-being. Older people who exercise regularly have better balance and greater bone density and are less likely than their sedentary peers to suffer injuries as a result of falls. Regular endurance training also substantially reduces the risk of many chronic and disabling diseases including heart disease, cancer, diabetes, osteoporosis, and dementia.

Other forms of exercise training are also beneficial for older adults. Resistance training is a safe and effective way to build strength and fat-free mass and can help people remain independent as they age. Lifting weights has also been shown to boost spirits in older people, perhaps because improvements in strength appear quickly and are easily applied to everyday tasks such as climbing stairs and carrying groceries. Flexibility exercises can improve the range of

motion in joints and also help people maintain functional independence as they age.

It's never too late to start exercising. Even in people over 80, beginning an exercise program can improve physical functioning and quality of life. Most older adults are able to participate in moderate walking and strengthening and stretching exercises, and modified programs can be created for people with chronic conditions and other special health concerns (see Chapter 7). The wellness benefits of exercise are available to people of all ages and levels of ability.

? QUESTIONS FOR CRITICAL THINKING AND REFLECTION

If you already follow an exercise program, how could you modify it to help improve your cellular metabolism? What specific activities (or changes to existing ones) could you incorporate into your program for this purpose?

Reduced Risk of Chronic Disease

Regular endurance exercise lowers your risk of many chronic, disabling diseases. It can also help people with those diseases improve their health (see the box "Benefits of Exercise for Older Adults"). The most significant health benefits occur when someone who is sedentary becomes moderately active.

Cardiovascular Diseases Sedentary living is a key contributor to **cardiovascular disease (CVD)**. CVD is a general category that encompasses several diseases of the heart and blood vessels, including coronary heart disease (which can cause heart attacks), stroke, and high blood pressure. Sedentary people are significantly more likely to die of CVD than are fit individuals.

Cardiorespiratory endurance exercise lowers your risk of CVD by doing the following:

- Promoting a healthy balance of fats in the blood. High concentrations of blood fats such as cholesterol and

triglycerides are linked to CVD. Exercise raises levels of "good cholesterol" (high-density lipoproteins, or HDL) and may lower levels of "bad cholesterol" (low-density lipoproteins, or LDL).

- Reducing high blood pressure, which is a contributing factor to several kinds of CVD.
- Enhancing the function of the cells that line the arteries (endothelial cells).
- Reducing inflammation.
- Preventing obesity and type 2 diabetes, both of which contribute to CVD.

Details on various types of CVD, their associated risk factors, and lifestyle factors that can reduce your risk for developing CVD are discussed in Chapter 11.

Cancer Although the findings are not conclusive, some studies have shown a relationship between increased physical activity and a reduction in a person's risk of cancer. Exercise reduces the risk of colon cancer in women, and it may reduce the risk of cancers of the breast and reproductive organs. Physical activity during the high school and college years may be particularly important

cardiovascular disease (CVD) Disease of the heart and blood vessels.

for preventing breast cancer later in life. Exercise may also reduce the risk of pancreatic cancer and prostate cancer. See Chapter 12 for more information on various types of cancer.

Type 2 Diabetes Regular exercise helps prevent the development of type 2 diabetes, the most common form of diabetes. Exercise metabolizes (burns) excess sugar and makes cells more sensitive to the hormone insulin, which is involved in the regulation of blood sugar levels. Obesity is a key risk factor for diabetes, and exercise helps keep body fat at healthy levels. But even without fat loss, exercise improves control of blood sugar levels in many people with diabetes, and physical activity is an important part of treatment. (See Chapter 6 for more on diabetes and insulin resistance.)

Osteoporosis A special benefit of exercise, especially for women, is protection against osteoporosis, a disease that results in loss of bone density and poor bone strength. Weight-bearing exercise—particularly weight training—helps build bone during the teens and twenties. People with denser bones can better endure the bone loss that occurs with aging. With stronger bones and muscles and better balance, fit people are less likely to experience debilitating falls and bone fractures. (See Chapter 8 for more on osteoporosis.)

Deaths from All Causes Physically fit people have a reduced risk of dying prematurely from all causes, with the greatest benefits found for people with the highest levels of fitness (see Figure 3.4 for the results of one study). Poor fitness is a good predictor of premature death and is as important a risk factor as smoking, high blood pressure, obesity, and diabetes.

Better Control of Body Fat

Too much body fat is linked to a variety of health problems, including CVD, cancer, and type 2 diabetes. Healthy body composition can be difficult to achieve and maintain because a diet that contains all essential nutrients can be relatively high in calories, especially for someone who is sedentary. Excess calories are stored in the body as fat. Regular exercise increases daily calorie expenditure so that a healthy diet is less likely to lead to weight gain. Endurance exercise burns calories directly and, if intense enough, continues to do so by raising resting metabolic

FIGURE 3.4 Cardiorespiratory fitness and risk of premature death. People with high levels of cardiorespiratory fitness have a substantially lower risk of premature death than unfit individuals.

SOURCE: Myers, J., et al. 2002. Exercise capacity and mortality among men referred for exercise testing. *New England Journal of Medicine* 346(11): 793–801.

rate for several hours following an exercise session. A higher metabolic rate means that it is easier for a person to maintain a healthy weight or to lose weight. Exercise alone cannot ensure a healthy body composition, however; as described in Chapters 6 and 9, you will lose more weight more rapidly and keep it off longer if you decrease your calorie intake and boost your calorie expenditure through exercise.

Improved Immune Function

Exercise can have either positive or negative effects on the immune system, the physiological processes that protect us from disease. Moderate endurance exercise boosts immune function, whereas overtraining (excessive training) depresses it. Physically fit people get fewer colds and upper respiratory tract infections than people who are not fit. Exercise affects immune function by influencing levels of specialized cells and chemicals involved in the immune response. In addition to regular moderate exercise, the immune system can be strengthened by eating a well-balanced diet, managing stress, and getting 7–8 hours of sleep every night.

MOTIVATION BOOSTER

Focus on benefits. Make a list of five benefits of endurance exercise that are particularly meaningful to you—reducing your risk of diabetes, for example, or being able to hike with friends. Put the list in a prominent location—on your mirror or refrigerator, for example—and use it as a motivational tool for beginning and maintaining your fitness program.

Improved Psychological and Emotional Well-Being

Most people who participate in regular endurance exercise experience social, psychological, and emotional

TERMS

endorphins Substances resembling morphine that are secreted by the brain and that decrease pain, suppress fatigue, and produce euphoria.

neurotransmitters Brain chemicals that transmit nerve impulses.

Exercise, Mood, and the Mind

Although much of the discussion of the benefits of exercise focuses on improvements to physical wellness, many people discover that the best reason to become and stay active is the boost that regular exercise provides to the nonphysical dimensions of wellness. The following are just some of the effects of regular physical activity.

- **Reduced anxiety.** Exercise reduces symptoms of anxiety such as worry and self-doubt both in people who are anxious most of the time (trait anxiety) and in people who become anxious in response to a particular experience (state anxiety). Exercise is associated with a lower risk for panic attacks, generalized anxiety disorder, and social anxiety disorder.

- **Reduced depression and improved mood.** Exercise relieves feelings of sadness and hopelessness and can be as effective as psychotherapy in treating mild-to-moderate cases of depression. Exercise improves mood and increases feelings of well-being in both depressed and nondepressed people.

- **Improved sleep.** Regular physical activity helps people fall asleep more easily; it also improves the quality of sleep, making it more restful.

- **Reduced stress.** Exercise reduces the body's overall response to all forms of stressors and helps people deal more effectively with the stress they do experience.

- **Enhanced self-esteem, self-confidence, and self-efficacy.** Exercise can boost self-esteem and self-confidence by providing opportunities for people to succeed and excel; it also improves body image (see Chapters 6 and 9). Sticking with an exercise program increases people's belief in their ability to be active, thereby boosting self-efficacy.

- **Enhanced creativity and intellectual functioning.** In studies of college students, physically active students score higher on tests of creativity than sedentary students. Exercise improves alertness and memory in the short term, and over time, exercise helps maintain reaction time, short-term memory, and nonverbal reasoning skills.

- **Improved work productivity.** Workers' quality of work, time-management abilities, and mental and interpersonal performance have been found to be better on days they exercise.

- **Increased opportunities for social interaction.** Exercise provides many opportunities for positive interaction with others.

How does exercise cause all these positive changes? A variety of mechanisms has been proposed. Physical activity stimulates the thought and emotion centers of the brain, producing improvements in mood and cognitive functioning. It increases alpha brain-wave activity, which is associated with a highly relaxed state. Exercise stimulates the release of chemicals such as **endorphins,** which may suppress fatigue, decrease pain, and produce euphoria, and phenylethylamine, which may boost energy, mood, and attention. Exercise decreases the secretion of hormones triggered by emotional stress and alters the levels of many other **neurotransmitters,** including serotonin, a brain chemical linked to mood.

Exercise also provides a distraction from stressful stimuli and an emotional outlet for feelings of stress, hostility, and aggression. Finally, exercise is a fun way to spend time!

---

benefits. Performing physical activities provides proof of skill mastery and self-control, thus enhancing self-image. Recreational sports provide an opportunity to socialize, have fun, and strive to excel. Endurance exercise lessens anxiety, depression, stress, anger, and hostility, thereby improving mood and boosting cardiovascular health. Regular exercise also improves sleep. For more on the wellness benefits of regular endurance exercise, see the box "Exercise, Mood, and the Mind."

ASSESSING CARDIORESPIRATORY FITNESS

The body's ability to maintain a level of exertion (exercise) for an extended time is a direct reflection of cardiorespiratory fitness. It is determined by the body's ability to take up, distribute, and use oxygen during physical activity. As explained earlier, the best quantitative measure of cardiorespiratory endurance is maximal oxygen consumption, expressed as $\dot{V}O_{2max}$, the amount of oxygen the body uses when a person reaches maximum ability to supply oxygen during exercise (measured in milliliters of oxygen used per minute for each kilogram of body weight). Maximal oxygen consumption can be measured precisely in an exercise physiology laboratory through analysis of the air a person inhales and exhales when exercising to a level of exhaustion (maximum intensity). This procedure can be expensive and time-consuming, making it impractical for the average person.

Choosing an Assessment Test

Fortunately, several simple assessment tests provide reasonably good estimates of maximal oxygen consumption (within ±10–15% of the results of a laboratory test). Three commonly used assessments are the following:

- **The 1-mile walk test.** This estimates your level of cardiorespiratory fitness (maximal oxygen consumption) based on the amount of time it takes you to complete

1 mile of brisk walking and your heart rate at the end of your walk. A fast time and a low heart rate indicate a high level of cardiorespiratory endurance.

• **_The 3-minute step test._** The rate at which the pulse returns to normal after exercise is also a good measure of cardiorespiratory capacity; heart rate remains lower and recovers faster in people who are more physically fit. For the step test, you step continually at a steady rate and then monitor your heart rate during recovery.

• **_The 1.5-mile run-walk test._** Oxygen consumption increases with speed in distance running, so a fast time on this test indicates high maximal oxygen consumption.

Lab 3.1 provides detailed instructions for each of these tests. To assess yourself, choose one of these methods based on your access to equipment, your current physical condition, and your own preference. Don't take any of these tests without checking with your physician if you are ill or have any of the risk factors for exercise discussed in Chapter 2 and Lab 2.1. Table 3.2 lists the fitness prerequisites and cautions recommended for each test.

Monitoring Your Heart Rate

Each time your heart beats, it pumps blood into your arteries; this surge of blood causes a pulse that you can feel by holding your fingers against an artery. Counting your pulse to determine your exercise heart rate is a key part of most assessment tests for maximal oxygen consumption. Heart rate can also be used to monitor exercise intensity during a workout. (Intensity is described in more detail in the next section.)

The two most common sites for monitoring heart rate are the carotid artery in the neck and the radial artery in the wrist (Figure 3.5). To take your pulse, press your index and middle fingers gently on the correct site. You may have to shift position several times to find the best place to feel your pulse. Don't use your thumb to check

When feeling for the carotid pulse under the angle of the jaw, use very light pressure.

The radial pulse is felt on the wrist just under the thumb.

FIGURE 3.5 Checking your pulse. The pulse can be taken at the carotid artery in the neck (top) or at the radial artery in the wrist (bottom).

your pulse; it has a pulse of its own that can confuse your count. Be careful not to push too hard, particularly when taking your pulse in the carotid artery (strong

Table 3.2	Fitness Prerequisites and Cautions for the Cardiorespiratory Endurance Assessment Tests

Note: The conditions for exercise safety given in Chapter 2 apply to all fitness assessment tests. If you answered yes to any question on the PAR-Q in Lab 2.1, see your physician before taking any assessment test. If you experience any unusual symptoms while taking a test, stop exercising and discuss your condition with your instructor.

Test	Fitness Prerequisites/Cautions
1-mile walk test	Recommended for anyone who meets the criteria for safe exercise. This test can be used by individuals who cannot perform other tests because of low fitness level or injury.
3-minute step test	If you suffer from joint problems in your ankles, knees, or hips or are significantly overweight, check with your physician before taking this test. People with balance problems or for whom a fall would be particularly dangerous, including older adults and pregnant women, should use special caution or avoid this test.
1.5-mile run-walk test	Recommended for people who are healthy and at least moderately active. If you have been sedentary, you should participate in a 4- to 8-week walk-run program before taking the test. Don't take this test in extremely hot or cold weather if you aren't used to exercising under those conditions.

Heart Rate Monitors

A heart rate monitor is an electronic device that checks the user's pulse, either continuously or on demand. These devices make it easy to monitor your heart rate before, during, and after exercise.

Wearable Monitors

Most consumer-grade monitors have two pieces—a strap that wraps around the user's chest and a wrist strap. The chest strap contains one or more small electrodes, which detect changes in the heart's electrical voltage. A transmitter in the chest strap sends this data to a receiver in the wrist strap. A small computer in the wrist strap calculates the wearer's heart rate and displays it on a small screen.

In a few low-cost monitors, the chest and wrist straps are connected together by a wire, but the most popular monitors use wireless technology to transmit data between the straps. In advanced wireless monitors, data is encoded so it cannot be read by any other monitors that may be nearby, as is often the case in a crowded gym. A one-piece (or "strapless") heart rate monitor does not include a chest strap; the wrist-worn device contains sensors that detect a pulse in the wearer's hand.

Monitors in Gym Equipment

Many pieces of workout equipment—including newer-model treadmills, stationary bikes, and elliptical trainers—feature built-in heart rate monitors. The monitor is usually mounted into the device's handles. To check your heart rate at any time while working out, simply grip the handles in the appropriate place; within a few seconds, your current heart rate will appear on the device's console.

Other Features

Heart rate monitors can do more than just check your pulse. For example, most monitors can tell you the following kinds of information:

- Highest and lowest heart rate during a session
- Average heart rate
- Target heart range, based on your age, weight, and other factors
- Time spent within the target range
- Number of calories burned during a session

Some monitors can upload their data to a computer, so information can be stored and analyzed. The analytical software can help you track your progress over a period of time or a number of workouts.

Advantages

Heart rate monitors are useful if very close tracking of heart rate is important in your program. They offer several advantages:

- They are accurate, and they reduce the risk of mistakes when checking your own pulse. (Note, however, that chest-strap monitors are considered more accurate than strapless models. If you use a monitor built into gym equipment, its accuracy will depend on how well the device is maintained.)
- They are easy to use, although a sophisticated, multifunction monitor may take some time to master.
- They do the monitoring for you, so you don't have to worry about checking your own pulse.

When shopping for a heart rate monitor, do your homework. Quality, reliability, and warranties vary. Ask personal trainers in your area for their recommendations, and look for product reviews in consumer magazines or online.

---

pressure on this artery may cause a reflex that slows the heart rate).

Heart rates are usually assessed in beats per minute (bpm). But counting your pulse for an entire minute isn't practical when you're exercising. And because heart rate slows rapidly when you stop exercising, it can give inaccurate results. It's best to do a shorter count—10 seconds—and then multiply the result by 6 to get your heart rate in beats per minute. (You can also use a heart rate monitor to check your pulse. See the box "Heart Rate Monitors" for more information.)

Interpreting Your Score

Once you've completed one or more of the assessment tests, use the table under "Rating Your Cardiovascular Fitness" at the end of Lab 3.1 to determine your current level of cardiorespiratory fitness. As you interpret your score,

remember that field tests of cardiorespiratory fitness are not precise scientific measurements and have up to a 10–15% margin of error.

You can use the assessment tests to monitor the progress of your fitness program by retesting yourself from time to time. Always compare scores for the *same* test: Your scores on different tests may vary considerably because of differences in skill and motivation and weaknesses in the tests themselves.

QUESTIONS FOR CRITICAL THINKING AND REFLECTION

Why do you think a relatively slow resting pluse rate is a sign of good cardiorespiratory fitness? What physical conditions or attributes are reflected in your pulse rate?

DEVELOPING A CARDIORESPIRATORY ENDURANCE PROGRAM

Cardiorespiratory endurance exercises are best for developing the type of fitness associated with good health, so they should serve as the focus of your exercise program. To create a successful endurance exercise program, follow these guidelines:

- Set realistic goals.
- Set your starting frequency, intensity, and duration of exercise at appropriate levels.
- Choose suitable activities.
- Warm up and cool down.
- Adjust your program as your fitness improves.

Setting Goals

You can use the results of cardiorespiratory fitness assessment tests to set a specific oxygen consumption goal for your cardiorespiratory endurance program. Your goal should be high enough to ensure a healthy cardiorespiratory system, but not so high that it will be impossible to achieve. Scores in the fair and good ranges for maximal oxygen consumption suggest good fitness; scores in the excellent and superior ranges indicate a high standard of physical performance.

Through endurance training, an individual may be able to improve maximal oxygen consumption ($\dot{V}O_{2max}$) by about 10–30%. The amount of improvement possible depends on genetics, age, health status, and initial fitness level; people who start at a very low fitness level can improve by a greater percentage than elite athletes because the latter are already at a much higher fitness level, one that may approach their genetic physical limits. If you are tracking $\dot{V}O_{2max}$ using the field tests described in this chapter, you may be able to increase your score by more than 30% due to improvements in other physical factors, such as muscle power, which can affect your performance on the tests.

Another physical factor you can track to monitor progress is resting heart rate—your heart rate at complete rest, measured in the morning before you get out of bed and move around. Resting heart rate may decrease by as much as 10–15 beats per minute in response to endurance training. Changes in resting heart rate may be noticeable after only about 4–6 weeks of training.

You may want to set other types of goals for your fitness program. For example, if you walk, jog, or cycle as part of your fitness program, you may want to set a time or distance goal—working up to walking 5 miles in one session, completing a 4-mile run in 28 minutes, or cycling a total of 35 miles per week. A more modest goal might be to achieve the Surgeon General's minimum activity level of doing at least 30 minutes of moderate activity on most days. Although it's best to base your program on "SMART" goals, you may also want to set more qualitative goals, such as becoming more energetic, sleeping better, and improving the fit of your clothes.

Applying the FITT Equation

As described in Chapter 2, you can use the acronym FITT to remember key parameters of your fitness program: Frequency, Intensity, Time (duration), and Type of activity.

Frequency of Training To build cardiorespiratory endurance, you should exercise 3–5 days per week. Beginners should start with 3 and work up to 5 days per week. Training more than 5 days per week can lead to injury and isn't necessary for the typical person on an exercise program designed to promote wellness. (It is safe to do moderate-intensity activity such as walking and gardening every day.) Training fewer than 3 days per week makes it difficult to improve your fitness (unless exercise intensity is very high) or to use exercise to lose weight. In addition, you risk injury because your body never gets a chance to fully adapt to regular exercise training.

Intensity of Training Intensity is the most important factor in achieving training effects. You must exercise intensely enough to stress your body so that fitness improves. Four methods of monitoring exercise intensity are described below; choose the method that works best for you. Be sure to make adjustments in your intensity levels for environmental or individual factors. For example, on a hot and humid day or on your first day back to your program after an illness, you should decrease your intensity level.

TARGET HEART RATE ZONE One of the best ways to monitor the intensity of cardiorespiratory endurance exercise is to measure your heart rate. It isn't necessary to exercise at your maximum heart rate to improve maximal oxygen consumption. Fitness adaptations occur at lower heart rates with a much lower risk of injury.

According to the American College of Sports Medicine, your **target heart rate zone**—rates at which you should exercise to experience cardiorespiratory benefits—is between 65% and 90% of your maximum heart rate. To calculate your target heart rate zone, follow these steps:

1. Estimate your maximum heart rate (MHR) by subtracting your age from 220, or have it measured precisely by undergoing an exercise stress test in a doctor's office, hospital, or sports medicine lab. (*Note:* The formula to estimate maximum heart rate carries an error of about ±10–15 beats per minute and can be very inaccurate for some people, particularly older adults and young children. If your exercise heart rate seems inaccurate—that is, exercise within your target zone seems either too easy or too difficult—then use the perceived exertion method described in the next section or have your maximum heart rate measured precisely.)

2. Multiply your MHR by 65% and 90% to calculate your target heart rate zone. (*Note:* Very unfit people should use 55% of MHR for their training threshold.)

For example, a 19-year-old would calculate her target heart rate zone as follows:

MHR = 220 − 19 = 201

65% training intensity = 0.65 × 201 = 131 bpm

90% training intensity = 0.90 × 201 = 181 bpm

To gain fitness benefits, the young woman in our example would have to exercise at an intensity that raises her heart rate to between 131 and 181 bpm.

An alternative method for calculating target heart rate range uses **heart rate reserve,** the difference between maximum heart rate and resting heart rate. Using this method, target heart rate is equal to resting heart rate plus between 50% (40% for very unfit people) and 85% of heart rate reserve. Although some people (particularly those with very low levels of fitness) will obtain more accurate results using this more complex method, both methods provide reasonable estimates of an appropriate target heart rate zone. Formulas for both methods of calculating target heart rate are given in Lab 3.2.

If you have been sedentary, start by exercising at the lower end of your target heart rate range (65% of maximum heart rate or 50% of heart rate reserve) for at least 4–6 weeks. Fast and significant gains in maximal oxygen consumption can be made by exercising closer to the top of the range, but you may increase your risk of injury and overtraining. You *can* achieve significant health benefits by exercising at the bottom of your target range, so don't feel pressured into exercising at an unnecessarily intense level. If you exercise at a lower intensity, you can increase the duration or frequency of training to obtain as much benefit to your health, as long as you are above the 65% training threshold. (For people with a very low initial level of fitness, a lower training intensity, 55–64% of maximum heart rate or 40–49% of heart rate reserve, may be sufficient to achieve improvements in maximal oxygen consumption, especially at the start of an exercise program. Intensities of 70–85% of maximum heart rate are appropriate for average individuals.)

By monitoring your heart rate, you will always know if you are working hard enough to improve, not hard enough, or too hard. As your program progresses and your fitness improves, you will need to jog, cycle, or walk faster in order to reach your target heart rate zone. To monitor your heart rate during exercise, count your pulse while you're still moving or immediately after you stop exercising. Count beats for 10 seconds, and then multiply that number by 6 to see if your heart rate is in your target zone. Table 3.3 shows target heart rate ranges and 10-second counts based on the maximum heart rate formula.

Table 3.3	Target Heart Rate Range and 10-Second Counts	
Age (years)	Target Heart Rate Range (bpm)*	10-Second Count (beats)*
20–24	127–180	21–30
25–29	124–176	20–29
30–34	121–171	20–28
35–39	118–167	19–27
40–44	114–162	19–27
45–49	111–158	18–26
50–54	108–153	18–25
55–59	105–149	17–24
60–64	101–144	16–24
65+	97–140	16–23

*Target heart rates lower than those shown here are appropriate for individuals with a very low initial level of fitness. Ranges are based on the following formula: Target heart rate = 0.65 to 0.90 of maximum heart rate, assuming maximum heart rate = 220 − age. The heart rate range values shown here correspond to ratings of perceived exertion (RPE) values of about 12–18.

target heart rate zone   The range of heart rates that should be reached and maintained during cardiorespiratory endurance exercise to obtain training effects.

heart rate reserve   The difference between maximum heart rate and resting heart rate; used in one method for calculating target heart rate range.

METS One way scientists describe fitness is in terms of the capacity to increase metabolism (energy usage level) above rest. Scientists use METs to measure the metabolic cost of an exercise. One **MET** represents the body's resting metabolic rate—that is, the energy requirement of the body at rest. Exercise intensity is expressed in multiples of resting metabolic rate. For example, an exercise intensity of 2 METs is 2 times the resting metabolic rate.

METs are used to describe exercise intensities for occupational activities and exercise programs. Exercise intensities of less than 3–4 METs are considered low. Household chores and most industrial jobs fall into this category. Exercise at these intensities does not improve fitness for most people, but it will improve fitness for people with low physical capacities. Activities that increase metabolism by 6–8 METs are classified as moderate-intensity exercises and are suitable for most people beginning an exercise program. Vigorous exercise increases metabolic rate by more than 10 METs. Fast running or cycling, as well as intense play in sports like racquetball, can place people in this category. Table 3.4 lists the MET ratings for various activities.

METs are intended to be only an approximation of exercise intensity. Skill, body weight, body fat, and

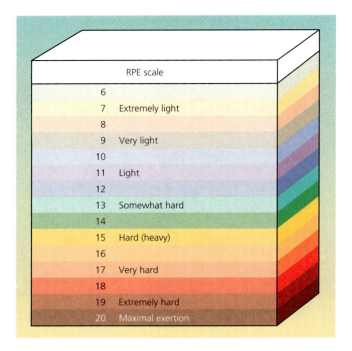

FIGURE 3.6 Ratings of perceived exertion (RPE). Experienced exercisers may use this subjective scale to estimate how near they are to their target heart rate zone. The scale was developed in the 1950s by Swedish exercise physiologist Gunnar Borg and is also known as the Borg scale.

SOURCE: *Psychology from Research to Practice* (1978), ed. H. L. Pick. Kluwer Academic/Plenum Publishing Corporation. With kind permission of Springer Science and Business Media and the author.

environment affect the accuracy of METs. As a practical matter, however, these limitations can be disregarded. METs are a good way to express exercise intensity because this system is easy for people to remember and apply.

RATINGS OF PERCEIVED EXERTION Another way to monitor intensity is to monitor your perceived level of exertion. Repeated pulse counting during exercise can become a nuisance if it interferes with the activity. As your exercise program progresses, you will probably become familiar with the amount of exertion required to raise your heart rate to target levels. In other words, you will know how you feel when you have exercised intensely enough. If this is the case, you can use the scale of **ratings of perceived exertion (RPE)** shown in Figure 3.6 to monitor the intensity of your exercise session without checking your pulse.

To use the RPE scale, select a rating that corresponds to your subjective perception of how hard you are exercising when you are training in your target heart rate zone. If your target zone is about 135–155 bpm, exercise intensely enough to raise your heart rate to that level, and then associate a rating—for example, "somewhat hard" or "hard" (14 or 15)—with how hard you feel you are working. To reach and maintain a similar intensity in future workouts,

Table 3.4	Approximate MET and Caloric Costs of Selected Activities for a 154-Pound Person	
Activity	**METs**	**Caloric Expenditure (kilocalories/min)**
Rest	1	1.2
Light housework	2–4	2.4–4.8
Bowling	2–4	2.5–5
Walking	2–7	2.5–8.5
Archery	3–4	3.7–5
Dancing	3–7	3.7–8.5
Hiking	3–7	3.7–8.5
Horseback riding	3–8	3.7–10
Cycling	3–8	3.7–10
Basketball (recreational)	3–9	3.7–11
Swimming	4–8	5–10
Tennis	4–9	5–11
Fishing (fly, stream)	5–6	6–7.5
In–line skating	5–8	6–10
Skiing (downhill)	5–8	6–10
Rock climbing	5–10	6–12
Scuba diving	5–10	6–12
Skiing (cross-country)	6–12	7.5–15
Jogging	8–12	10–15

NOTE: Intensity varies greatly with effort, skill, and motivation.

SOURCE: Adapted from American College of Sports Medicine. 2006. *ACSM's Guidelines for Exercise Testing and Prescription*, 7th ed. Philadelphia: Lippincott Williams and Wilkins.

exercise hard enough to reach what you feel is the same level of exertion. You should periodically check your RPE against your target heart rate zone to make sure it's correct. RPE is an accurate means of monitoring exercise intensity, and you may find it easier and more convenient than pulse counting.

TALK TEST Another easy method of monitoring exercise exertion—in particular, to prevent overly intense exercise—is the talk test. Although your breathing rate will increase during cardiorespiratory endurance exercise, you should not work out so intensely that you cannot speak comfortably. The talk test is an effective gauge of intensity for many types of activities.

Time (Duration) of Training

A total duration of 20–60 minutes is recommended; exercise can take place in a single session or in multiple sessions lasting 10 or more minutes. The total duration of exercise depends on its intensity. To improve cardiorespiratory endurance during a low- to moderate-intensity activity such as walking or slow swimming, you should exercise for 45–60 minutes. For high-intensity exercise performed at the top of your target heart rate zone, a duration of 20 minutes is sufficient. Some studies have shown that 5–10 minutes of extremely intense exercise (greater than 90% of maximal oxygen consumption) improves cardiorespiratory endurance. However, training at high intensity, particularly during high-impact activities, increases the risk of injury. Also, because of the discomfort of high-intensity exercise, you are more likely to discontinue your exercise program. Longer-duration, low- to moderate-intensity activities generally result in more gradual gains in maximal oxygen consumption. In planning your program, start with less vigorous activities and gradually increase intensity.

Type of Activity

Cardiorespiratory endurance exercises include activities that involve the rhythmic use of large-muscle groups for an extended period of time, such as jogging, walking, cycling, aerobic dancing and other forms of group exercise, cross-country skiing, and swimming. (For a discussion of the benefits of walking and running, see the box "Should I Walk or Run for Fitness?" on p. 74.) Start-and-stop sports, such as tennis and racquetball, also qualify, as long as you have enough skill to play continuously and intensely enough to raise your heart rate to target levels.

Having fun is a strong motivator; select a physical activity that you enjoy, and it will be easier to stay with your program. Exercising with a friend can also be helpful as a motivator. Consider whether you prefer competitive or individual sports and whether starting something new would be best. Other important considerations are access to facilities, expense, equipment, and the time required to achieve an adequate skill level and workout.

Warming Up and Cooling Down

It's important to warm up before every session of cardiorespiratory endurance exercise and to cool down afterward. Because the body's muscles work better when their temperature is slightly above resting level, warming up enhances performance and decreases the chance of injury. It gives the body time to redirect blood to active muscles and the heart time to adapt to increased demands. Warming up also helps spread **synovial fluid** throughout the joints, which helps protect their surfaces from injury.

As mentioned in Chapter 2, a warm-up session should include low-intensity, whole-body movements similar to those in the activity that will follow. Low-intensity movements might include walking slowly before beginning a brisk walk, hitting forehands and backhands before a tennis match, and running a 12-minute mile before progressing to an 8-minute one. An active warm-up of 5–10 minutes is adequate for most types of exercise. However, warm-up time will depend on your level of fitness, experience, and individual preferences.

If you like to stretch before exercising, experts recommend that you stretch after the active part of your warm-up, when your body temperature has been elevated (see Chapter 5). Studies have found that stretching prior to exercise can decrease performance, so some experts recommend that stretching be done *after* a workout.

Cooling down after exercise is important for returning the body to a nonexercising state. A cool-down helps maintain blood flow to the heart and brain and redirects blood from working muscles to other areas of the body; it helps prevent a large drop in blood pressure, dizziness, and other potential cardiovascular complications. A cool-down, consisting of 5–10 minutes of reduced activity, should follow every workout to allow heart rate, breathing, and circulation to return to normal. Decrease the intensity of exercise gradually during your cool-down. For example, following a running workout, begin your cool-down by jogging at half speed for 30 seconds to a minute; then do several minutes of walking, reducing your speed slowly. A good rule of thumb is to cool down at least until your heart rate

MET A unit of measure that represents the body's resting metabolic rate—that is, the energy requirement of the body at rest.

ratings of perceived exertion (RPE) A system of monitoring exercise intensity based on assigning a number to the subjective perception of target intensity.

synovial fluid Fluid produced within many joints that provides lubrication and nutrients for the joints.

Should I Walk or Run for Fitness?

Which exercise is more beneficial for fitness—walking or running? Enthusiasts have been debating this question for years, and experts say the answer is a complicated one, at least in technical terms. Each has its advantages and drawbacks, but both walking and running can be excellent forms of exercise.

Common Benefits

Walking and running (or jogging) both allow you to burn calories and build cardiorespiratory fitness. They are both affordable, since all you need is a good pair of shoes. They are also highly accessible for most people because you can run or walk just about anywhere, as long as you choose a route that is safe.

Big Differences

As forms of exercise, the main difference between walking and running is the way they allow your body to burn calories. All things being equal, running burns more calories than walking—that is, until you factor in the duration of your exercise.

For example, if you run a mile, your body will primarily burn carbohydrates for energy because you are exercising at a relatively high intensity for a relatively short amount of time. If you walk a mile, however, your body will metabolize more fat because you are exercising for a longer amount of time. Because of walking's potential as a fat-burning exercise, some experts say that it is more effective to walk briskly for 45 minutes than to run for 20 minutes. However, running increases post-exercise metabolism more than walking, which contributes to the energy cost of exercise.

In terms of cardiorespiratory fitness, evidence varies, but experts say that brisk walking (up to a speed of about 5 mph) produces the same or better fitness benefits compared to running. Your results will depend on factors such as your age and weight, the pace at which you move, and the distance or amount of time you run or walk.

Because running and walking differ in these ways, many fitness experts say the best approach is to combine them. If your workouts include long, brisk walks interspersed with short, intense bursts of running, you can maximize your fat burning and your cardiorespiratory fitness.

The other main difference between walking and running is the risks they pose. Walking is gentler on the joints than running and carries a much lower likelihood of injury. Running is considered a high-impact form of exercise that can take a severe toll on the joints (especially the knees), ankles, and feet. Running also carries a higher risk of sudden cardiac arrest or failure, although this risk is low in healthy people who are used to running and who exercise within their limits.

How To Choose?

Instead of trying to figure out which exercise is "better," physicians and fitness authorities say you should simply do the exercise with which you are most comfortable. Here are two points that can help you decide:

• If you have been sedentary a long time or have a health problem that prevents you from running comfortably (or that might make running dangerous), then walking is probably the better option. If you are concerned that exercising might pose a risk to your health, however, talk to your physician before starting *any* kind of exercise program.

• If your exercise time is limited, running (or a combination of brisk walking and running) may suit your schedule, as it allows you to burn more calories in less time than walking. However, if you are new to running, start with a walking program and work your way into running.

See Chapter 7 for detailed information on setting up a personalized walking, running, or combination program.

---

drops below 100 beats per minute. Doing stretching exercises at the end of a workout is an excellent strategy: Your muscles are warm, allowing you to stretch farther with less risk of injury; in addition, there is no danger of decreased performance.

The general pattern of a safe and successful workout for cardiorespiratory fitness is illustrated in Figure 3.7.

> **MOTIVATION BOOSTER**
>
> **Enlist support.** Studies of college students have found that social support is a key factor influencing whether students exercise. Do your friends and family members actively support your fitness goals and program? If not, enlist their help and encouragement—it can make a big difference.

Building Cardiorespiratory Fitness

Building fitness is as much an art as a science. Your rate of progress will depend on your age, health status, genetics, initial level of fitness, and motivation. Your fitness improves when you overload your body. However, you must increase the intensity, frequency, and duration of exercise carefully to avoid injury and overtraining.

For the initial stage of your program, which may last anywhere from 3 to 6 weeks, exercise at the low end of your target heart rate zone. Begin with a frequency of 3–4 days per week, and choose a duration appropriate for your fitness level: 12–15 minutes if you are very unfit, 20 minutes if you are sedentary but otherwise healthy, and 30–40 minutes if you are an experienced exerciser. Use this stage of your program to allow both your body and your schedule to adjust to your new exercise routine. Once you can exercise at the upper

Warm-up 5–10 minutes | Endurance exercise 20–60 minutes | Cool-down 5–10 minutes

90% Training intensity

Target Heart Rate Zone

65% Training intensity

Heart rate (bpm): 180, 170, 160, 150, 140, 130, 120, 110, 100, 90, 80, 70

Resting heart rate

Frequency: 3–5 days per week

Intensity: 55/65–90% of maximum heart rate, 40/50–85% of heart rate reserve plus resting heart rate, or an RPE rating of about 12–18 (lower intensities—55–64% of maximum heart rate and 40–49% of heart rate reserve—are applicable to people who are quite unfit; for average individuals, intensities of 70–85% of maximum heart rate are appropriate)

Time (duration): 20–60 minutes (one session or multiple sessions lasting 10 or more minutes)

Type of activity: Cardiorespiratory endurance exercises, such as walking, jogging, biking, swimming, cross-country skiing, and rope skipping

FIGURE 3.7   The FITT principle for a cardiorespiratory endurance workout. Longer-duration exercise at lower intensities can often be as beneficial for promoting health as shorter-duration, high-intensity exercise.

Table 3.5	Sample Progression for an Endurance Program		
Stage/Week	Frequency (days/ week)	Intensity* (beats/ minute)	Time (duration in minutes)
Initial stage			
1	3	120–130	15–20
2	3	120–130	20–25
3	4	130–145	20–25
4	4	130–145	25–30
Improvement stage			
5–7	3–4	145–160	25–30
8–10	3–4	145–160	30–35
11–13	3–4	150–165	30–35
14–16	4–5	150–165	30–35
17–20	4–5	160–180	35–40
21–24	4–5	160–180	35–40
Maintenance stage			
25+	3–5	160–180	20–60

*The target heart rates shown here are based on calculations for a healthy 20-year-old with a resting heart rate of 60 beats per minute; the program progresses from an initial target heart rate of 50% to a maintenance range of 70–85% of heart rate reserve.

SOURCE: Adapted from American College of Sports Medicine. 2006. *ACSM's Guidelines for Exercise Testing and Prescription,* 7th ed. Philadelphia: Lippincott Williams and Wilkins. Reprinted with permission from the publisher.

levels of frequency (4–5 days per week) and duration (30–40 minutes) without excessive fatigue or muscle soreness, you are ready to progress.

The next phase of your program is the improvement stage, lasting from 4 to 6 months. During this phase, slowly and gradually increase the amount of overload until you reach your target level of fitness (see the sample training progression in Table 3.5). Take care not to increase overload too quickly. It is usually best to avoid increasing intensity and duration during the same session or all three training variables in 1 week. Increasing duration in increments of 5–10 minutes every 2–3 weeks is usually appropriate. Signs that you are increasing overload too quickly include muscle aches and pains, lack of usual interest in exercise, extreme fatigue, and inability to complete a workout. Keep an exercise log or training diary to help you monitor your workouts and progress.

Maintaining Cardiorespiratory Fitness

You will not improve your fitness indefinitely. The more fit you become, the harder you have to work to improve. There are limits to the level of fitness you can achieve, and if you increase intensity and duration indefinitely,

you are likely to become injured or overtrained. After an improvement stage of 4–6 months, you may reach your goal of an acceptable level of fitness. You can then maintain fitness by continuing to exercise at the same intensity at least 3 nonconsecutive days every week. If you stop exercising, you lose your gains in fitness fairly rapidly. If you take time off for any reason, start your program again at a lower level and rebuild your fitness in a slow and systematic way.

When you reach the maintenance stage, you may want to set new goals for your program and make some adjustments to maintain your motivation. Adding variety to your program can be a helpful strategy. Engaging in multiple types of endurance activities, an approach known as **cross-training**, can help boost enjoyment and prevent some types of injuries. For example, someone who has been jogging 5 days a week may change her program so that she jogs 3 days a week, plays tennis 1 day a week, and goes for a bike ride 1 day a week.

cross-training   Alternating two or more activities to improve a single component of fitness (for example, walking 2 days per week and swimming 2 days per week to build cardiorespiratory endurance).

TERMS

WEB

Exercise in Hot Weather

Following a few simple principles can minimize the problems associated with exercising in the heat. To help alert people about weather conditions that could increase the risk of heat illness, the U.S. Weather Service developed the **heat index**—a measure that incorporates both temperature and relative humidity. For example, a temperature of 95 degrees combined with a relative humidity of 50% has a heat index of 107.

Prolonged exposure or physical activity when the heat index is 80–90 can cause fatigue; at a heat index of 90 or above, heat cramps, heat exhaustion, and heatstroke become more likely. Reduce and avoid exercise when the heat index is 90 or above.

A complete chart of heat index values can be found on the *Fit and Well* Online Learning Center. Local heat index information is available from the National Weather Service (http://www.weather.gov).

To avoid the risk of heat illness, follow these guidelines:

- Be in good physical condition. Exercise training can help the body adapt to heat by increasing the sweat rate.
- Use caution when exercising in extreme heat or humidity (over 80°F and/or 60% humidity).
- Slow exercise or add rest breaks to maintain your prescribed target heart rate; as you become acclimatized, you can gradually increase intensity and duration.
- Exercise in the early morning or evening, when temperatures are lowest.

- Drink 2 cups of fluids 2 hours before you begin exercising, and drink 4–8 ounces of fluid every 10–15 minutes during exercise (more frequently during high-intensity activities). Plan for regular water breaks. For an exercise session lasting longer than 60–90 minutes, choose a sports beverage that is cold (8–13°C; 46–55°F), low in sugar (less than 8 grams per 100 milliliters), and contains a small amount of electrolytes.
- During a period of hot weather, weigh yourself every day before exercising. If your weight has decreased by 3% or more from the previous day, don't exercise without first rehydrating.
- Avoid supplements and beverages containing stimulants like ephedra and caffeine when exercising in the heat; they can promote heat-induced illness. Do not use salt pills.
- Wear clothing that breathes, allowing air to circulate and cool the body. Wearing white or light colors will help by reflecting, rather than absorbing, heat. A hat can help keep direct sun off your face. Do not wear rubber, plastic, or other nonporous clothing. "Sauna suits" cause loss of body water, not fat, and don't improve body composition.
- Rest frequently in the shade.
- Slow down or stop if you begin to feel uncomfortable. Watch for the signs of heat disorders; if they occur, act appropriately.

QUESTIONS FOR CRITICAL THINKING AND REFLECTION

Suppose you want to start a new cardiorespiratory exercise program. How do your age, health status, and current level of fitness affect the kind of program you design for yourself? For the first few weeks, how often would you exercise, at what intensity (heart rate), and for how long?

EXERCISE SAFETY AND INJURY PREVENTION

Exercising safely and preventing injuries are two important challenges for people who engage in cardiorespiratory endurance exercise. This section provides basic safety guidelines that can be applied to a variety of fitness activities; visit the *Fit and Well* Online Learning Center for more detailed information about the prevention and care of exercise injuries and safe exercise in challenging environmental conditions. Chapters 4 and 5 include additional advice specific to strength training and flexibility training.

Hot Weather and Heat Stress

Human beings require a relatively constant body temperature to survive. A change of just a few degrees in body temperature can quickly lead to distress and even death. If you lose too much water or if your body temperature gets too high, you may suffer from heat stress. Problems associated with heat stress include dehydration, heat cramps, heat exhaustion, and heatstroke.

In a high-temperature environment, exercise safety depends on the body's ability to dissipate heat and maintain blood flow to active muscles. The body releases heat from exercise through the evaporation of sweat. This process cools the skin and the blood circulating near the body's surface. Sweating is an efficient process as long as the air is relatively dry. As humidity increases, however, the sweating mechanism becomes less efficient because extra moisture in the air inhibits the evaporation of sweat from the skin. This is why it takes longer to cool down in humid weather than in dry weather.

You can avoid significant heat stress by staying fit, avoiding overly intense or prolonged exercise for which you are not prepared, drinking adequate fluids before and during exercise, and wearing clothes that allow heat to dissipate. For additional tips, see the box "Exercise in Hot Weather."

Dehydration   Your body needs water to carry out many chemical reactions and to regulate body temperature. Sweating during exercise depletes your body's water supply and can lead to **dehydration** if fluids aren't replaced. Although dehydration is most common in hot weather, it can occur in even comfortable temperatures if fluid intake is insufficient.

Dehydration increases body temperature and decreases sweat rate, plasma volume, cardiac output, maximal oxygen consumption, exercise capacity, muscular strength, and stores of liver glycogen. You may begin to feel thirsty when you have a fluid deficit of about 1% of total body weight.

Drinking fluids before and during exercise is important to prevent dehydration and enhance performance. Thirst receptors in the brain make you want to drink fluids, but during heavy or prolonged exercise or exercise in hot weather, thirst alone isn't a good indication of how much you need to drink. As a rule of thumb, drink at least 2 cups (16 ounces) of fluid 2 hours before exercise, and then drink enough during exercise to match fluid loss in sweat. Drink at least 1 cup of fluid for every 20–30 minutes of exercise, more in hot weather or if you sweat heavily. To determine if you're drinking enough fluid, weigh yourself before and after an exercise session—any weight loss is due to fluid loss that needs to be replaced.

Very rarely, athletes consume too much water and develop *hyponatremia,* a condition characterized by lung congestion, muscle weakness, and nervous system problems. Following the guidelines presented here can help prevent this condition.

Bring a water bottle when you exercise so you can replace your fluids when they're being depleted. For exercise sessions lasting less than 60–90 minutes, cool water is an excellent fluid replacement. For longer workouts, choose a sports drink that contains water and small amounts of electrolytes (sodium, potassium, and magnesium) and simple carbohydrates ("sugar," usually in the form of sucrose, glucose, lactate, or glucose polymers). Electrolytes, which are lost from the body in sweat, are important because they help regulate the balance of fluids in body cells and the bloodstream. The carbohydrates in typical sports drinks are rapidly digestible and can thus help maintain blood glucose levels. Choose a beverage with no more than 8 grams of simple carbohydrate per 100 milliliters. See Chapter 8 for more on diet and fluid recommendations for active people.

Heat Cramps   Involuntary cramping and spasms in the muscle groups used during exercise are sometimes called **heat cramps.** While depletion of sodium and potassium from the muscles is involved with the problem, the primary cause of cramps is muscle fatigue. Children are particularly susceptible to heat cramps, but the condition can also occur in adults, even those who are fit. The best treat-ment for heat cramps is a combination of gentle stretching, replacement of fluid and electrolytes, and rest.

Heat Exhaustion   Symptoms of **heat exhaustion** include the following:

- A rapid, weak pulse
- Low blood pressure
- Headache
- Faintness, weakness, dizziness
- Profuse sweating
- Pale face
- Psychological disorientation (in some cases)
- Normal or slightly elevated core body temperature

Heat exhaustion occurs when an insufficient amount of blood returns to the heart because so much of the body's blood volume is being directed to working muscles (for exercise) and to the skin (for cooling). Treatment for heat exhaustion includes resting in a cool area, removing excess clothing, applying cool or damp towels to the body, and drinking fluids. An affected individual should rest for the remainder of the day and drink plenty of fluids for the next 24 hours.

Heatstroke   **Heatstroke** is a major medical emergency involving the failure of the brain's temperature regulatory center. The body does not sweat enough, and body temperature rises dramatically to extremely dangerous levels. In addition to high body temperature, symptoms can include the following:

- Hot, flushed skin (dry or sweaty), red face
- Chills, shivering
- Very high or very low blood pressure
- Confusion, erratic behavior
- Convulsions, loss of consciousness

A heatstroke victim should be cooled as rapidly as possible and immediately transported to a hospital. To lower body temperature, get out of the heat, remove excess

heat index   A measure of how hot it feels; the temperature that would have the same heating effect on a person as a given combination of temperature and relative humidity.

dehydration   Excessive loss of body fluid.

heat cramps   Sudden development of muscle spasms and pain associated with intense exercise in hot weather.

heat exhaustion   Heat illness related to dehydration resulting from exertion in hot weather.

heatstroke   A severe and often fatal heat illness produced by exposure to very high temperatures, especially when combined with intense exercise; characterized by significantly elevated core body temperature.

clothing, drink cold fluids, and apply cool or damp towels to the body or immerse the body in cold water.

Cold Weather

In extremely cold conditions, problems can occur if a person's body temperature drops or if particular parts of the body are exposed. If the body's ability to warm itself through shivering or exercise can't keep pace with heat loss, the core body temperature begins to drop. This condition, known as **hypothermia**, depresses the central nervous system, resulting in sleepiness and a lower metabolic rate. As metabolic rate drops, body temperature declines even further, and coma and death can result.

Frostbite—the freezing of body tissues—is another potential danger of exercise in extremely cold conditions. Frostbite most commonly occurs in exposed body parts like earlobes, fingers, and toes, and it can cause permanent circulatory damage. Hypothermia and frostbite both require immediate medical treatment.

What can you do to exercise safely in cold conditions? First of all, don't stay out in very cold temperatures for too long. Take both the temperature and the wind into account when planning your exercise session. Frostbite within 30 minutes is possible in calm conditions when the temperature is colder than −5°F or in windy conditions (30 mph) if the temperature is below 10°F. **Wind chill** values that reflect both the temperature and the wind speed are available as part of a local weather forecast and from the National Weather Service (http://www.weather.gov); a complete wind chill chart is available on the *Fit and Well* Online Learning Center.

Appropriate clothing provides insulation and helps trap warm air next to the skin. Dress in layers so you can remove them as you warm up and can put them back on if you get cold. A substantial amount of heat loss comes from the head and neck, so keep these areas covered. In subfreezing temperatures, protect the areas of your body most susceptible to frostbite—fingers, toes, ears, nose, and cheeks—with warm socks, mittens or gloves, and a cap, hood, or ski mask. Wear clothing that breathes and will wick moisture away from your skin to avoid being cooled or overheated by trapped perspiration. Many types of comfortable, lightweight clothing that provide good insulation are available. It's also important to warm up thoroughly and to drink plenty of fluids.

Poor Air Quality

Air pollution can decrease exercise performance and negatively affect health, particularly if you have respiratory problems such as asthma, bronchitis, or emphysema, or if you smoke. The effects of smog are worse during exercise than at rest because air enters the lungs faster. Polluted air may also contain carbon monoxide, which displaces oxygen in the blood and reduces the amount of oxygen available to working muscles. In a 2007 study, the ACSM found that exercise in polluted air could decrease lung function to the same extent as heavy smoking. Symptoms of poor air quality include eye and throat irritations, difficulty breathing, and possibly headache and malaise.

Do not exercise outdoors during a smog alert or if air quality is very poor. If you have any type of cardiorespiratory difficulty, you should also avoid exertion outdoors when air quality is poor. You can avoid some smog and air pollution by exercising in indoor facilities, in parks, near water (riverbanks, lakeshores, and ocean beaches), or in residential areas with less traffic (areas with stop-and-go traffic will have lower air quality than areas where traffic moves quickly). Air quality is also usually better in the early morning and late evening, before and after the commute hours.

Exercise Injuries

Most injuries are annoying rather than serious or permanent. However, an injury that isn't cared for properly can escalate into a chronic problem, sometimes serious enough to permanently curtail the activity. It's important to learn how to deal with injuries so they don't derail your fitness program. Strategies for the care of common exercise injuries and discomforts appear in Table 3.6; some general guidelines are given below.

When to Call a Physician   Some injuries require medical attention. Consult a physician for the following:

- Head and eye injuries
- Possible ligament injuries
- Broken bones
- Internal disorders: chest pain, fainting, elevated body temperature, intolerance to hot weather

Also seek medical attention for ostensibly minor injuries that do not get better within a reasonable amount of time. You may need to modify your exercise program for a few weeks to allow an injury to heal.

Managing Minor Exercise Injuries   For minor cuts and scrapes, stop the bleeding and clean the wound. Treat

hypothermia   Low body temperature due to exposure to cold conditions.

frostbite   Freezing of body tissues characterized by pallor, numbness, and a loss of cold sensation.

wind chill   A measure of how cold it feels based on the rate of heat loss from exposed skin caused by cold and wind; the temperature that would have the same cooling effect on a person as a given combination of temperature and wind speed.

Table 3.6 Care of Common Exercise Injuries and Discomforts

Injury	Symptoms	Treatment
Blister	Accumulation of fluid in one spot under the skin	Don't pop or drain it unless it interferes too much with your daily activities. If it does pop, clean the area with antiseptic and cover with a bandage. Do not remove the skin covering the blister.
Bruise (contusion)	Pain, swelling, and discoloration	R-I-C-E: rest, ice, compression, elevation.
Fracture and/or dislocation	Pain, swelling, tenderness, loss of function, and deformity	Seek medical attention, immobilize the affected area, and apply cold.
Joint sprain	Pain, tenderness, swelling, discoloration, and loss of function	R-I-C-E. Apply heat when swelling has disappeared. Stretch and strengthen affected area.
Muscle cramp	Painful, spasmodic muscle contractions	Gently stretch for 15–30 seconds at a time and/or massage the cramped area. Drink fluids and increase dietary salt intake if exercising in hot weather.
Muscle soreness or stiffness	Pain and tenderness in the affected muscle	Stretch the affected muscle gently; exercise at a low intensity; apply heat. Nonsteroidal anti-inflammatory drugs, such as ibuprofen, help some people.
Muscle strain	Pain, tenderness, swelling, and loss of strength in the affected muscle	R-I-C-E; apply heat when swelling has disappeared. Stretch and strengthen the affected area.
Plantar fasciitis	Pain and tenderness in the connective tissue on the bottom of your feet	Apply ice, take nonsteroidal anti-inflammatory drugs, and stretch. Wear night splints when sleeping.
Shin splint	Pain and tenderness on the front of the lower leg; sometimes also pain in the calf muscle	Rest; apply ice to the affected area several times a day and before exercise; wrap with tape for support. Stretch and strengthen muscles in the lower legs. Purchase good-quality footwear and run on soft surfaces.
Side stitch	Pain on the side of the abdomen	Stretch the arm on the affected side as high as possible; if that doesn't help, try bending forward while tightening the abdominal muscles.
Tendinitis	Pain, swelling, and tenderness of the affected area	R-I-C-E; apply heat when swelling has disappeared. Stretch and strengthen the affected area.

injuries to soft tissue (muscles and joints) with the R-I-C-E principle: Rest, Ice, Compression, and Elevation.

- **Rest:** Stop using the injured area as soon as you experience pain. Avoid any activity that causes pain.

- **Ice:** Apply ice to the injured area to reduce swelling and alleviate pain. Apply ice immediately for 10–20 minutes, and repeat every few hours until the swelling disappears. Let the injured part return to normal temperature between icings, and do not apply ice to one area for more than 20 minutes. An easy method for applying ice is to freeze water in a paper cup, peel some of the paper away, and rub the exposed ice on the injured area. If the injured area is large, you can surround it with several bags of crushed ice or ice cubes, or bags of frozen vegetables. Place a thin towel between the bag and your skin. If you use a cold gel pack, limit application time to 10 minutes. Apply ice regularly for 36–48 hours or until the swelling is gone; it may be necessary to apply ice for a week or more if swelling persists.

- **Compression:** Wrap the injured area firmly with an elastic or compression bandage between icings. If the area starts throbbing or begins to change color, the bandage may be wrapped too tightly. Do not sleep with the wrap on.

- **Elevation:** Raise the injured area above heart level to decrease the blood supply and reduce swelling. Use pillows, books, or a low chair or stool to raise the injured area.

The day after the injury, some experts recommend also taking an over-the-counter medication such as aspirin, ibuprofen, or naproxen to decrease inflammation. To rehabilitate your body, follow the steps listed in the box "Rehabilitation Following a Minor Athletic Injury" on p. 80.

Preventing Injuries The best method for dealing with exercise injuries is to prevent them. If you choose activities for your program carefully and follow the training guidelines described here and in Chapter 2, you should be able to avoid most types of injuries. Important guidelines for preventing athletic injuries include the following:

- Train regularly and stay in condition.
- Gradually increase the intensity, duration, or frequency of your workouts.
- Avoid or minimize high-impact activities; alternate them with low-impact activities.
- Get proper rest between exercise sessions.
- Drink plenty of fluids.
- Warm up thoroughly before you exercise and cool down afterward.

Rehabilitation Following a Minor Athletic Injury

• Reduce the initial inflammation using the R-I-C-E principle (see text).

• After 36–48 hours, apply heat *if the swelling has completely disappeared.* Immerse the affected area in warm water or apply warm compresses, a hot water bottle, or a heating pad. As soon as it's comfortable, begin moving the affected joints slowly. If you feel pain, or if the injured area begins to swell again, reduce the amount of movement. Continue stretching and moving the affected area until you have regained normal range of motion.

• Gradually begin exercising the injured area to build strength and endurance. Depending on the type of injury, weight training, walking, and resistance training with a partner can all be effective.

• Gradually reintroduce the stress of an activity until you can return to full intensity. Don't progress too rapidly or you'll reinjure yourself. Before returning to full exercise participation, you should have a full range of motion in your joints, normal strength and balance among your muscles, normal coordinated patterns of movement (with no injury compensation movements, such as limping), and little or no pain.

• Achieve and maintain a good level of flexibility.

• Use proper body mechanics when lifting objects or executing sports skills.

• Don't exercise when you are ill or overtrained.

• Use proper equipment, particularly shoes, and choose an appropriate exercise surface. If you exercise on a grass field, soft track, or wooden floor, you are less likely to be injured than on concrete or a hard track. (For information on athletic shoes, see the box "Choosing Exercise Footwear.")

• Don't return to your normal exercise program until any athletic injuries have healed. Restart your program at a lower intensity and gradually increase the amount of overload.

QUESTIONS FOR CRITICAL THINKING AND REFLECTION

Have you ever suffered an injury while exercising? If so, how did you treat the injury? Compare your treatment with the guidelines given in this chapter. Did you do the right things? What can you do to avoid such injuries in the future?

SUMMARY

• The cardiorespiratory system consists of the heart, blood vessels, and respiratory system; it picks up and transports oxygen, nutrients, and waste products.

• The body takes chemical energy from food and uses it to produce ATP and fuel cellular activities. ATP is stored in the body's cells as the basic form of energy.

• During exercise, the body supplies ATP and fuels cellular activities by combining three energy systems: immediate, for short periods of activity; nonoxidative (anaerobic), for intense activity; and oxidative (aerobic), for prolonged activity. Which

TIPS FOR TODAY AND THE FUTURE

Regular, moderate exercise, even in short bouts spread through the day, can build and maintain cardiorespiratory fitness.

RIGHT NOW YOU CAN

■ Assess your cardiorespiratory fitness by using one of the methods discussed in this chapter and in Lab 3.1.

■ Do a short bout of endurance exercise: 10–15 minutes of walking, jogging, cycling, or another endurance activity.

■ If you have physical activity planned for later in the day, drink some fluids now to make sure you are fully hydrated for your workout.

■ Consider the exercise equipment, including shoes, you currently have on hand. If you need new equipment, start gathering the information you'll need to get the best equipment you can afford.

■ Contact someone you know who engages in regular endurance exercise. Ask what strategies she or he uses to find time for exercise and to stay motivated.

IN THE FUTURE YOU CAN

■ Graduate to a different, more challenging fitness assessment as your cardiorespiratory fitness improves.

■ Incorporate different types of exercises into your cardiorespiratory endurance training to keep yourself challenged and motivated.

---

energy system predominates depends on the duration and intensity of the activity.

• Cardiorespiratory endurance exercise improves cardiorespiratory functioning and cellular metabolism; it reduces the risk of chronic diseases such as heart disease, cancer, type 2 diabetes, obesity, and osteoporosis; and it improves immune function and psychological and emotional well-being.

• Cardiorespiratory fitness is measured by determining how well the cardiorespiratory system transports and uses oxygen.

(continued on p. 83)

Choosing Exercise Footwear

Footwear is perhaps the most important item of equipment for almost any activity. Shoes protect and support your feet and improve your traction. When you jump or run, you place as much as six times more force on your feet than when you stand still. Shoes can help cushion against the stress that this additional force places on your lower legs, thereby preventing injuries. Some athletic shoes are also designed to help prevent ankle rollover, another common source of injury.

General Guidelines

When choosing athletic shoes, first consider the activity you've chosen for your exercise program. Shoes appropriate for different activities have very different characteristics. For example, running shoes typically have highly cushioned midsoles, rubber outsoles with elevated heels, and a great deal of flexibility in the forefoot. The heels of walking shoes tend to be lower, less padded, and more beveled than those designed for running. For aerobic dance, shoes must be flexible in the forefoot and have straight, nonflared heels to allow for safe and easy lateral movements. Court shoes also provide substantial support for lateral movements; they typically have outsoles made from white rubber that will not damage court surfaces.

Also consider the location and intensity of your workouts. If you plan to walk or run on trails, you should choose shoes with water-resistant, highly durable uppers and more outsole traction. If you work out intensely or have a relatively high body weight, you'll need thick, firm midsoles to avoid bottoming-out the cushioning system of your shoes.

Foot type is another important consideration. If your feet tend to roll inward excessively, you may need shoes with additional stability features on the inner side of the shoe to counteract this movement. If your feet tend to roll outward excessively, you may need highly flexible and cushioned shoes that promote foot motion. For aerobic dancers whose feet tend to roll inward or outward, mid- or high-cut shoes may be more appropriate than low-cut aerobic shoes or cross-trainers (shoes designed to be worn for several different activities). Compared to men, women have narrower feet overall and narrower heels relative to the forefoot. Most women will get a better fit if they choose shoes that are specifically designed for women's feet rather than shoes that are downsized versions of men's shoes.

Successful Shopping

For successful shoe shopping, keep the following strategies in mind:

- Shop at an athletic shoe or specialty store that has personnel trained to fit athletic shoes and a large selection of styles and sizes.

- Shop late in the day or, ideally, following a workout. Your foot size increases over the course of the day and after exercise.

- Wear socks like those you plan to wear during exercise. If you have an old pair of athletic shoes, bring them with you. The wear pattern on your old shoes can help you select a pair with extra support or cushioning in the places you need it the most.

- Ask for help. Trained salespeople know which shoes are designed for your foot type and your level of activity. They can also help fit your shoes properly.

- Don't insist on buying shoes in what you consider to be your typical shoe size. Sizes vary from shoe to shoe. In addition, foot sizes change over time, and many people have one foot that is larger or wider than the other. Try several sizes in several widths, if necessary. Don't buy shoes that are too small.

- Try on both shoes and wear them around for 10 or more minutes. Try walking on a noncarpeted surface. Approximate the movements of your activity: walk, jog, run, jump, and so on.

- Check the fit and style carefully:

    Is the toe box roomy enough? Your toes will spread out when your foot hits the ground or you push off. There should be at least one thumb's width of space from the longest toe to the end of the toe box.

    Do the shoes have enough cushioning? Do your feet feel supported when you bounce up and down? Try bouncing on your toes and on your heels.

    Do your heels fit snugly into the shoe? Do they stay put when you walk, or do they rise up?

    Are the arches of your feet right on top of the shoes' arch supports?

    Do the shoes feel stable when you twist and turn on the balls of your feet? Try twisting from side to side while standing on one foot.

    Do you feel any pressure points?

- If the shoes are not comfortable in the store, don't buy them. Don't expect athletic shoes to stretch over time in order to fit your feet properly.

- If you exercise at dawn or dusk, choose shoes with reflective sections for added visibility and safety.

- Replace athletic shoes about every 3 months or 300–500 miles of jogging or walking.

Q **What kind of clothing should I wear during exercise?**

A Exercise clothing should be comfortable, let you move freely, and allow your body to cool itself. Avoid clothing that constricts normal blood flow or is made from nylon or rubberized fabrics that prevent evaporation of perspiration. Cotton is an excellent material for facilitating the evaporation of sweat. If you sweat heavily when you exercise and find that too much moisture accumulates in cotton clothing, try fabrics containing synthetic materials such as polypropylene that wick moisture away from the skin. Socks made with moisture-wicking compounds may be particularly helpful for people whose feet sweat heavily.

A sports bra is a key piece of clothing for women. A good sports bra should be made of a breathable fabric to allow for evaporation of sweat; it should fit well and have comfortable seams and closures. Try on several styles and sizes to see what fits best, and try the jump test to make sure the bra will provide enough support for your activities. Find a bra that emphasizes function over fashion.

Q **Do I need a special diet for my endurance exercise program?**

A No. For most people, a nutritionally balanced diet contains all the energy and nutrients needed to sustain an exercise program. Don't waste your money on unnecessary supplements. (Chapter 8 has information about putting together a healthy diet.)

Q **How can I measure how far I walk or run?**

A The simplest and cheapest way to measure distance is with a pedometer, which counts your steps. A pedometer's accuracy depends on how precisely you measure your stride length; follow the instructions that come with your pedometer to set this measure. Although stride length varies among individuals, 2000 steps typically equals about 1 mile, and 10,000 steps equals about 5 miles. To track your distance and your progress using a pedometer, follow the guidelines in Lab 2.3. For advice on purchasing a pedometer that meets your needs, check consumer and fitness magazines and Web sites. More tips on using pedometers are provided on the Online Learning Center.

Q **How can I safely increase exercise intensity to build fitness?**

A For both athletes and nonathletes, it is extremely important to increase intensity very gradually and to rest between exercise sessions. If you train too hard and/or don't rest enough, you are more likely to be injured—and be discouraged from continuing with your fitness program. For endurance training, overload techniques such as interval training and wind sprints can help you build fitness quickly but also pose a greater risk of injury or overtraining. Start off with a few high-intensity bouts of exercise and build up gradually. Don't practice interval training or wind sprints more than 2–3 days per week unless you have a high fitness level.

Increase intensity or duration by about 1–3% in a single workout; rest the following day and then do your typical workout. Repeat the more difficult workout after another day of rest. Adjust your progress according to how you feel. You can't increase fitness in a few days. Be patient—with gradual increases in intensity and plenty of rest between workouts, you will be able to move to a higher level of fitness without injury.

Q **If I plan to include both cardiorespiratory endurance training and strength training in a single workout, which should I do first?**

A It depends on your goals. If your primary goal is cardiorespiratory conditioning, then do your endurance workout first. If your fitness program is focused on large gains in strength and you plan to lift relatively heavy weights, then do your strength training workout first. You are likely to make the most rapid gains in fitness in whichever activity you engage in first, when you are fresh.

Q **Is it all right to participate in cardiorespiratory endurance exercise while menstruating?**

A Yes. There is no evidence that exercise during menstruation is unhealthy or that it has negative effects on performance. If you have headaches, backaches, and abdominal pain during menstruation, you may not feel like exercising; for some women, exercise helps relieve these symptoms. Listen to your body, and exercise at whatever intensity is comfortable for you.

Q **Will high altitude affect my ability to exercise?**

A At high altitudes (above 1500 meters or about 4900 feet), there is less oxygen available in the air than at lower altitudes. High altitude doesn't affect anaerobic exercise, such as stretching and weight lifting, but it does affect aerobic activities—that is, any type of cardiovascular endurance exercise—because the heart and lungs have to work harder, even when the body is at rest, to deliver enough oxygen to body cells. The increased cardiovascular strain of exercise reduces endurance. To play it safe when at high altitudes, avoid heavy exercise—at least for the first few days—and drink plenty of water. And don't expect to reach your normal lower altitude exercise capacity.

For more Common Questions Answered about endurance training, visit the Online Learning Center.

The upper limit of this measure is called maximal oxygen consumption, or $\dot{V}O_{2max}$.

- $\dot{V}O_{2max}$ can be measured precisely in a laboratory, or it can be estimated reasonably well through less expensive assessment tests.

- To have a successful exercise program, set realistic goals; choose suitable activities; begin slowly; always warm up and cool down; and, as fitness improves, exercise more often, longer, and/or harder.

- Intensity of training can be measured through target heart rate zone, METs, ratings of perceived exertion, or the "talk test."

- With careful attention to fluid intake, clothing, duration of exercise, and exercise intensity, endurance training can be safe in hot and cold weather conditions.

- Serious injuries require medical attention. Application of the R-I-C-E principle (rest, ice, compression, elevation) is appropriate for treating many types of muscle or joint injuries.

FOR FURTHER EXPLORATION

BOOKS

American College of Sports Medicine. 2003. *ACSM Fitness Book.* 3rd ed. Champaign, Ill.: Human Kinetics. *Includes fitness assessment tests and advice on creating a complete fitness program.*

Barough, N. 2004. *Walking for Fitness.* New York: DK. *Provides advice on putting together a walking program that matches your fitness goals.*

Beim, G., and R. Winter. 2003. *The Female Athlete's Body Book: How to Prevent and Treat Sports Injuries in Women and Girls.* New York: McGraw-Hill/Contemporary. *Provides detailed information on the prevention and treatment of athletic injuries in women and girls.*

Caron, M. 2007. *Walking for Fitness: The Beginner's Handbook.* Vancouver, B.C.: Greystone Books. *Features two complete programs for walking your way to fitness, with advice on shoes, motivation, and nutrition.*

Fenton, M. 2008. *The Complete Guide to Walking, New and Revised: For Health, Weight Loss, and Fitness.* Guilford, Conn.: Lyons Press. *Discusses walking as a fitness method and a way to avoid diseases such as diabetes.*

Gotlin, R. 2007. *Sports Injuries Guidebook.* Champaign, Ill.: Human Kinetics. *Provides information and care instructions on many types of sports-related injuries.*

Hewitt, B., ed. 2005. *New Cyclist Handbook.* Emmaus, Penn.: Rodale. *Includes information on buying and caring for a bicycle as well as on increasing fitness.*

Juba, K. 2002. *Swimming for Fitness.* New York: Lyons Press. *Provides step-by-step instructions for setting up a swimming fitness program, including advice on technique and avoiding injury and overtraining.*

Nieman, D.C. 2007. *Exercise Testing and Prescription: A Health-Related Approach,* 6th ed. New York: McGraw-Hill. *A comprehensive discussion of the effect of exercise and exercise testing and prescription.*

Noakes, T. 2003. *Lore of Running,* 4th ed. Champaign, Ill.: Human Kinetics. *Provides detailed information on physiology, training, racing, and injury prevention.*

ORGANIZATIONS AND WEB SITES

American Academy of Orthopaedic Surgeons. Provides fact sheets on many fitness and sports topics, including how to begin a program, how to choose equipment, and how to prevent and treat many types of injuries.
http://orthoinfo.aaos.org

American Heart Association. Provides information on cardiovascular health and disease, including the role of exercise in maintaining heart health and exercise tips for people of all ages.
800-AHA-USA1
http://www.americanheart.org

Dr. Pribut's Running Injuries Page. Provides information about running and many types of running injuries.
http://www.drpribut.com/sports/spsport.html

Federal Trade Commission: Consumer Protection—Diet, Health, and Fitness. Provides several brochures with consumer advice about purchasing exercise equipment.
http://www.ftc.gov/bcp/menus/consumer/health.shtm

The Human Heart. An online museum exhibit with information on the structure and function of the heart, blood vessels, and respiratory system.
http://www.fi.edu/learn/heart/index.html

MedlinePlus: Exercise and Physical Fitness. Provides links to news and reliable information about fitness from government agencies and professional associations.
http://www.nlm.nih.gov/medlineplus/exerciseandphysicalfitness.html

Physician and Sportsmedicine. Provides many articles with easy-to-understand advice about exercise injuries.
http://ww.postgradmed.com/index.html

Runner's World Online. Contains a wide variety of information about running, including tips for beginning runners, advice about training, and a shoe buyer's guide.
http://www.runnersworld.com

University of Florida: Keeping Fit. Provides useful information about fitness in a question-and-answer format; an extensive set of links is also provided.
http://www.hhp.ufl.edu/faculty/pbird/keepingfit

Women's Sports Foundation. Provides information and links about training and about many specific sports activities.
http://www.womenssportsfoundation.org

Yahoo/Recreation. Contains links to many sites with practical advice on many sports and activities.
http://dir.yahoo.com/recreation/sports

See also the listings in Chapters 2 and 11.

SELECTED BIBLIOGRAPHY

Adler, P. A., and B. L. Roberts. 2006. The use of Tai Chi to improve health in older adults. *Orthopedic Nursing* 25(2): 122–126.

American College of Sports Medicine. 2006. *ACSM's Guidelines for Exercise Testing and Prescription,* 7th ed. Philadelphia: Lippincott Williams and Wilkins.

American College of Sports Medicine. 2006. *ACSM's Resource Manual for Guidelines for Exercise Testing and Prescription,* 5th ed. Philadelphia: Lippincott Williams and Wilkins.

Brooks, G. A., et al. 2005. *Exercise Physiology: Human Bioenergetics and Its Applications,* 4th ed. New York: McGraw-Hill.

Campbell, K. L., and A. McTiernan. 2007. Exercise and biomarkers for cancer prevention studies. *The Journal of Nutrition* 137(1 Suppl.): 161S–169S.

Carnethon, M. R., et al. 2005. A longitudinal study of physical activity and heart rate recovery: CARDIA, 1987–1993. *Medicine and Science in Sports and Exercise* 37: 606–612.

Colcombe, S., et al. 2006. Aerobic exercise training increases brain volume in aging humans. *The Journals of Gerontology Series A: Biological Sciences and Medical Sciences* 61(11): 1166–1170.

Duscha, B. D., et al. 2005. Effects of exercise training amount and intensity on peak oxygen consumption in middle-age men and women at risk for cardiovascular disease. *Chest* 128(4): 2788–2793.

Federal Trade Commission. 2007. *Weightloss and Fitness* (http://www.ftc.gov/bcp/menus/consumer/health/weight.shtm; retrieved November 5, 2007).

Ferrara, C. M., et al. 2006. Effects of aerobic and resistive exercise training on glucose disposal and skeletal muscle metabolism in older men. *The Journals of Gerontology Series A: Biological Sciences and Medical Sciences* 61(5): 480–487.

Fogelholm, M. 2006. Exercise, substrate oxidation and energy balance. *International Journal of Obesity* 30(6): 1022.

Hagstromer, M., et al. 2006. The International Physical Activity Questionnaire (IPAQ): A study of concurrent and construct validity. *Public Health Nutrition* 9(6): 755–762.

Hew-Butler, T., et al. 2005. Consensus statement of the 1st International Exercise-Associated Hyponatremia Consensus Development Conference, Cape Town, South Africa, 2005. *Clinical Journal of Sports Medicine* 15(4): 208–213.

Interval training: More benefit, less fatigue. 2005. *Consumer Reports,* May.

John, E. M., P. L. Horn-Ross, and J. Koo. 2004. Lifetime physical activity and breast cancer risk in a multiethnic population. *Cancer Epidemiology, Biomarkers, and Prevention* 12(11 Pt. 1): 1143–1152.

Karavatas, S. G., and K. Tavakol. 2005. Concurrent validity of Borg's rating of perceived exertion in African-American young adults, employing heart rate as the standard. *Internet Journal of Allied Health Sciences and Practice* 3(January).

Ko, G. T., et al. 2006. A 10-week Tai-Chi program improved the blood pressure, lipid profile and SF-36 scores in Hong Kong Chinese women. *Medical Science Monitor: International Medical Journal of Experimental and Clinical Research* 12(5): CR196–CR199.

Kondo, N., et al. 2005. Association of inflammatory marker and highly sensitive C-reactive protein with aerobic exercise capacity, maximum oxygen uptake and insulin resistance in healthy middle-aged volunteers. *Circulation Journal* 69: 452–457.

Lambert, C. P., and W. J. Evans. 2005. Adaptations to aerobic and resistance exercise in the elderly. *Reviews in Endocrine and Metabolic Disorders* 6: 137–143.

Laughlin, M. H. 2004. Joseph B. Wolfe Memorial Lecture. Physical activity in prevention and treatment of coronary disease: The battle line is in exercise vascular cell biology. *Medicine and Science in Sports and Exercise* 36: 352–362.

Luebbers, P. E. 2005. Running and walking form. *ACSM Fit Society Page,* Summer.

Macfarlane, D. J., et al. 2006. Very short intermittent vs. continuous bouts of activity in sedentary adults. *Preventive Medicine* 43(4): 332–336.

National Weather Service. 2005. *Heat Index* (http://www.crh.noaa.gov/arx/heatindex.php; retrieved November 5, 2007).

Nieman, D. C. 2005. Can exercise help me sleep better? *ACSM's Health & Fitness Journal* 9(3): 6.

Nurmi-Lawton, J. A., et al. 2004. Evidence of sustained skeletal benefits from impact-loading exercise in young females. *Journal of Bone and Mineral Research* 19(2): 314–322.

Okura, T., et al. 2006. Effect of regular exercise on homocysteine concentrations: The HERITAGE Family Study. *European Journal of Applied Physiology* 98(4): 394–401.

Persinger, R., et al. 2004. Consistency of the talk test for exercise prescription. *Medicine and Science in Sports and Exercise* 36(9): 1632–1636.

Peterson, J. A. 2005. 10 common mistakes made by individuals who engage in aerobic exercises. *ACSM's Health & Fitness Journal* 9(3): 44.

Rixon K. P., et al. 2006. Analysis of the assessment of caloric expenditure in four modes of aerobic dance. *Journal of Strength and Conditioning Research* 20(3): 593–596.

Roberpgs, R. A., et al. 2004. Biochemistry of exercise-induced metabolic acidosis. *American Journal of Physiology: Regulatory, Integrative and Comparative Physiology* 287(3): R502–R516.

Robinson, D. L. 2007. Bicycle helmet legislation: Can we reach a consensus? *Accident Analysis and Prevention* 39(1): 86–93.

Scott, S. 2005. Combating depression with exercise. *ACSM's Health & Fitness Journal* 9(4): 31.

Shaibi, G. Q., et al. 2006. Aerobic fitness among Caucasian, African–American, and Latino youth. *Ethnic Diseases* 16(1): 120–125.

Shaw, K., et al. 2006. Exercise for overweight or obesity. *Cochrane Database of Systematic Reviews Online* Oct. 18(4): CD003817.

Slentz, C. A., et al. 2005. Inactivity, exercise, and visceral fat. STRRIDE: A randomized, controlled study of exercise intensity and amount. *Journal of Applied Physiology* 99(4): 1613–1618.

Suominen, H. 2006. Muscle training for bone strength. *Aging Clinical and Experimental Research* 18(2): 85–93.

Swain, D. P. 2005. Moderate or vigorous intensity exercise: Which is better for improving aerobic fitness? *Preventive Cardiology* 8: 55–58.

Tunceli, K., et al. 2006. Long-term effects of obesity on employment and work limitations among U.S. Adults, 1986 to 1999. *Obesity* 14(9): 1637–1646.

Wellman, N. S., et al. 2007. Eat better and move more: A community-based program designed to improve diets and increase physical activity among older Americans. *American Journal of Public Health* 97(4): 710–717.

Yamashita, S., et al. 2006. Effects of music during exercise on RPE, heart rate and the autonomic nervous system. *The Journal of Sports Medicine and Physical Fitness* 46(3): 425–430.

LAB 3.1 Assessing Your Current Level of Cardiorespiratory Endurance

Before taking any of the cardiorespiratory endurance assessment tests, refer to the fitness prerequisites and cautions given in Table 3.2. Choose one of the following three tests presented in this lab:

- 1-mile walk test
- 3-minute step test
- 1.5-mile run-walk test

For best results, don't exercise strenuously or consume caffeine the day of the test, and don't smoke or eat a heavy meal within about 3 hours of the test.

The 1-Mile Walk Test

Equipment

1. A track or course that provides a measurement of 1 mile
2. A stopwatch, clock, or watch with a second hand
3. A weight scale

Preparation

Measure your body weight (in pounds) before taking the test.

Body weight: _____ lb

Instructions

1. Warm up before taking the test. Do some walking, easy jogging, or calisthenics and some stretching exercises.
2. Cover the 1-mile course as quickly as possible. Walk at a pace that is brisk but comfortable. You must raise your heart rate above 120 beats per minute (bpm).
3. As soon as you complete the distance, note your time and take your pulse for 10 seconds.

   Walking time: _____ min _____ sec

   10-second pulse count: _____ beats
4. Cool down after the test by walking slowly for several minutes.

Determining Maximal Oxygen Consumption

1. Convert your 10-second pulse count into a value for exercise heart rate by multiplying it by 6.

   Exercise heart rate: $\underset{\text{10-sec pulse count}}{\underline{\hspace{2cm}}} \times 6 = $ _____ bpm
2. Convert your walking time from minutes and seconds to a decimal figure. For example, a time of 14 minutes and 45 seconds would be 14 + (45/60), or 14.75 minutes.

   Walking time: _____ min + (_____ sec ÷ 60 sec/min) = _____ min
3. Insert values for your age, gender, weight, walking time, and exercise heart rate in the following equation, where

   W = your weight (in pounds)

   A = your age (in years)

   G = your gender (male = 1; female = 0)

   T = your time to complete the 1-mile course (in minutes)

   H = your exercise heart rate (in beats per minute)

   $\dot{V}O_{2max} = 132.853 - (0.0769 \times W) - (0.3877 \times A) + (6.315 \times G) - (3.2649 \times T) - (0.1565 \times H)$

For example, a 20-year-old, 190-pound male with a time of 14.75 minutes and an exercise heart rate of 152 bpm would calculate maximal oxygen consumption as follows:

$$\dot{V}O_{2max} = 132.853 - (0.0769 \times 190) - (03877 \times 20) + (6.315 \times 1) - (3.2649 \times 14.75) - (0.1565 \times 152) = 45\ ml/kg/min$$

$$\dot{V}O_{2max} = 132.853 - (0.0769 \times \underset{\text{weight (lb)}}{\underline{\hspace{2cm}}}) - (0.3877 \times \underset{\text{age (years)}}{\underline{\hspace{2cm}}}) + (6.315 \times \underset{\text{gender}}{\underline{\hspace{2cm}}})$$

$$- (3.2649 \times \underset{\text{walking time (min)}}{\underline{\hspace{2cm}}}) - (0.1565 \times \underset{\text{exercise heart rate (bpm)}}{\underline{\hspace{2cm}}}) = \underline{\hspace{2cm}}\ ml/kg/min$$

4. Copy this value for $\dot{V}O_{2max}$ into the appropriate place in the chart on the final page of this lab.

The 3-Minute Step Test

Equipment

1. A step, bench, or bleacher step that is 16.25 inches from ground level

2. A stopwatch, clock, or watch with a second hand

3. A metronome

Preparation

Practice stepping up onto and down from the step before you begin the test. Each step has four beats: up-up-down-down. Males should perform the test with the metronome set for a rate of 96 beats per minute, or 24 steps per minute. Females should set the metronome at 88 beats per minute, or 22 steps per minute.

Instructions

1. Warm up before taking the test. Do some walking, easy jogging, and stretching exercises.

2. Set the metronome at the proper rate. Your instructor or a partner can call out starting and stopping times; otherwise, have a clock or watch within easy viewing during the test.

3. Begin the test and continue to step at the correct pace for 3 minutes.

4. Stop after 3 minutes. Remain standing and count your pulse for the 15-second period from 5 to 20 seconds into recovery.

   15-second pulse count: _____ beats

5. Cool down after the test by walking slowly for several minutes.

Determining Maximal Oxygen Consumption

1. Convert your 15-second pulse count to a value for recovery heart rate by multiplying by 4.

   Recovery heart rate: $\underset{\text{15-sec pulse count}}{\underline{\hspace{3cm}}} \times 4 = \underline{\hspace{2cm}}\ bpm$

2. Insert your recovery heart rate in the equation below, where

   H = recovery heart rate (in beats per minute)

   Males: $\dot{V}O_{2max} = 111.33 - (0.42 \times H)$

   Females: $\dot{V}O_{2max} = 65.81 - (0.1847 \times H)$

   For example, a man with a recovery heart rate of 162 bpm would calculate maximal oxygen consumption as follows:

   $$\dot{V}O_{2max} = 111.33 - (0.42 \times 162) = 43\ ml/kg/min$$

   Males: $\dot{V}O_{2max} = 111.33 - (0.42 \times \underset{\text{recovery heart rate (bpm)}}{\underline{\hspace{3cm}}}) = \underline{\hspace{2cm}}\ ml/kg/min$

   Females: $\dot{V}O_{2max} = 65.81 - (0.1847 \times \underset{\text{recovery heart rate (bpm)}}{\underline{\hspace{3cm}}}) = \underline{\hspace{2cm}}\ ml/kg/min$

3. Copy this value for $\dot{V}O_{2max}$ into the appropriate place in the chart on the final page of this lab.

The 1.5-Mile Run-Walk Test

Equipment

1. A running track or course that is flat and provides exact measurements of up to 1.5 miles
2. A stopwatch, clock, or watch with a second hand

Preparation

You may want to practice pacing yourself prior to taking the test to avoid going too fast at the start and becoming prematurely fatigued. Allow yourself a day or two to recover from your practice run before taking the test.

Instructions

1. Warm up before taking the test. Do some walking, easy jogging, and stretching exercises.
2. Try to cover the distance as fast as possible without overexerting yourself. If possible, monitor your own time, or have someone call out your time at various intervals of the test to determine whether your pace is correct.
3. Record the amount of time, in minutes and seconds, it takes you to complete the 1.5-mile distance.

   Running-walking time: _____ min _____ sec
4. Cool down after the test by walking or jogging slowly for about 5 minutes.

Determining Maximal Oxygen Consumption

1. Convert your running time from minutes and seconds to a decimal figure. For example, a time of 14 minutes and 25 seconds would be 14 + (25/60), or 14.4 minutes.

   Running-walking time: _____ min + (_____ sec ÷ 60 sec/min) = _____ min
2. Insert your running time into the equation below, where

   T = running time (in minutes)

   $\dot{V}O_{2max} = (483 \div T) + 3.5$

   For example, a person who completes 1.5 miles in 14.4 minutes would calculate maximal oxygen consumption as follows:

   $\dot{V}O_{2max} = (483 \div 14.4) + 3.5 = 37$ *ml/kg/min*

   $\dot{V}O_{2max} = (483 \div \underset{\text{run-walk time (min)}}{\underline{\hspace{2cm}}}) + 3.5 = \underline{\hspace{2cm}}$ **ml/kg/min**
3. Copy this value for $\dot{V}O_{2max}$ into the appropriate place in the chart on the final page of this lab.

Rating Your Cardiovascular Fitness

Record your $\dot{V}O_{2max}$ score(s) and the corresponding fitness rating from the table below.

Women	Very Poor	Poor	Fair	Good	Excellent	Superior
Age: 18–29	Below 31.6	31.6–35.4	35.5–39.4	39.5–43.9	44.0–50.1	Above 50.1
30–39	Below 29.9	29.9–33.7	33.8–36.7	36.8–40.9	41.0–46.8	Above 46.8
40–49	Below 28.0	28.0–31.5	31.6–35.0	35.1–38.8	38.9–45.1	Above 45.1
50–59	Below 25.5	25.5–28.6	28.7–31.3	31.4–35.1	35.2–39.8	Above 39.8
60–69	Below 23.7	23.7–26.5	26.6–29.0	29.1–32.2	32.3–36.8	Above 36.8
Men						
Age: 18–29	Below 38.1	38.1–42.1	42.2–45.6	45.7–51.0	51.1–56.1	Above 56.1
30–39	Below 36.7	36.7–40.9	41.0–44.3	44.4–48.8	48.9–54.2	Above 54.2
40–49	Below 34.6	34.6–38.3	38.4–42.3	42.4–46.7	46.8–52.8	Above 52.8
50–59	Below 31.1	31.1–35.1	35.2–38.2	38.3–43.2	43.3–49.6	Above 49.6
60–69	Below 27.4	27.4–31.3	31.4–34.9	35.0–39.4	39.5–46.0	Above 46.0

SOURCE: Ratings based on norms from The Cooper Institute of Aerobic Research, Dallas, Texas; from *The Physical Fitness Specialist Manual*, Revised 2002. Used with permission.

	$\dot{V}O_{2max}$	Cardiovascular Fitness Rating
1-mile walk test		
3-minute step test		
1.5-mile run-walk test		

Using Your Results

How did you score? Are you surprised by your rating for cardiovascular fitness? Are you satisfied with your current rating?

If you're not satisfied, set a realistic goal for improvement: _____

Are you satisfied with your current level of cardiovascular fitness as evidenced in your daily life—your ability to walk, run, bicycle, climb stairs, do yard work, engage in recreational activities?

If you're not satisfied, set some realistic goals for improvement, such as completing a 5K run or 25-mile bike ride:

What should you do next? Enter the results of this lab in the Preprogram Assessment column in Appendix D. If you've set goals for improvement, begin planning your cardiorespiratory endurance exercise program by completing the plan in Lab 3.2. After several weeks of your program, complete this lab again, and enter the results in the Postprogram Assessment column of Appendix D. How do the results compare? (Remember, it's best to compare $\dot{V}O_{2max}$ scores for the same test.)

SOURCES: Kline, G. M., et al. 1987. Estimation of $\dot{V}O_{2max}$ from a one-mile track walk, gender, age, and body weight. *Medicine and Science in Sports and Exercise* 19(3): 253–259. McArdle, W. D., F. I. Katch, and V. L. Katch. 1991. *Exercise Physiology: Energy, Nutrition, and Human Performance.* Philadelphia: Lea and Febiger, pp. 225–226. Brooks, G. A., and T. D. Fahey. 1987. *Fundamentals of Human Performance.* New York: Macmillan.

LAB 3.2 Developing an Exercise Program for Cardiorespiratory Endurance

1. *Goals.* List goals for your cardiorespiratory endurance exercise program. Your goals can be specific or general, short or long term. In the first section, include specific, measurable goals that you can use to track the progress of your fitness program. These goals might be things like raising your cardiorespiratory fitness rating from fair to good or swimming laps for 30 minutes without resting. In the second section, include long-term and more qualitative goals, such as improving self-confidence and reducing your risk for chronic disease.

   Specific Goals: Current Status   Final Goals

   _____   _____

   _____   _____

   _____   _____

   Other goals: _____

   _____

2. *Type of Activities.* Choose one or more endurance activities for your program. These can include any activity that uses large-muscle groups, can be maintained continuously, and is rhythmic and aerobic in nature. Examples include walking, jogging, cycling, group exercise such as aerobic dance, rowing, rope skipping, stair-climbing, cross-country skiing, swimming, skating, and endurance game activities such as soccer and tennis. Choose activities that are both convenient and enjoyable. Fill in the activity names on the program plan.

3. *Frequency.* On the program plan, fill in how often you plan to participate in each activity; the ACSM recommends participating in cardiorespiratory endurance exercise 3–5 days per week.

Program Plan

Type of Activity	Frequency (check ✓)							Intensity (bpm or RPE)	Time (min)
	M	T	W	Th	F	Sa	Su		

4. *Intensity.* Determine your exercise intensity using one of the following methods, and enter it on the program plan. Begin your program at a lower intensity and slowly increase intensity as your fitness improves, so select a range of intensities for your program.

   a. Target heart rate zone: Calculate target heart rate zone in beats per minute and then calculate the corresponding 10-second exercise count by dividing the total count by 6. For example, the 10-second exercise counts corresponding to a target heart rate zone of 122–180 bpm would be 20–30 beats.

   Maximum heart rate: 220 − _____ = _____ bpm

                                     age (yeas)

   Maximum Heart Rate Method

   65% training intensity = _____ bpm × 0.65 = _____ bpm

                                 maximum heart rate

   90% training intensity = _____ bpm × 0.90 = _____ bpm

                                 maximum heart rate

   Target heart rate zone = _____ to _____ bpm   10-second count = _____ to _____

Heart Rate Reserve Method

Resting heart rate: _____ bpm (taken after 10 minutes of complete rest)

Heart rate reserve = _____ bpm − _____ bpm = _____ bpm

maximum heart rate   resting heart rate

50% training intensity = (_____ bpm × 0.50) + _____ bpm = _____ bpm

heart rate reserve   resting heart rate

85% training intensity = (_____ bpm × 0.85) + _____ bpm = _____ bpm

heart rate reserve   resting heart rate

Target heart rate zone = _____ to _____ bpm   10-second count = _____ to _____

b. Ratings of perceived exertion (RPE): If you prefer, determine an RPE value that corresponds to your target heart rate range (see p. 72 and Figure 3.6).

5. *Time (Duration).* A total time of 20–60 minutes is recommended; your duration of exercise will vary with intensity. For developing cardiorespiratory endurance, higher-intensity activities can be performed for a shorter duration; lower intensities require a longer duration. Enter a duration (or a range of duration) on the program plan.

6. *Monitoring Your Program.* Complete a log like the one below to monitor your program and track your progress. Note the date on top, and fill in the intensity and time (duration) for each workout. If you prefer, you can also track other variables such as distance. For example, if your cardiorespiratory endurance program includes walking and swimming, you may want to track miles walked and yards swum in addition to the duration of each exercise session. For more extensive sets of logs, refer to the Daily Fitness and Nutrition Journal that accompanies your text.

Activity/Date														
1	Intensity													
	Time													
	Distance													
2	Intensity													
	Time													
	Distance													
3	Intensity													
	Time													
	Distance													
4	Intensity													
	Time													
	Distance													

7. *Making Progress.* Follow the guidelines in the chapter and Table 3.5 to slowly increase the amount of overload in your program. Continue keeping a log, and periodically evaluate your progress.

Progress Checkup: Week _____ of program

Goals: Original Status   Current Status

_____   _____

_____   _____

_____   _____

List each activity in your program and describe how satisfied you are with the activity and with your overall progress. List any problems you've encountered or any unexpected costs or benefits of your fitness program so far.

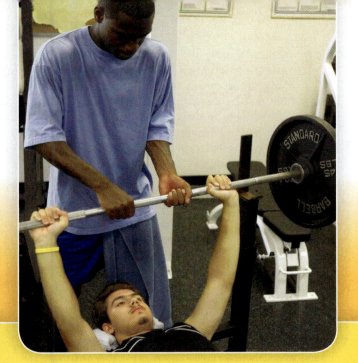

LOOKING AHEAD>>>>>

AFTER READING THIS CHAPTER, YOU SHOULD BE ABLE TO:

- Describe the basic physiology of muscles and how strength training affects muscles
- Define muscular strength and endurance, and describe how they relate to wellness
- Explain how muscular strength and endurance can be assessed
- Apply the FITT principle to create a safe and successful strength training program
- Describe the effects of supplements and drugs that are marketed to active people and athletes
- Explain how to safely perform common strength training exercises using free weights and weight machines

MUSCULAR STRENGTH AND ENDURANCE

4

TEST YOUR KNOWLEDGE

1. **For women, weight training typically results in which of the following?**

   a. bulky muscles
   b. significant increases in body weight
   c. improved body image

2. **To maximize strength gains, it is a good idea to hold your breath as you lift a weight.**

   True or false?

3. **Regular strength training is associated with which of the following benefits?**

   a. denser bones
   b. reduced risk of heart disease
   c. improved body composition
   d. fewer injuries

ANSWERS

1. **c.** Because the vast majority of women have low levels of testosterone, they do not develop large muscles or gain significant amounts of weight in response to a moderate weight training program. Men have higher levels of testosterone, so they can build large muscles more easily.

2. **FALSE.** Holding one's breath while lifting weights, called the Valsalva maneuver, can significantly (and possibly dangerously) elevate blood pressure; it also reduces blood flow to the heart and may cause faintness. You should breathe smoothly and normally while weight training. Some experts recommend that you exhale during the most difficult part of each exercise (the "sticking point").

3. **ALL FOUR.** Regular strength training has many benefits for lifetime wellness for both men and women.

FIT AND WELL ONLINE LEARNING CENTER www.mhhe.com/fahey

Visit the *Fit and Well* Online Learning Center for resources that will help you get the most out of your course!

- Study and review aids include practice quizzes, glossary flashcards, chapter summaries, learning objectives, PowerPoint presentations, Common Questions Answered, student handouts, crossword puzzles, Internet activities, and links to wellness Web sites.
- Behavior change tools include a daily fitness and nutrition journal, a behavior change workbook, sample behavior change plans, and blank behavior change logs to print and use.
- Chapter 4 resources also include video clips showing how to do all the exercises described and illustrated in the chapter (look for the video icon)—using free weights, weight machines, resistance bands, stability balls, and no equipment.

uscles make up more than 40% of your body mass. You depend on them for movement, and, because of their mass, they are the site of a large portion of the energy reactions (metabolism) that take place in your body. Strong, well-developed muscles help you perform daily activities with greater ease, protect you from injury, and enhance your well-being in other ways.

As described in Chapter 2, muscular strength is the amount of force a muscle can produce with a single maximum effort; muscular endurance is the ability to resist fatigue while holding or repeating a muscular contraction. This chapter explains the benefits of strength training (also called *resistance training*) and describes methods of assessing muscular strength and endurance. It then explains the basics of weight training and provides guidelines for setting up your own strength training program.

BASIC MUSCLE PHYSIOLOGY AND THE EFFECTS OF STRENGTH TRAINING

Muscles move the body and enable it to exert force because they move the skeleton. When a muscle contracts (shortens), it moves a bone by pulling on the tendon that attaches the muscle to the bone, as shown in Figure 4.1. When a muscle relaxes (lengthens), the tension placed on the tendon is released and the bone moves back to—or closer to—its starting position.

Muscle Fibers

Muscles consist of individual muscle cells, or **muscle fibers,** connected in bundles (see Figure 4.1). A single muscle is made up of many bundles of muscle fibers and is covered by layers of connective tissue that hold the

fibers together. Muscle fibers, in turn, are made up of smaller protein structures called **myofibrils.**

Strength training causes the size of individual muscle fibers to increase by increasing the number of myofibrils. Larger muscle fibers mean a larger and stronger muscle. The development of large muscle fibers is called **hypertrophy;** inactivity causes **atrophy,** the reversal of this process. In some species, muscles can increase in size through a separate process called **hyperplasia,** which involves an increase in the number of muscle fibers rather than the size of muscle fibers. In humans, hyperplasia is not thought to play a significant role in determining muscle size.

Muscle fibers are classified as slow-twitch or fast-twitch fibers according to their strength, speed of contraction, and energy source.

- **Slow-twitch fibers** are relatively fatigue-resistant, but they don't contract as rapidly or strongly as fast-twitch fibers. The principal energy system that fuels slow-twitch fibers is aerobic (oxidative). Slow-twitch muscle fibers are typically reddish in color.

- **Fast-twitch fibers** contract more rapidly and forcefully than slow-twitch fibers but fatigue more quickly. Although oxygen is important in the energy system that fuels fast-twitch fibers, they rely more on anaerobic (nonoxidative) metabolism than do slow-twitch fibers (see Chapter 3 for a discussion of energy systems). Fast-twitch muscle fibers are typically whitish in color.

Most muscles contain a mixture of slow-twitch and fast-twitch fibers. The proportion of the types of fibers varies significantly among different muscles and different individuals, and that proportion is largely fixed at birth, although fibers can contract faster or slower following a period of training or a period of inactivity. The type of fiber that acts during a particular activity depends on the type of work required. Endurance activities like jogging tend to use slow-twitch fibers, whereas strength and

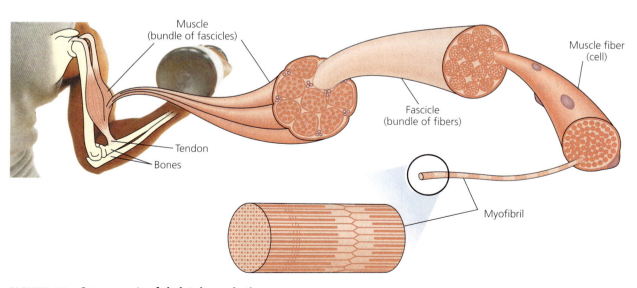

FIGURE 4.1 Components of skeletal muscle tissue.

FIGURE 4.2 Motor unit recruitment during muscle contraction. The number and size of motor units recruited for muscle contraction depends on the load (amount of resistance) and the speed of the movement. For light resistance, a small number of small motor units, made up primarily of slow-twitch fibers, are recruited. To move against heavy resistance or to move a light object very fast, a large number of motor units are recruited, including both small and large motor units. Large motor units contain a high proportion of fast-twitch fibers.

Number and size of motor units recruited — Large / Small

Resistance and/or speed — Low / High

power activities like sprinting use fast-twitch fibers. Strength training can increase the size and strength of both fast-twitch and slow-twitch fibers, although fast-twitch fibers are preferentially increased.

Motor Units

To exert force, the body recruits one or more motor units to contract. A **motor unit** is made up of a nerve connected to a number of muscle fibers. The number of muscle fibers in a motor unit varies from two to hundreds. Small motor units contain slow-twitch fibers, while large motor units contain fast-twitch fibers. When a motor nerve calls on its fibers to contract, all fibers contract to their full capacity. The number of motor units recruited depends on the amount of strength required: When a person picks up a small weight, he or she uses fewer and smaller motor units than when picking up a large weight (Figure 4.2).

Strength training improves the body's ability to recruit motor units—a phenomenon called **muscle learning**—which increases strength even before muscle size increases. The physiological changes and benefits that result from strength training are summarized in Table 4.1.

BENEFITS OF MUSCULAR STRENGTH AND ENDURANCE

Enhanced muscular strength and endurance can lead to improvements in the areas of performance, injury prevention, body composition, self-image, lifetime muscle and bone health, and chronic disease prevention.

Improved Performance of Physical Activities

A person with a moderate-to-high level of muscular strength and endurance can perform everyday tasks— such as climbing stairs and carrying groceries—with ease. Increased strength can enhance your enjoyment of recreational sports by making it possible to achieve high levels of performance and to handle advanced techniques. Strength training also results in modest improvements in maximal oxygen consumption. People with poor muscle strength tire more easily and are less effective in both everyday and recreational activities.

Injury Prevention

Increased muscular strength and endurance help protect you from injury in two key ways:

- By enabling you to maintain good posture
- By encouraging proper body mechanics during everyday activities such as walking and lifting

TERMS WEB

muscle fiber   A single muscle cell, usually classified according to strength, speed of contraction, and energy source.

myofibrils   Protein structures that make up muscle fibers.

hypertrophy   An increase in the size of muscle fibers, usually stimulated by muscular overload, as occurs during strength training.

atrophy   A decrease in the size of muscle fibers.

hyperplasia   An increase in the number of muscle fibers.

slow-twitch fibers   Red muscle fibers that are fatigue-resistant but have a slow contraction speed and a lower capacity for tension; usually recruited for endurance activities.

fast-twitch fibers   White muscle fibers that contract rapidly and forcefully but fatigue quickly; usually recruited for actions requiring strength and power.

power   The ability to exert force rapidly.

motor unit   A motor nerve (one that initiates movement) connected to one or more muscle fibers.

muscle learning   The improvement in the body's ability to recruit motor units, brought about through strength training.

Table 4.1	Physiological Changes and Benefits from Strength Training
Change	**Benefits**
Increased muscle mass*	Increased muscular strength
	Improved body composition
	Higher rate of metabolism
	Toned, healthy-looking muscles
Increased utilization of motor units during muscle contractions	Increased muscular strength and power
Improved coordination of motor units	Increased muscular strength and power
Increased strength of tendons, ligaments, and bones	Lower risk of injury to these tissues
Increased storage of fuel in muscles	Increased resistance to muscle fatigue
Increased size of fast-twitch muscle fibers (from a high-resistance program)	Increased muscular strength and power
Increased size of slow-twitch muscle fibers (from a high-repetition program)	Increased muscular endurance
Increased blood supply to muscles (from a high-repetition program)	Increased delivery of oxygen and nutrients
	Increased elimination of wastes
Biochemical improvements (for example, increased sensitivity to insulin)	Enhanced metabolic health
Improved blood fat levels	Reduced risk of heart disease

*Due to genetic and hormonal differences, men will build more muscle mass than women, but both genders make about the same percent gains in strength through a good program.

Good muscle strength and, particularly, endurance in the abdomen, hips, lower back, and legs support the back in proper alignment and help prevent low-back pain, which afflicts more than 85% of Americans at some time in their lives. (Prevention of low-back pain is discussed in Chapter 5.)

Training for muscular strength and endurance also makes the **tendons**, **ligaments**, and cartilage cells stronger and less susceptible to injury. Resistance exercise prevents injuries best when the strength training program is gradual and progressive and builds all the major muscle groups.

Improved Body Composition

As Chapter 2 explained, healthy body composition means that the body has a high proportion of fat-free mass (primarily composed of muscle) and a relatively small proportion of fat. Strength training improves body composition by increasing muscle mass, thereby tipping the body composition ratio toward fat-free mass and away from fat.

Building muscle mass through strength training also helps with losing fat because metabolic rate is related to muscle mass: the more muscle mass, the higher the metabolic rate. A high metabolic rate means that a nutritionally sound diet coupled with regular exercise will not lead to an increase in body fat. Strength training can boost resting metabolic rate by 0–15%, depending on how hard you train. Resistance exercise also increases muscle temperature, which in turn slightly increases the rate at which you burn calories over the hours following a weight training session.

Enhanced Self-Image and Quality of Life

Strength training leads to an enhanced self-image in both men and women by providing stronger, firmer-looking muscles and a toned, healthy-looking body. Women tend to lose inches, increase strength, and develop greater muscle definition. Men tend to build larger, stronger muscles. The larger muscles in men combine with high levels of the hormone **testosterone** for a strong tissue-building effect; see the box "Gender Differences in Muscular Strength."

Because strength training involves measurable objectives (pounds lifted, repetitions accomplished), a person can easily recognize improved performance, leading to greater self-confidence and self-esteem. Strength training also improves quality of life by increasing energy, preventing injuries, and making daily activities easier and more enjoyable.

Improved Muscle and Bone Health with Aging

Research has shown that good muscular strength helps people live healthier lives. A lifelong program of regular strength training prevents muscle and nerve degeneration that can compromise the quality of life and increase the risk of hip fractures and other potentially life-threatening injuries.

In the general population, people begin to lose muscle mass after age 30, a condition called *sarcopenia*. At first they may notice that they cannot play sports as well as they could in high school. After more years of inactivity and strength loss, people may have trouble performing even the simple movements of daily life, such as walking up a flight of stairs or doing yard work. By age 75, about 25% of men and 75% of women cannot lift more than 10 pounds overhead. Although aging contributes to decreased strength, inactivity causes most of the loss. Poor strength makes it much more likely that a person will be injured during everyday activities.

DIMENSIONS OF DIVERSITY

Gender Differences in Muscular Strength

Men are generally stronger than women because they typically have larger bodies and a larger proportion of their total body mass is made up of muscle. But when strength is expressed per unit of cross-sectional area of muscle tissue, men are only 1–2% stronger than women in the upper body and about equal to women in the lower body. (Men have a larger proportion of muscle tissue in the upper body, so it's easier for them to build upper-body strength than it is for women.) Individual muscle fibers are larger in men, but the metabolism of cells within those fibers is the same in both sexes.

Two factors that help explain these disparities are testosterone levels and the speed of nervous control of muscle. Testosterone is responsible for the development of secondary sex characteristics in males (facial hair, deep voice, etc.). Testosterone also promotes the growth of muscle tissue in both males and females. Testosterone levels are about 5–10 times higher in men than in women, so men tend to have larger

muscles. Also, because the male nervous system can activate muscles faster, men tend to have more power.

Some women are concerned that they will develop large muscles from strength training. Because of hormonal differences, most women do not develop big muscles unless they train intensely over many years or take anabolic steroids. Women do gain muscle and improve body composition through strength training, but they don't develop bulky muscles or gain significant amounts of weight: A study of average women who weight trained 2–3 days per week for 8 weeks found that the women gained about 1.75 pounds of muscle and lost about 3.5 pounds of fat.

Losing muscle over time is a much greater health concern for women than small gains in muscle weight, especially because any gains in muscle weight are typically more than balanced by loss of fat weight. Both men and women lose muscle mass and power as they age, but because men start out with more muscle and don't lose power as quickly, older

women tend to have greater impairment of muscle function than older men. This may partially account for the higher incidence of life-threatening falls in older women.

The bottom line is that both men and women can increase strength through strength training. Women may not be able to lift as much weight as men, but pound for pound of muscle, they have nearly the same capacity to gain strength as men. Strength training is particularly beneficial for women because it helps prevent bone and muscle loss with aging and maintains fat-free weight during weight control programs.

SOURCES: Fahey, T. D. 2006. *Weight Training for Men and Women,* 6th ed. New York: McGraw-Hill. IDEA. 2006. *Fitness Tip—Why Women Need Weight Training* (http://www.ideafit.com/articles/women_training.asp; retrieved November 19, 2007). Krivickas, L. S., et al. 2001. Age and gender-related differences in maximum shortening velocity of skeletal muscle fibers. *American Journal of Physical Medicine and Rehabilitation* 80: 447–455.

As a person ages, motor nerves can become disconnected from the portion of muscle they control. By age 70, 15% of the motor nerves in most people are no longer connected to muscle tissue. Aging and inactivity also cause muscles to become slower and therefore less able to perform quick, powerful movements. Strength training helps maintain motor nerve connections and the quickness of muscles.

Osteoporosis (bone loss) is common in people over age 55, particularly postmenopausal women. Osteoporosis leads to fractures that can be life-threatening. Hormonal changes from aging account for much of the bone loss that occurs, but lack of bone mass due to inactivity and a poor diet are contributing factors. Strength training can lessen bone loss even if it is taken up later in life, and if practiced regularly, strength training may even build bone mass in postmenopausal women and older men. Increased muscle strength can also help prevent falls, which are a major cause of injury in people with osteoporosis. (Additional strategies for preventing osteoporosis are described in Chapter 8.)

MOTIVATION BOOSTER

Inspire yourself. Make a list of five benefits of muscular strength and endurance that are particularly meaningful to you—reducing your risk of back pain, for example, or improving your tennis game. Post the list in a prominent location and use it as a motivational tool for beginning and maintaining your strength training program.

TERMS

tendon   A tough band of fibrous tissue that connects a muscle to a bone or other body part and transmits the force exerted by the muscle.

ligament   A tough band of tissue that connects the ends of bones to other bones or supports organs in place.

testosterone   The principal male hormone, responsible for the development of secondary sex characteristics and important in increasing muscle size.

QUESTIONS FOR CRITICAL THINKING AND REFLECTION

What benefits of strength training are most important to you? Are you more interested in improved physical performance? Better body composition and appearance? Long-term health benefits? How can you define your goals so they are most meaningful and motivating for you?

Prevention of Chronic Disease

Strength training helps prevent and manage both CVD and diabetes by:

- Improving glucose metabolism.
- Increasing maximal oxygen consumption.
- Reducing blood pressure.
- Increasing HDL cholesterol and reducing LDL cholesterol (in some people).

Stronger muscles reduce the demand on the heart during ordinary daily activities such as lifting and carrying objects. The benefits of resistive exercise to the heart are so great that the American Heart Association recommends that healthy adults and many low-risk cardiac patients do strength training 2–3 days per week. Resistance training is not appropriate for people with some types of heart disease.

ASSESSING MUSCULAR STRENGTH AND ENDURANCE

Muscular strength is usually assessed by measuring the maximum amount of weight a person can lift one time. This single maximum effort is called a **repetition maximum (RM).** You can assess the strength of your major muscle groups by taking the one–repetition maximum (1 RM) test for the bench press and by taking functional leg strength tests. You can measure 1 RM directly or estimate it by doing multiple repetitions with a sub-maximal (lighter) weight. It is best to train for at least several weeks before attempting a direct 1 RM test; once you have a baseline value, you can retest after 6–12 weeks to check your progress. Refer to Lab 4.1 for guidelines on taking these tests. For more accurate results, avoid any strenuous weight training for 48 hours beforehand.

Muscular endurance is usually assessed by counting the maximum number of **repetitions** of a muscular contraction a person can do (such as in push-ups) or the maximum amount of time a person can hold a muscular contraction (such as in the flexed-arm hang). You can test the muscular endurance of major muscle groups in your body by taking the curl-up test, the push-up test, and the squat endurance test. Refer to Lab 4.2 for complete instructions on taking these assessment tests.

CREATING A SUCCESSFUL STRENGTH TRAINING PROGRAM

Strength training develops muscular strength and endurance in the same way that endurance exercise develops cardiovascular fitness: When the muscles are stressed by a greater load than they are used to, they adapt and improve their function. The type of adaptation that occurs depends on the type of stress applied. To get the most out of your strength training program, design it to achieve maximum fitness benefits with minimum risk of injury. Before you begin, seriously consider the type and amount of training that's right for you.

Static Versus Dynamic Strength Training Exercises

Strength training exercises are generally classified as static or dynamic. Each involves a different way of using and strengthening muscles.

Static Exercise   Also called **isometric** exercise, **static exercise** involves a muscle contraction without a change in the length of the muscle or the angle in the joint on which the muscle acts. In isometrics, the muscle contracts, but there is no movement. To perform an isometric exercise, a person can use an immovable object like a wall to provide resistance, or simply tighten a muscle while remaining still (for example, tightening the abdominal muscles while sitting at a desk). The spine extension and the side bridge, shown on p. 114–115, are both isometric exercises.

Static exercises are not as widely used as dynamic exercises because they don't develop strength throughout a joint's entire range of motion. However, static exercises are useful in strengthening muscles after an injury or surgery, when movement of the affected joint could delay healing. Isometrics are also used to overcome weak points in an individual's range of motion. Statically strengthening a muscle at its weakest point will allow more weight to be lifted with that muscle during dynamic exercise. Certain types of calisthenics and Pilates exercises (described in more detail later in the chapter) also involve static contractions. For maximum strength gains, hold the isometric contraction maximally for 6 seconds; do 5–10 repetitions.

Dynamic Exercise   Also called **isotonic** exercise, **dynamic exercise** involves a muscle contraction with a change in the length of the muscle. (*Isotonic* means "same tension," which does not accurately describe the way muscles contract, but the term is widely used to describe

A concentric contraction.   An eccentric contraction.

dynamic exercises.) Dynamic exercises are the most popular type of exercises for increasing muscle strength and seem to be most valuable for developing strength that can be transferred to other forms of physical activity. They can be performed with weight machines, free weights, or a person's own body weight (as in curl-ups or push-ups).

There are two kinds of dynamic muscle contractions:

• A **concentric muscle contraction** occurs when the muscle applies enough force to overcome resistance and shortens as it contracts.

• An **eccentric muscle contraction** (also called a *pliometric contraction*) occurs when the resistance is greater than the force applied by the muscle and the muscle lengthens as it contracts.

For example, in an arm curl, the biceps muscle works concentrically as the weight is raised toward the shoulder and eccentrically as the weight is lowered.

CONSTANT AND VARIABLE RESISTANCE Two of the most common dynamic exercise techniques are constant resistance exercise and variable resistance exercise.

• **Constant resistance exercise** uses a constant load (weight) throughout a joint's entire range of motion. Training with free weights is a form of constant resistance exercise. A problem with this technique is that, because of differences in leverage, there are points in a joint's range of motion where the muscle controlling the movement is stronger and points where it is weaker. The amount of weight a person can lift is limited by the weakest point in the range.

• In **variable resistance exercise**, the load is changed to provide maximum load throughout the entire range of motion. This form of exercise uses machines that place more stress on muscles at the end of the range of motion, where a person has better leverage and can exert more force. The Nautilus pull-over machine is an example of a variable resistance exercise machine.

Constant and variable resistance exercises are both extremely effective for building strength and endurance.

OTHER DYNAMIC EXERCISE TECHNIQUES Athletes use four other kinds of isotonic techniques, primarily for training and rehabilitation.

• **Eccentric (pliometric) loading** involves placing a load on a muscle as it lengthens. The muscle contracts eccentrically in order to control the weight. Eccentric loading is practiced during most types of resistance training. For example, you are performing an eccentric movement as you lower the weight to your chest during a bench press in preparation for the active movement. You can also perform exercises designed specifically to overload muscle eccentrically, a technique called *negatives*.

• **Plyometrics** is the sudden eccentric loading and stretching of muscles followed by a forceful concentric contraction. An example would be the action of the lower-body muscles when jumping from a bench to the ground and then jumping back onto the bench. This type of exercise is used to develop explosive strength; it also helps build and maintain bone density.

• **Speed loading** involves moving a weight as rapidly as possible in an attempt to approach the speeds used in movements like throwing a softball or sprinting. In the bench press, for example, speed loading might involve

repetition maximum (RM) The maximum amount of resistance that can be moved a specified number of times.

repetitions The number of times an exercise is performed during one set.

static (isometric) exercise Exercise involving a muscle contraction without a change in the length of the muscle.

dynamic (isotonic) exercise Exercise involving a muscle contraction with a change in the length of the muscle.

concentric muscle contraction A dynamic contraction in which the muscle gets shorter as it contracts.

eccentric muscle contraction A dynamic contraction in which the muscle lengthens as it contracts; also called a *pliometric contraction*.

constant resistance exercise A type of dynamic exercise that uses a constant load throughout a joint's entire range of motion.

variable resistance exercise A type of dynamic exercise that uses a changing load, providing a maximum load throughout the joint's entire range of motion.

eccentric (pliometric) loading Loading the muscle while it is lengthening; sometimes called *negatives*.

plyometrics Rapid stretching of a muscle group that is undergoing eccentric stress (the muscle is exerting force while it lengthens), followed by a rapid concentric contraction.

speed loading Moving a load as rapidly as possible.

TERMS WEB

Exercise Machines Versus Free Weights

Exercise Machines		Free Weights	
Advantages	**Disadvantages**	**Advantages**	**Disadvantages**
• Are safe and convenient	• Have limited availability	• Allow dynamic movements	• Are not as safe
• Don't require spotters	• Are inappropriate for performing dynamic movements	• Allow user to develop control of weights	• Require spotters
• Don't require lifter to balance bar	• Allow limited number of exercises	• Allow greater variety of exercises	• Require more skill
• Provide variable resistance	• Train muscles rather than movements	• Are widely available, inexpensive, and convenient for home use	• Cause more blisters and calluses
• Require less skill	• Place minimal stress on core stabilizing muscles (those in torso)	• Train core stabilizing muscles	
• Make it easy to move from one exercise to next		• Are better for building power	
• Allow easy isolation of muscles and muscle groups		• Are truer to real-life situations—strength transfers to daily activities	
• Support back (on many machines)			

doing 5 repetitions as fast as possible using a weight that is half the maximum load you can lift. You can gauge your progress by timing how fast you can perform the repetitions. Speed loading is not recommended for most people because of the risk of injury.

• **Isokinetic** exercise involves exerting force at a constant speed against an equal force exerted by a special strength training machine. The isokinetic machine provides variable resistance at different points in the joint's range of motion, matching the effort applied by the individual while keeping the speed of the movement constant. Isokinetic exercises are excellent for building strength and endurance, but the equipment is expensive and less commonly available than other kinds of weight machines.

Comparing Static and Dynamic Exercise Static exercises require no equipment, so they can be done virtually anywhere. They build strength rapidly and are useful for rehabilitating injured joints. On the other hand, they have to be performed at several different angles for each joint to improve strength throughout the joint's entire range of motion. Dynamic exercises can be performed without equipment (calisthenics) or with equipment (weight training). They are excellent for building strength and endurance,

and they tend to build strength through a joint's full range of motion. Most people develop muscular strength and endurance using dynamic exercises. Ultimately, the type of exercise a person chooses depends on individual goals, preferences, and access to equipment.

Weight Machines Versus Free Weights

Your muscles will get stronger if you make them work against a resistance. Resistance can be provided by free weights, by your own body weight, or by sophisticated exercise machines. Weight machines are preferred by many people because they are safe, convenient, and easy to use. You just set the resistance (usually by placing a pin in the weight stack), sit down at the machine, and start working. Machines make it easy to isolate and work specific muscles. You don't need a **spotter**—someone who stands by to assist when free weights are used—and you don't have to worry about dropping a weight on yourself.

Free weights require more care, balance, and coordination to use, but they strengthen your body in ways that are more adaptable to real life. They are also more popular with athletes for developing explosive strength for sports. Unless you are training seriously for a sport that requires a great deal of strength, training on machines is probably safer, more convenient, and just as effective as training with free weights. However, you can increase strength with either weight machines or free weights. Information listed in the box "Exercise Machines Versus Free Weights" can help you make a decision about which equipment you may prefer.

TERMS

isokinetic The application of force at a constant speed against an equal force.

spotter A person who assists with a weight training exercise done with free weights.

Remember, you don't need a fitness center or expensive equipment to strength train. If you prefer to train at home or like low-cost alternatives, consider the following.

Resistance Bands   Resistance or exercise bands are elastic strips or tubes of rubber material that are inexpensive, lightweight, and portable. They are available in a variety of styles and levels of resistance; some are sold with instructional guides or DVDs, and classes may be offered at fitness centers. Many free weight exercises can be adapted for resistance bands. For example, you can do biceps curls by standing on the center of the band and holding one end of the band in each hand; resistance is provided when you stretch the band to perform the curl.

Special guidelines for using resistance bands safely include examining them regularly for flaws and tears and taking care to avoid snapping the bands. Keeping a firm grip on the bands may require wrapping or looping the band; some people find bands with preformed handles easier to grasp.

Exercise (Stability) Balls   The exercise or stability ball is an extra-large inflatable ball. It was originally developed for use in physical therapy but has become a popular piece of exercise equipment for use in the home or gym. It can be used to work the entire body, but it is particularly effective for working the so-called stability muscles ("the core") in the abdomen, chest, and back—muscles that are important for preventing back problems. The ball's instability forces the exerciser to use the stability muscles to balance the body—even when a person simply sits on the ball. Moves such as crunches have been found to be more effective when they are performed with an exercise ball.

When choosing a ball, make sure that your thighs are parallel to the ground when you sit on it; if you are a beginner or have back problems, choose a larger ball so that your thighs are at an angle, with hips higher than knees. Beginners should use caution until they feel comfortable with the movements and take care to avoid poor form due to fatigue.

Although stability ball exercises are generally safe, poor technique can cause falls. It is a good idea to take a class or get help from a trainer to learn proper technique and create an effective stability program.

Pilates   Pilates (*pil LAH teez*) was developed by German gymnast and boxer Joseph Pilates early in the twentieth century. It often involves the use of specially designed resistance training devices, although some classes feature just mat or floor work. Pilates focuses on strengthening and stretching the core muscles in the back, abdomen, and buttocks to create a solid base of

Resistance for strength training can be provided by many different techniques and types of equipment. Shown here are resistance bands (top), a stability ball (center), and a Pilates mat exercise that uses body weight for resistance.

support for whole-body movement; the emphasis is on concentration, control, movement flow, and breathing. Mat exercises can be done at home, but because there are hundreds of Pilates exercises, some of them strenuous, it is best to begin with some qualified instruction. The Pilates Method Alliance (www.pilatesmethodalliance. com) offers advice on finding a qualified teacher.

No-Equipment Calisthenics   You can use your own body weight as resistance for strength training. Exercises such as curl-ups, push-ups, squats, step-ups, heel raises, chair dips, and lunges can be done anywhere.

Video clips showing exercises with resistance bands, stability balls, and no equipment can be found on the Online Learning Center.

Applying the FITT Principle: Selecting Exercises and Putting Together a Program

A complete weight training program works all the major muscle groups. It usually takes about 8–10 different exercises to get a complete full-body workout. Use the FITT principle—frequency, intensity, time, and type—to set the parameters of your program.

Frequency of Exercise   For general fitness, the American College of Sports Medicine (ACSM) recommends a frequency of at least two days per week for weight training. Allow your muscles at least 1 day of rest between workouts; if you train too often, your muscles won't be able to work with enough intensity to improve their fitness, and soreness and injury are more likely to result. If you enjoy weight training and want to train more often, try working different muscle groups on alternate days—a training plan called a *split routine*. For example, work your arms and upper body one day, work your lower body the next day, and then return to upper-body exercises on the third day.

Intensity of Exercise: Amount of Resistance   The amount of weight (resistance) you lift in weight training exercises is equivalent to intensity in cardiorespiratory endurance training. It determines how your body will adapt to weight training and how quickly these adaptations will occur.

Choose weights based on your current level of muscular fitness and your fitness goals. Choose a weight heavy enough to fatigue your muscles but light enough for you to complete the repetitions with good form. To build strength rapidly, you should lift weights as heavy as 80% of your maximum capacity (1 RM). If you're more interested in building endurance, choose a lighter weight (perhaps 40–60% of 1 RM) and do more repetitions.

For example, if your maximum capacity for the leg press is 160 pounds, you might lift 130 pounds to build

strength and 80 pounds to build endurance. For a general fitness program to develop both strength and endurance, choose a weight in the middle of this range, perhaps 70% of 1 RM. Or you can create a program that includes both higher-intensity exercise (80% of 1 RM for 8–10 repetitions) and lower-intensity exercise (60% of 1 RM for 15–20 repetitions); this routine will develop both fast-twitch and slow-twitch muscle fibers.

As noted previously, women do not have to worry about developing bulky muscles from weight training. Increases in muscle size are determined largely by testosterone levels, and college-age women have only about one-fifth the testosterone of college-age men.

Because it can be tedious and time-consuming to continually reassess your maximum capacity for each exercise, you might find it easier to choose a weight based on the number of repetitions of an exercise you can perform with a given resistance.

Time of Exercise: Repetitions and Sets   To improve fitness, you must do enough repetitions of each exercise to fatigue your muscles. The number of repetitions needed to cause fatigue depends on the amount of resistance: the heavier the weight, the fewer repetitions to reach fatigue. In general, a heavy weight and a low number of repetitions (1–5) build strength and overload primarily fast-twitch fibers, whereas a light weight and a high number of repetitions (15–20) build endurance and overload primarily slow-twitch fibers (Figure 4.3).

For a general fitness program to build both strength and endurance, try to do about 8–12 repetitions of each exercise; a few exercises, such as abdominal crunches and calf raises, may require more. To avoid injury, older (approximately age 50–60 and above) and frailer people

FIGURE 4.3   Training for strength versus training for endurance.

should perform more repetitions (10–15) using a lighter weight.

In weight training, a **set** refers to a group of repetitions of an exercise followed by a rest period. To develop strength and endurance for general fitness, you can make gains doing a single set of each exercise, provided you use enough resistance to fatigue your muscles. (You should just barely be able to complete the 8–12 repetitions—using good form—for each exercise.) Doing more than 1 set of each exercise will increase strength development, and most serious weight trainers do at least 3 sets of each exercise (see the section "More Advanced Strength Training Programs" for guidelines on more advanced programs).

If you perform more than 1 set of an exercise, you need to rest long enough between sets to allow your muscles to work with enough intensity to increase fitness. The length of the rest interval depends on the amount of resistance. In a program to develop a combination of strength and endurance for wellness, a rest period of 1–3 minutes between sets is appropriate; if you are lifting heavier loads to build maximum strength, rest 3–5 minutes between sets. You can save time in your workouts if you alternate sets of different exercises. Each muscle group can rest between sets while you work on other muscles.

Overtraining—doing more exercise than your body can recover from—can occur in response to heavy resistance training. Possible signs of overtraining include lack of progress or decreased performance, chronic fatigue, decreased coordination, and chronic muscle soreness. The best remedy for overtraining is rest; add more days of recovery between workouts. With extra rest, chances are you'll be refreshed and ready to train again. Adding variety to your program, as discussed later in the chapter, can also help you avoid overtraining with resistance exercise.

Type or Mode of Exercise   For overall fitness, you need to include exercises for your neck, upper back, shoulders, arms, chest, abdomen, lower back, thighs, buttocks, and calves—about 8–10 exercises in all. If you are also training for a particular sport, include exercises to strengthen the muscles important for optimal performance *and* the muscles most likely to be injured. A weight training program for general fitness is presented later in this chapter, on pp. 111–119.

It is important to balance exercises between **agonist** and **antagonist** muscle groups. (When a muscle contracts, it is known as the agonist; the opposing muscle, which must relax and stretch to allow contraction by the agonist, is known as the antagonist.) Whenever you do an exercise that moves a joint in one direction, also select an exercise that works the joint in the opposite direction. For example, if you do knee extensions to develop the muscles on the front of your thighs, also do leg curls to develop the antagonistic muscles on the back of your thighs.

The order of exercises can also be important. Do exercises for large-muscle groups or for more than one joint before you do exercises that use small-muscle groups or single joints. This allows for more effective overload of the larger, more powerful muscle groups. Small-muscle groups fatigue more easily than larger ones, and small-muscle fatigue limits your capacity to overload large-muscle groups. For example, lateral raises, which work the shoulder muscles, should be performed after bench presses, which work the chest and arms in addition to the shoulders. If you fatigue your shoulder muscles by doing lateral raises first, you won't be able to lift as much weight and effectively fatigue all the key muscle groups used during the bench press.

Also, order exercises so that you work agonist and antagonist muscle groups in sequence, one after the other. For example, follow biceps curls, which work the biceps, with triceps extensions, which exercise the triceps—the antagonist muscle to the biceps.

The Warm-Up and Cool-Down

As with cardiorespiratory endurance exercise, you should warm up before every weight training session and cool down afterward (Figure 4.4). You should do both a general warm-up—several minutes of walking or easy jogging—and a warm-up for the weight training exercises you plan to perform. For example, if you plan to do 1 or more sets of 10 repetitions of bench presses with 125 pounds, you might do 1 set of 10 repetitions with 50 pounds as a warm-up. Do similar warm-up exercises for each exercise in your program.

? **QUESTIONS FOR CRITICAL THINKING AND REFLECTION**
Considering your lifestyle and the physical activities you most commonly do, which is more important to you—muscular strength or muscular endurance? Do you think this will always be the case, or do you think your patterns of activity, exercise, recreation, and sport might change in the future? For example, are there recreational activities you would like to try out at some point in your life, such as kayaking or rock climbing?

set   A group of repetitions followed by a rest period.

agonist   A muscle in a state of contraction, opposed by the action of another muscle, its *antagonist*.

antagonist   A muscle that opposes the action of another muscle, its *agonist*.

Warm-up 5–10 minutes	Strength training exercises for major muscle groups (8–10 exercises)		Cool-down 5–10 minutes
	Sample program		
	Exercise	*Muscle group developed*	
	Bench press	Chest, shoulders, triceps	
	Pull-ups	Lats, biceps	
	Shoulder press	Shoulders, trapezius, triceps	
	Upright rowing	Deltoids, trapezius	
	Biceps curls	Biceps	
	Lateral raises	Shoulders	
	Squats	Gluteals, quadriceps	
	Heel raises	Calves	
	Abdominal curls	Abdominals	
	Spine extensions	Low- and mid-back spine extensors	
Start	Side bridges	Obliques, quadratus lumborum	**Stop**

Frequency: At least 2 days per week

Intensity/Resistance: Weights heavy enough to cause muscle fatigue when exercises are performed with good form for the selected number of repetitions

Time: Repetitions: 8–12 of each exercise (10–15 with a lower weight for people over age 50–60); **Sets:** 1 (doing more than 1 set per exercise may result in faster and greater strength gains); rest 1–2 minutes between exercises.

Type of activity: 8–10 strength training exercises that focus on major muscle groups

FIGURE 4.4   The FITT principle for a strength training workout.

To cool down after weight training, relax for 5–10 minutes after your workout. Although this is controversial, a few studies have suggested that including a period of postexercise stretching may help prevent muscle soreness; warmed-up muscles and joints make this a particularly good time to work on flexibility.

Getting Started and Making Progress

The first few sessions of weight training should be devoted to learning the exercises. You need to learn the movements, and your nervous system needs to practice communicating with your muscles so you can develop strength effectively. To start, choose a weight that you can move easily through 8–12 repetitions, do only 1 set of each exercise, and rest 1–2 minutes between exercises. Gradually add weight and (if you want) sets to your program over the first few weeks until you are doing 1–3 sets of 8–12 repetitions of each exercise.

Knowing how much resistance to add and when to add it is as much an art as a science. As you progress, add weight according to the "two-for-two" rule: When you can perform two additional repetitions with a given weight on two consecutive training sessions, increase the load. For example, if your target is to perform 8–10 repetitions per exercise, and you performed 12 repetitions in your previous two workouts, it would be appropriate to increase your load. If adding weight means you can do only 7 or 8 repetitions, stay with that weight until you can again complete 12 repetitions per set. If you can do only 4–6 repetitions after adding weight, or if you can't maintain good form, you've added too much and should take some off.

You can add more resistance in large-muscle exercises, such as squats and bench presses, than you can in small-muscle exercises, such as curls. For example, when you can complete 12 repetitions of squats with good form, you may be able to add 10–20 pounds of additional resistance; for curls, on the other hand, you might add only 3–5 pounds. As a general guideline, try increases of approximately 5%, which is half a pound of additional weight for each 10 pounds you are currently lifting.

You can expect to improve rapidly during the first 6–10 weeks of training: a 10–30% increase in the amount of weight lifted. Gains will then come more slowly. Your rate of improvement will depend on how hard you work and how your body responds to resistance training. There will be individual differences in the rate of improvement. Factors such as age, gender, motivation, and heredity will affect your progress.

After you achieve the level of strength and muscularity you want, you can maintain your gains by training 2–3 days per week. You can monitor the progress of your program by recording the amount of resistance and the number of repetitions and sets you perform on a workout card like the one shown in Figure 4.5.

More Advanced Strength Training Programs

The weight training program just described is sufficient to develop and maintain muscular strength and endurance for general fitness. If you have a different goal, you may need to adjust your program accordingly. As mentioned previously, performing more sets and fewer repetitions with a heavier load will cause greater increases in strength. A program designed to build strength might include 3–5 sets of 4–6 repetitions each; the load used should be heavy enough to cause fatigue with the smaller number of repetitions. Rest long enough after a set (3–5 minutes) to allow your muscles to recover and to work intensely during the next set.

Experienced weight trainers often engage in some form of cycle training, also called *periodization,* in which the exercises, number of sets and repetitions, and intensity

WORKOUT CARD FOR   Sara Lopez

Exercise/Date		9/14	9/16	9/18	9/21	9/23	9/25	9/28	9/30	10/2	10/5	10/7	10/9	10/12	10/14	10/16					
Bench press	Wt.	45	45	45	50	50	50	60	60	60	60	65	65	70	70	70					
	Sets	1	1	1	1	1	1	1	1	1	1	1	1	1	1	1					
	Reps.	10	12	12	10	12	12	10	9	12	12	12	12	9	9	10					
Pull-ups (assisted)	Wt.	–	–	–	–	–	–	–	–	–	–	–	–	–	–	–					
	Sets	1	1	1	1	1	1	1	1	1	1	1	1	1	1	1					
	Reps.	5	5	5	6	6	6	7	7	7	8	8	8	9	9	10					
Shoulder press	Wt.	20	20	20	25	25	25	30	30	30	30	30	30	35	35	35					
	Sets	1	1	1	1	1	1	1	1	1	1	1	1	1	1	1					
	Reps.	10	12	12	10	12	12	8	10	9	10	12	12	10	10	10					
Upright rowing	Wt.	5	5	10	10	10	10	12	12	12	12	15	15	15	15	15					
	Sets	1	1	1	1	1	1	1	1	1	1	1	1	1	1	1					
	Reps.	12	12	8	10	11	12	9	10	12	12	8	8	8	9	10					
Biceps curls	Wt.	15	15	15	20	20	20	25	25	25	25	25	25	30	30	30					
	Sets	1	1	1	1	1	1	1	1	1	1	1	1	1	1	1					
	Reps.	10	10	10	10	12	12	8	10	10	10	12	12	9	10	12					
Lateral raise	Wt.	5	5	5	5	5	5	7.5	7.5	7.5	7.5	7.5	7.5	10	10	10					
	Sets	1	1	1	1	1	1	1	1	1	1	1	1	1	1	1					
	Reps.	8	8	10	10	12	12	8	10	10	10	12	12	8	8	9					
Squats	Wt.	–	–	–	45	45	45	55	55	55	65	65	65	75	75	75					
	Sets	1	1	1	1	1	1	1	1	1	1	1	1	1	1	1					
	Reps.	10	12	15	8	12	12	8	12	12	10	13	12	8	10	10					
Heel raises	Wt.	–	–	–	45	45	45	55	55	55	65	65	65	75	75	75					
	Sets	1	1	1	1	1	1	1	1	1	1	1	1	1	1	1					
	Reps.	15	15	15	8	12	12	10	12	12	10	12	12	10	9	12					
Abdominal curls	Wt.	–	–	–	–	–	–	–	–	–	–	–	–	–	–	–					
	Sets	1	1	1	1	1	1	1	1	1	1	1	1	1	1	1					
	Reps.	20	20	20	20	20	20	25	25	25	25	25	25	25	25	25					
Spine extensions	Wt.	–	–	–	–	–	–	–	–	–	–	–	–	–	–	–					
	Sets	1	1	1	1	1	1	1	1	1	1	1	1	1	1	1					
	Reps.	5	5	5	8	8	8	10	10	10	10	10	10	11	12	12					
Side bridge	Wt.	–	–	–	–	–	–	–	–	–	–	–	–	–	–	–					
	Sets	1	1	1	1	1	1	1	1	1	1	1	1	1	1	1					
	Seconds	60	60	60	65	65	70	70	70	70	76	75	80	80	80	80					

FIGURE 4.5   A sample workout card for a general fitness strength training program.

are varied within a workout and/or between workouts. For example, you might do a particular exercise more intensely during some sets or on some days than others; you might also vary the exercises you perform for particular muscle groups. Several sample cycle training programs are described in a Student Handout on the *Fit and Well* Online Learning Center. For more detailed information on these more advanced training techniques, consult a strength coach certified by the National Strength and Conditioning Association or another reliable source. If you decide to adopt a more advanced training regimen, start off slowly to give your body a chance to adjust and to minimize the risk of injury.

Weight Training Safety

Injuries happen in weight training. Maximum physical effort, elaborate machinery, rapid movements, and heavy weights can combine to make the weight room a dangerous place if proper precautions aren't taken. To help ensure that your workouts are safe and productive, follow the guidelines in the box "Safe Weight Training" and the following suggestions.

Use Proper Lifting Technique   Every exercise has a proper technique that is important for obtaining maximum benefits and preventing injury. Your instructor or weight room attendant can help explain the specific techniques for different exercises and weight machines.

Perform exercises smoothly and with good form. The ACSM suggests a moderate rate for each repetition—a 3-second concentric contraction and a 3-second eccentric contraction. Lift or push the weight forcefully during the active phase of the lift and then lower it slowly with control. Perform all lifts through the full range of motion.

Use Spotters and Collars with Free Weights   Spotters are necessary when an exercise has potential for danger; a weight that is out of control or falls can cause a serious injury. A spotter can assist you if you cannot complete a lift or if the weight tilts. A spotter can also help you move a weight into position before a lift and provide help or additional resistance during a lift. Spotting requires practice and coordination between the lifter and the spotter(s).

Collars are devices that secure weights to a barbell or dumbbell. Although people lift weights without collars,

Safe Weight Training

General Guidelines

• When beginning a program or trying new exercises or equipment, ask an instructor to show you how to do exercises safely and correctly.

• Lift weights from a stabilized body position; keep weights as close to your body as possible.

• Protect your back by maintaining control of your spine and avoiding dangerous positions. Don't twist your body while lifting.

• Observe proper lifting techniques and good form at all times. If you have to alter your technique to complete a repetition, you are probably lifting too much weight. Don't lift beyond the limits of your strength.

• Don't hold your breath while doing weight training exercises. Holding your breath, called the Valsalva maneuver, causes a decrease in blood returning to the heart and can make you become dizzy and faint. It can also increase blood pressure to dangerous levels. Exhale when exerting the greatest force, and inhale when moving the weight into position for the active phase of the lift. Breathe smoothly and steadily.

• Be aware of what's going on around you. Stay away from other people when they're doing exercises, and don't get distracted. If you bump into someone, you could cause an injury.

• Don't use defective equipment. Be aware of broken collars or bolts, frayed cables, broken chains, or loose cushions. Report equipment damage or malfunctions immediately.

• Don't chew gum when exercising; you could choke on the gum or bite your tongue.

• Don't exercise if you're ill, injured, or overtrained. Do not try to work through the pain.

• When returning to training after an illness or layoff, start with lighter weights than you were using before the break in training.

Free Weights

• Make sure the bar is loaded evenly on both sides and that weights are secured with collars.

• When you pick a weight up from the ground, keep your back straight and your head level. Don't bend at the waist with straight legs.

• Lift weights smoothly and slowly; don't jerk them. Control the weight through the entire range of motion. Lifting a weight too fast can increase the force output to dangerous levels.

• Do most of your lifting with your legs. Keep your hips and buttocks back. When doing standing lifts, maintain a good posture so that you protect your back. Bend at the hips, not with the spine. Feet should be shoulder-width apart, heels and balls of the feet in contact with the floor, and knees slightly bent.

• Don't bounce weights against your body during an exercise.

• When lifting barbells and dumbbells, wrap your thumbs around the bar when gripping it. You can easily drop a weight when using a "thumbless" grip.

Spotting

• Use spotters for free weights exercises in which the bar crosses the face or head (e.g., the bench press), is placed on the back (e.g., squats), or is racked in front of the chest (e.g., over-head press from the rack).

• Spotters should be at least as tall and as strong as the lifter.

• If one spotter is used, the spotter should stand behind the lifter; if two spotters are used, one spotter should stand at each end of the barbell.

• For squats with heavy resistance, use at least three spotters—one behind the lifter (hands near lifter's hips, waist, or torso) and one on each side of the bar. Squatting in a power rack will increase safety during this exercise.

• Spot dumbbell exercises at the forearms, as close to the weights as possible.

• For over-the-face and over-the-head lifts, the spotter should hold the bar with an alternate grip (one palm up and one palm down) inside the lifter's grip.

• When providing a handoff, the spotter should make sure that the lifter has control of the weight before moving away.

• Ensure good communication between spotter and lifter by agreeing on verbal signals before the exercise.

• Spotters should pay attention and be ready to act quickly to assist a person having trouble. Lifters should tell spotters to take the bar if they can no longer contribute to making the lift.

Weight Machines

• Keep away from moving weight stacks. Pay attention when you're changing weights.

• Adjust each machine for your body so that you don't have to work in an awkward position. Lock everything in place before you begin.

• Make sure the machines are clean. Carry a towel around with you, and place it on the machine where you will sit or lie down.

doing so is dangerous. It is easy to lose your balance or to raise one side of the weight faster than the other. Without collars, the weights on one side of the bar will slip off, and the weights on the opposite side will crash to the floor.

Be Alert for Injuries   Report any obvious muscle or joint injuries to your instructor or physician, and stop exercising the affected area. Training with an injured joint or muscle can lead to a more serious injury. Make sure you get the necessary first aid. Even minor injuries heal faster if you use the R-I-C-E principle of treating injuries described in Chapter 3.

Consult a physician if you have any unusual symptoms during exercise or if you're uncertain whether weight training is a proper activity for you. Conditions such as heart disease and high blood pressure can be aggravated during weight training. Immediately report symptoms such as headaches; dizziness; labored breathing; numbness; vision disturbances; and chest, neck, or arm pains.

MOTIVATION BOOSTER

Graph your total workout. If you want an easy overall measure of your progress, calculate the total amount of weight you lift during each workout. For each exercise, multiply the amount of resistance by the number of repetitions and the number of sets; for example, if you do 1 set of 11 repetitions of the bench press with 60 pounds of resistance, your total for the bench press would be $1 \times 11 \times 60 = 660$ pounds. Next, add up the amounts for each exercise to get your workout total. Graph the total amount of weight lifted during each workout to measure your progress and boost your motivation.

A Caution About Supplements and Drugs

Many active people use a wide variety of nutritional supplements and drugs in the quest for improved performance and appearance. (Table 4.2 lists a selective summary of "performance aids" along with their potential side effects.) Most of these substances are ineffective and expensive, and many are dangerous (see the box "Dietary Supplements: A Consumer Dilemma" on p. 108). A balanced diet should be your primary nutritional strategy.

QUESTIONS FOR CRITICAL THINKING AND REFLECTION

Do you think athletes should be allowed to use drugs and supplements to improve their sports performance? Would you be tempted to use a banned performance-enhancing drug if you thought you could get away with it? Why or why not?

WEIGHT TRAINING EXERCISES

A general book on fitness and wellness cannot include a detailed description of all weight training exercises. Here we present a basic program for developing muscular strength and endurance for general fitness using free weights and weight machines. Instructions for each exercise are accompanied by photographs and a listing of the muscles being trained. Table 4.3 on p. 109 lists alternative and additional exercises that can be performed on various machines or with free weights. If you are interested in learning how to do these exercises, ask your instructor or coach for assistance. An illustration of the muscular system is shown in Figure 4.6 on p. 110.

Labs 4.2 and 4.3 will help you assess your current level of muscular endurance and design your own weight training program. If you want to develop strength for a particular activity, your program should contain exercises for general fitness, exercises for the muscle groups most important for the activity, and exercises for muscle groups most often injured. Regardless of the goals of your program or the type of equipment you use, your program should be structured so that you obtain maximum results without risking injury.

TIPS FOR TODAY AND THE FUTURE

You don't need a complicated or heavy training program to improve strength: Just 1 set of 8–12 repetitions of 8–10 exercises, done at least 2 days per week, is enough for general fitness.

RIGHT NOW YOU CAN

- Do a set of static (isometric) exercises. If you're sitting, try tightening your abdominal muscles as you press your lower back into the seat or work your arms by placing the palms of your hands on top of your thighs and pressing down. Hold the contraction for 6 seconds and do 5–10 repetitions; don't hold your breath.
- Think of three things you've done in the past 24 hours that would have been easier or more enjoyable if you increased your level of muscular strength and endurance. Examples might be carrying your books, climbing stairs, or playing recreational sports. Begin to visualize improvements in your quality of life that could come from increased muscular strength and endurance.

IN THE FUTURE YOU CAN

- Make an appointment with a trainer at your campus or neighborhood fitness facility. A trainer can help you put together an appropriate weight training program and introduce you to the equipment at the facility.
- Invest in an inexpensive set of free weights, a stability ball, or a resistance band. Then make a regular appointment with yourself to use your new equipment.

Table 4.2   Performance Aids Marketed to Weight Trainers

Substance	Supposed Effects	Actual Effects	Selected Potential Side Effects
Adrenal androgens, such as dehydroepiandrosterone (DHEA), androstenedione	Increased testosterone, muscle mass, and strength; decreased body fat	Increased testosterone, strength, and fat-free mass; decreased fat in older subjects (more studies needed in younger people)	Gonadal suppression, prostate hypertrophy, breast development in males, masculinization in women and children; long-term effects unknown
Amino acids	Increased muscle mass	No effects if dietary protein intake is adequate; consuming before or after training may improve performance	Minimal side effects; unbalanced amino acid intake can cause problems with protein metabolism
Amphetamines	Prevention of fatigue; increased confidence and training intensity	Increased arousal, wakefulness, and confidence; feeling of enhanced decision-making ability	Depression and fatigue (after drug wears off), extreme confusion; neural and psychological effects including aggressiveness, paranoia, hallucinations, compulsive behavior, restlessness, irritability, heart arrhythmia, high blood pressure, and chest pain
Anabolic steroids	Increased muscle mass, strength, power, psychological aggressiveness, and endurance	Increased strength, power, fat-free mass, and aggression; no effects on endurance	Liver damage and tumors, decrease in high-density lipoprotein (good cholesterol), depressed sperm and testosterone production, high blood pressure, depressed immune function, problems with sugar metabolism, psychological disturbances, gonadal suppression, liver disease, acne, breast development in males, masculinization in women and children, heart disease, thicker blood, and increased risk of cancer; steroids are controlled substances*
Beta-agonists, such as clenbuterol, salmeterol, terbutaline	Enhanced performance; prevention of muscle atrophy; increased fat-free weight; decreased body fat	Used to treat asthma, including exercise-induced asthma	Insomnia, heart arrhythmia, anxiety, anorexia, nausea, heart enlargement, heart attack (particularly if used with steroids), and heart failure
Chromium picolinate	Increased muscle mass, decreased body fat; improved blood sugar control	Well-controlled studies show no significant effect on fat-free mass or body fat	Moderate doses (50–200 µg) appear safe; higher doses may cause DNA damage and other serious effects; long-term effects unknown
Creatine monohydrate	Increased creatine phosphate levels in muscles, muscle mass, and capacity for high-intensity exercise	Increased muscle mass and performance in some types of high-intensity exercise	Minimal side effects; long-term effects unknown
Dinitrophenol (DPN)	Weight loss	Weight loss; releases food energy as heat	Increased body temperature, leading to heat injury and death; banned by the FDA
Diuretics	Promotes loss of body fluid	Promotes loss of body fluid to accentuate muscle definition; often taken with potassium supplements and very-low-calorie diets	Muscle cell destruction, low blood pressure, blood chemistry abnormalities, and heart problems
Ephedra	Decreased body fat; increased training intensity due to stimulant effect	Decreased appetite, particularly when taken with caffeine; some evidence for increased training intensity	Abnormal heart rhythms, nervousness, headache, gastrointestinal distress, and heatstroke; banned by the FDA

| Table 4.2 | Performance Aids Marketed to Weight Trainers *(continued)* |

Substance	Supposed Effects	Actual Effects	Selected Potential Side Effects
Erythropoietin, darbepoetin	Enhanced performance during endurance events	Stimulated growth of red blood cells; enhanced oxygen uptake and endurance	Increased blood viscosity (thickness); can cause potentially fatal blood clots
Ginseng	Decreased effects of physical and emotional stress; increased oxygen consumption	Most well-controlled studies show no effect on performance	No serious side effects; high doses can cause high blood pressure, nervousness, and insomnia
Growth hormone	Increased muscle mass, strength, and power; decreased body fat	Increased muscle mass and strength; decreased fat mass; studies show no effect on muscle or exercise performance	Elevated blood sugar, high insulin levels, and carpal tunnel syndrome; enlargement of the heart and other organs; acromegaly (disease characterized by increased growth of bones in hands and face); diseases of the heart, nerves, bones, and joints; an extremely expensive controlled substance*
Human chorionic gonadotrophin (HCG)	Increased testosterone production; prevention of muscle atrophy during steroid withdrawal	Increased testosterone production	Interferes with normal testosterone regulation; banned in most sports
Beta-hydroxy beta-methylbutyrate (HMB)	Increased strength and muscle mass; decreased body fat	Some studies show increased fat-free mass and decreased fat; more research needed	No reported side effects; long-term effects unknown
Insulin	Increased muscle mass	Effectiveness in stimulating muscle growth unknown	Insulin shock (characterized by extremely low blood sugar), which can lead to unconsciousness and death
Insulin-like growth factor (IGF)	Increased muscle mass; improved cellular function	Actual effects in healthy, active people unknown	Similar to side effects of growth hormone; long-term use promotes cancer
"Metabolic-optimizing" meals for athletes	Increased muscle mass and energy supply; decreased body fat	No proven effects beyond those of balanced meals	No reported side effects; extremely expensive
Over-the-counter stimulants, such as caffeine, phenylpropanolamine (PPA)	Weight loss; improved endurance; stimulant effect	Can be used for weight control; may improve endurance; does not appear to enhance short-term maximal exercise capacity	Increased risk of heart attack and stroke in some people (in high doses); increased incidence of abnormal heart rhythm and insomnia; caffeine is addictive
Prescription appetite suppressants, such as diethylproprion, phentermine, sibutramine, rimonabant	Weight control, weight loss	Weight loss; typically prescribed only for short-term use	Restlessness, anxiety, dizziness, depression, tremors, increased urination, diarrhea, constipation, vomiting, high blood pressure, swelling of legs or ankles, insomnia, seizures, fast or irregular heartbeat, heart palpitations, blurred vision, rashes, and difficulty breathing; can be habit-forming
Protein, amino acids, polypeptide supplements	Increased muscle mass and growth hormone release; accelerated muscle develop-ment; decreased body fat	No effects if dietary protein intake is adequate; may promote protein synthesis if taken immediately before or after weight training	Can be dangerous for people with liver or kidney disease; substituting amino acid or polypeptide supplements for protein-rich food can cause nutrient deficiencies

*Possession of a controlled substance is illegal without a prescription, and physicians are not allowed to prescribe controlled substances for the improvement of athletic performance. In addition, the use of anabolic steroids, growth hormone, or any of several other substances listed in this table is banned for athletic competition.

SOURCES: Brooks, G. A., et al. 2005. *Exercise Physiology: Human Bioenergetics and Its Applications*, 4th ed. New York: McGraw-Hill. Sports-supplement dangers. 2001. *Consumer Reports,* June. U.S. National Library of Medicine, National Institutes of Health. 2007. *MedlinePlus Medical Encyclopedia* (http://www.nlm.nih.gov/medlineplus/encyclopedia.html; retrieved November 19, 2007).

Dietary Supplements: A Consumer Dilemma

Wading through manufacturers' claims can be tricky when you are considering taking a dietary supplement. While drugs and food products undergo stringent government testing, dietary supplements can be freely marketed without testing for safety or effectiveness. There is no guarantee that advertisements about dietary supplements are accurate or true.

What's the difference between a drug—which must be approved by the Food and Drug Administration (FDA)—and a dietary supplement? In some cases, the only real difference is in how the product is marketed. Some dietary supplements are as potentially dangerous as potent prescription drugs. But because they have a different classification, dietary supplements do not have to prove they are safe and effective before being sold; the FDA can, however, take action against any unsafe supplement product after it reaches the market. This is what occurred in two high-profile cases in 2004 when the FDA acted against popular dietary supplements— androstenedione (andro) and ephedra.

Androstenedione

The male hormone testosterone is a powerful drug with many adverse effects; it is closely regulated by the FDA. Androstenedione, a hormone converted in the body to testosterone (and estrogen), was widely available without a prescription as a dietary supplement. Andro disrupts the hormonal balance of its users and can increase the risk of heart disease. Teens who take andro are at risk for early closure of bone growth centers, which could limit their adult height. (See Table 4.2 for some of andro's many other side effects.)

Advertisements for andro claimed that it would increase muscle size, strength, and performance, but there are actually few good studies of andro's effects on humans. The two best studies showed no significant difference in muscle growth and strength in andro users compared with nonusers. Most medical experts believe that andro is neither safe nor effective—yet it has been used by thousands of athletes, most of whom are unaware of the risks. In 2004, the FDA stated that andro was potentially dangerous and should not be marketed as a supplement; it ordered manufacturers to stop selling supplements containing andro.

Ephedra

Ephedra was a common ingredient of dietary supplements, often touted as an "energy booster" and a "fat burner." Because ephedra was marketed as a natural herbal product and available without a prescription, consumers assumed that it was free from serious side effects. However, the drug can cause severe high blood pressure, heart attacks, strokes, seizures, and heat illness, and it has been linked to a number of deaths. It may be especially risky in users who are dehydrated and/or fatigued or when it is combined with other stimulants such as caffeine.

Many sports organizations banned the use of ephedra because of safety concerns, and following the publication of additional studies and reports, the FDA acted to remove ephedra-containing products from the market. (Chapter 9 has more information about ephedra and other dietary supplements marketed for weight loss.)

Do You Need Supplements?

Supplement manufacturers often make glowing claims about their products, such as "Builds lean muscle fast" or "Burns fat and gives you energy." With all the hype, how can you determine if a particular supplement might be helpful? Ask yourself the following questions:

- **Do you really need a supplement at all?** Nutritional authorities agree that most athletes and young adults can obtain all the necessary ingredients for health and top athletic performance by eating a well-balanced diet and training appropriately. There is no dietary supplement that outperforms wholesome food and a good training regimen.

- **Is the product safe and effective?** The fact that a dietary supplement is available in your local store is no guarantee of safety. As described earlier, the FDA doesn't regulate supplements in the same way as drugs. The only way to determine if a supplement really works is to perform carefully controlled research on human subjects. Testimonials from individuals who claim to have benefited from the product don't count. Few dietary supplements have undergone careful human testing, so it is difficult to tell which of them may actually work.

- **Can you be sure that the specific product is of high quality?** There is no official agency that ensures the quality of dietary supplements. There is no guarantee that a supplement contains the desired ingredient, that dosages are appropriate, that potency is standardized, or that the product is free from contaminants. (See Chapter 8 for more information on dietary supplement labeling.)

A recent study of 12 over-the-counter brands of supplements containing androstenedione and related steroids found that 1 brand contained more and 11 brands contained less than the amount stated on the label; in addition, one brand contained a significant amount of a controlled steroid. The International Olympic Committee issued a warning to athletes based on a test of 634 different nutritional supplements: Researchers had found that 15% of the supplements tested contained unlabled substances that would cause an athlete to fail a drug test.

Many dietary supplements are ineffective and/or unsafe, but it is extremely difficult for consumers to get the information they need to make an informed decision. Reliable resources for information on dietary supplements include the FDA Center for Food Safety and Applied Nutrition (http://www.cfsan.fda. gov/~dms/supplmnt.html) and the USDA's Dietary Supplements page (http://fnic.nal.usda.gov/nal_display/index. php?info_center=4&tax_level=1&tax_subject=274).

Once you have gathered the best information you can find, consider whether the potential benefits of the supplement appear to outweigh the risks and the cost. When in doubt, it's best to avoid the product. Remember that no supplement eliminates the need for proper training, and no supplement has been shown to be safe and effective in long-term weight loss. A product that is marginally effective, not proven safe, and expensive to boot is probably not worth the money or the risk.

Table 4.3

Weight Training Exercises for Machines, Free Weights, Exercise Bands, and No Equipment

Company	Legs	Arms	Shoulders and Chest	Torso
Cybex	Hip abduction	Arm curl	Chest press	Ab crunch
	Hip adduction	Triceps extension	Incline press	Pull-down
	Leg extension		Overhead press	Torso rotation
	Leg press			
	Leg curl			
	Rotary calf			
Hammer	Abductor	Behind-neck press	Bench press	Behind-neck pull-down
	Adductor	Bench press	Flat back chest	Bilateral row
	Calf	Flat back chest	Iso wide chest	Dead lift
	H squat	Front military press	Lateral raise	Front pull-down
	Iso leg curl	Incline press	Rear deltoid	High row
	Iso leg extension	Iso behind-neck press	Rotator cuff	Iso pullover
	Iso lateral leg press	Iso incline press	Seated dip	Low row
	Leg curl	Iso wide chest		Pullover
	Leg extension	Seated bicep		Row
	Leg press	Seated triceps		Shrug
	Seated calf raise			
Nautilus	Calf raise	Biceps curl	10-degree chest	Abdominal
	Leg curl	Preacher curl	50-degree chest	Compound row
	Leg extension	Triceps extension	Bench press	Hip and back
	Leg press		Incline press	Hip flexion
			Lateral raise	Lat pull-down
			Military press	Pullover
			Seated dip	Rotary torso
Universal Gym	Abductor kick	Biceps curl	Bench press	Bent-over row
	Adductor kick	Dips	Front raise	Crunch
	Calf raises (leg press)	Lat pull	Incline press	Lat pull
	Knee extension		Rip-up	Pullover
	Knee flexion		Shoulder press	Pull-up
	Leg press		Upright row	Side bend
Free weights	Back squat	Barbell curl	Bench press	Abdominal crunch
	Front squat	Dumbbell curl	Decline press	Abdominal sit-ups
	Hack squat	French curl	Dumbbell back raise	Bent-over row
	Leg curl	Preacher curl	Dumbbell flys	Dead lift
	Leg extension		Dumbbell front raise	Incline lever row
	Leg press		Dumbbell lateral raise	Lat pull-down
	Lunges		Incline press	Pullover
	Seated calf		Overhead press	Seated row
	Smith machine			Shrug
	Step-ups			Upright row
Exercise bands	Squats	Biceps curls	Chest press	Trunk curl
	Lunges	Triceps extensions	Shoulder press	Reverse crunch
	Hamstring curls		Lateral raise	Sit backs
	Leg abduction		Seated row	Back extensions
	Leg adduction			Lat pull-down
	Kick backs			
Exercises without weights	Squats	Isometric curls	Push-ups	Curl-ups
	Overhead squats	Isometric triceps	Pull-ups	Bicycles
	Lunges	extensions	Handstand press	Knee raises from bar
	Side lunges	Chair dips	against wall	Side bends
	Rear lunges	90° Bent-arm bar hang,		Twists
	Wall sits	supine grip		
	Step-ups			

SOURCE: Adapted from Fahey., T. D., 2007. *Basic Weight Training for Men and Women*, 6th ed. Copyright © 2007. The McGraw-Hill Companies, Inc. Reprinted with permission of The McGraw-Hill Companies, Inc.

Anterior view

Temporalis
Masseter
[Scalenus}
Sternocleidomastoid
Trapezius
Pectoralis major
[Pectoralis minor]
Deltoid
Biceps brachius
Brachialis
Brachioradialis

Brachialis
Triceps brachius

External oblique

[Transverse abdominis]

Rectus abdominis

Adductor longus
Sartorius

Patella
(kneecap)

Gastrocnemius
(calf)
Soleus

Tibialis anterior

Rectus femoris
[Vastus intermedius]   Quadriceps
Vastus lateralis
Vastus medialis

Posterior view

Brachioradialis
Biceps brachius
[Rhomboid]

Splenius capitis
[Splenius cervicis]

Trapezius

Deltoid
Teres minor
Teres major
Latissimus dorsi
[Erector spinae]

Triceps brachius
Flexor carpi radialis
Flexor carpi ulnaris

External oblique
[Internal oblique]
[Quadratus
lumborum]
Gluteus maximus
(buttock)

Biceps femoris
Hamstrings   Semitendinosus
Semimembranosus

Gastrocnemius
(calf)

Tendo calcaneus
(Achilles tendon)

FIGURE 4.6   The muscular system. The muscle names enclosed in brackets refer to deep muscles.

Exercise 1 — Bench Press

Instructions: (a) Lying on a bench on your back with your feet on the floor, grasp the bar with palms upward and hands shoulder-width apart. If the weight is on a rack, move the bar carefully from the supports to a point over the middle of your chest or slightly above it (at the lower part of the sternum). **(b)** Lower the bar to your chest. Then press it in a straight line to the starting position. Don't arch your back or bounce the bar off your chest.

Muscles developed: Pectoralis major, triceps, deltoids

Front   Back

a

b

Note: *To allow an optimal view of exercise technique, a spotter does not appear in these demonstration photographs; however, spotters should be used for most exercises with free weights. Video clips illustrating spotting technique can be found on the* Fit and Well *Online Learning Center.*

Exercise 2 — Pull-Up

a

b

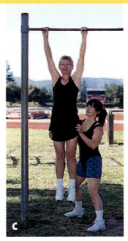

c

Assisted pull-up: (c) This is done as described for a pull-up, except that a spotter assists the person by pushing upward at the waist, hips, or legs during the exercise.

Front

Back

Muscles developed: Latissimus dorsi, biceps

Instructions: (a) Begin by grasping the pull-up bar with both hands, palms facing forward and elbows extended fully. **(b)** Pull yourself upward until your chin goes above the bar. Then return to the starting position.

Exercise 3 — Shoulder Press (Overhead or Military Press)

Instructions: This exercise can be done standing or seated, with dumbbells or a barbell. The shoulder press begins with the weight at your chest, preferably on a rack. **(a)** Grasp the weight with your palms facing away from you. **(b)** Push the weight overhead until your arms are extended. Then return to the starting position (weight at chest). Be careful not to arch your back excessively.

If you are a more advanced weight trainer, you can "clean" the weight (lift it from the floor to your chest). The clean should be attempted only after instruction from a knowledgeable coach; otherwise, it can lead to injury.

Front   Back

Muscles developed:
Deltoids, triceps, trapezius

Exercise 4 — Upright Rowing

Instructions: From a standing position with arms extended fully, grasp a barbell with a close grip (hands about 6–12 inches apart) and palms toward the body. Raise the bar to about the level of your collarbone, keeping your elbows above bar level at all times. Return to the starting position.

This exercise can be done using dumbbells, a weighted bar (shown), or a barbell.

Front   Back

Muscles developed:
Trapezius, deltoids, biceps

Exercise 5 — Biceps Curl

Instructions: **(a)** From a standing position, grasp the bar with your palms upward and your hands shoulder-width apart. **(b)** Keeping your upper body rigid, flex (bend) your elbows until the bar reaches a level slightly below the collarbone. Return the bar to the starting position.

This exercise can be done using dumbbells, a curl bar (shown), or a barbell; some people find that using a curl bar places less stress on the wrists.

Front

Muscles developed:
Biceps, brachialis

Exercise 6 — Lateral Raise

Instructions: (a) Stand with feet shoulder-width apart and a dumbbell in each hand. Hold the dumbbells parallel to each other. **(b)** With elbows slightly bent, slowly lift both weights until they reach shoulder level. Keep your wrists in a neutral position, in line with your forearms. Return to the starting position.

Front   Back

Muscles developed:
Deltoids

Exercise 7 — Squat

Instructions: If the bar is racked, place the bar on the fleshy part of your upper back and grasp the bar at shoulder width. Keeping your back straight and head level, remove the bar from the rack and take a step back. Stand with feet slightly more than shoulder-width apart and toes pointed slightly outward. **(a)** Rest the bar on the back of your shoulders, holding it there with hands facing forward. **(b)** Keeping your head level and lower back straight and pelvis back, squat down until your thighs are below parallel with the floor. Let your thighs move laterally (outward) so that you "squat between your legs." This will help keep your back straight and keep your heels on the floor. Drive upward toward the starting position, hinging at the hips and keeping your back in a fixed position throughout the exercise.

Front   Back

Back

Muscles developed:
Quadriceps, gluteus maximus, hamstrings, gastrocnemius

Exercise 8 — Heel Raise

Instructions: Stand with feet shoulder-width apart and toes pointed straight ahead. **(a)** Rest the bar on the back of your shoulders, holding it there with hands facing forward. **(b)** Press down with your toes while lifting your heels. Return to the starting position.

Back

Muscles developed:
Gastrocnemius, soleus

Exercise 9   Curl-Up or Crunch

Instructions: (a) Lie on your back on the floor with your arms folded across your chest and your feet on the floor or on a bench. **(b)** Curl your trunk up and forward by raising your head and shoulders from the ground. Lower to the starting position. Focus on using your abdominal muscles rather than the muscles in your shoulders, chest, and neck.

This exercise can also be done using an exercise ball (see p. 99).

Front

Muscles developed:
Rectus abdominis, obliques

a

b

Exercise 10   Spine Extension (Isometric Exercises)

Instructions: Begin on all fours with your knees below your hips and your hands below your shoulders.

Unilateral spine extension:
(a) Extend your right leg to the rear and reach forward with your right arm. Keep your spine neutral and your raised arm and leg in line with your torso. Don't arch your back or let your hip or shoulder sag. Hold this position for 10–30 seconds. Repeat with your left leg and left arm.

Bilateral spine extension:
(b) Extend your left leg to the rear and reach forward with your right arm. Keep your spine neutral and your raised arm and leg in line with your torso. Don't arch your back or let your hip or shoulder sag. Hold this position for 10–30 seconds. Repeat with your right leg and left arm.

Front   Back   Back

Muscles developed: Erector spinae, gluteus maximus, hamstrings, deltoids

You can make this exercise more difficult by making box patterns with your arms and legs.

a

b

Exercise 11 — Isometric Side Bridge

Instructions: Lie on the floor on your side with your knees bent and your top arm lying alongside your body. Lift your hips so that your weight is supported by your forearm and knee. Hold this position for 10 seconds, breathing normally. Repeat on the other side. Work up to a 60-second hold; perform one or more repetitions on each side.

Variation: You can make the exercise more difficult by keeping your legs straight and supporting yourself with your feet and forearm (see Lab 5.3) or with your feet and hand (with elbow straight). You can also do this exercise on an exercise ball.

Front   Back

Muscles developed: Obliques, quadratus lumborum

WEIGHT TRAINING EXERCISES: WEIGHT MACHINES

Exercise 1 — Bench Press (Chest or Vertical Press)

Instructions: Sit or lie on the seat or bench, depending on the type of machine and the manufacturer's instructions. Your back, hips, and buttocks should be pressed against the machine pads. Place your feet on the floor or the foot supports.

Front   Back

Muscles developed: Pectoralis major, anterior deltoids, triceps

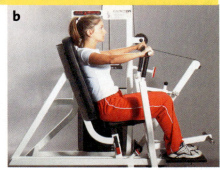

(a) Grasp the handles with your palms facing away from you; the handles should be aligned with your armpits.

(b) Push the bars until your arms are fully extended, but don't lock your elbows. Return to the starting position.

Exercise 2 — Lat Pull

Instructions: Begin in a seated or kneeling position, depending on the type of lat machine and the manufacturer's instructions.

Note: *This exercise focuses on the same major muscles as the assisted pull-up (Exercise 3); choose an appropriate exercise for your program based on your preferences and equipment availability.*

Front   Back

Muscles developed: Latissimus dorsi, biceps

(a) Grasp the bar of the machine with arms fully extended.

(b) Slowly pull the weight down until it reaches the top of your chest. Slowly return to the starting position.

Exercise 3   Assisted Pull-Up

Instructions: Set the weight according to the amount of assistance you need to complete a set of pull-ups—the heavier the weight, the more assistance provided.

(a) Stand or kneel on the assist platform, and grasp the pull-up bar with your elbows fully extended and your palms facing away. **(b)** Pull up until your chin goes above the bar and then return to the starting position.

Front   Back

Muscles developed: Latissimus dorsi, biceps

a   b

Exercise 4   Overhead Press (Shoulder Press)

Instructions: Adjust the seat so that your feet are flat on the ground and the hand grips are slightly above your shoulders.

(a) Sit down, facing away from the machine, and grasp the hand grips with your palms facing forward.

(b) Press the weight upward until your arms are extended. Return to the starting position.

Front   Back

Muscles developed: Deltoids, trapezius, triceps

a   b

Exercise 5   Biceps Curl

Instructions: (a) Adjust the seat so that your back is straight and your arms rest comfortably against the top and side pads. Place your arms on the support cushions and grasp the hand grips with your palms facing up.

(b) Keeping your upper body still, flex (bend) your elbows until the hand grips almost reach your collarbone. Return to the starting position.

Front

Muscles developed: Biceps, brachialis

a   b

Exercise 6   Pullover

Instructions: Adjust the seat so your shoulders are aligned with the cams. Push down on the foot pads with your feet to bring the bar forward until you can place your elbows on the pads. Rest your hands lightly on the bar. If possible, place your feet flat on the floor. **(a)** To get into the starting position, let your arms go backward as far as possible. **(b)** Pull your elbows forward until the bar almost touches your abdomen. Return to the starting position.

Front   Back

Muscles developed:
Latissimus dorsi, pectoralis major and minor, triceps, abdominals

Exercise 7   Lateral Raise

Instructions: (a) Adjust the seat so the pads rest just above your elbows when your upper arms are at your sides, your elbows are bent, and your forearms are parallel to the floor. Lightly grasp the handles. **(b)** Push outward and up with your arms until the pads are at shoulder height. Lead with your elbows rather than trying to lift the bars with your hands. Return to the starting position.

Front   Back

Muscles developed:
Deltoids, trapezius

Exercise 8   Triceps Extension

Note: *This exercise focuses on some of the same muscles as the assisted dip (Exercise 9); choose an appropriate exercise for your program based on your preferences and equipment availability.*

Instructions: (a) Adjust the seat so that your back is straight and your arms rest comfortably against the top and side pads. Place your arms on the support cushions and grasp the hand grips with palms facing inward.

(b) Keeping your upper body still, extend your elbows as much as possible. Return to the starting position.

Back

Muscles developed:
Triceps

Exercise 9 — Assisted Dip

Instructions: Set the weight according to the amount of assistance you need to complete a set of dips—the heavier the weight, the more assistance provided. **(a)** Stand or kneel on the assist platform with your body between the dip bar. With your elbows fully extended and palms facing your body, support your weight on your hands. **(b)** Lower your body until your upper arms are approximately parallel with the bars. Then push up until you reach the starting position.

Front   Back

Muscles developed:
Triceps, deltoids, pectoralis major

Exercise 10 — Leg Press

Instructions: Sit or lie on the seat or bench, depending on the type of machine and the manufacturer's instructions. Your head, back, hips, and buttocks should be pressed against the machine pads. Loosely grasp the handles at the side of the machine. **(a)** Begin with your feet flat on the foot platform about shoulder-width apart. Extend your legs but do not forcefully lock your knees. **(b)** Slowly lower the weight by bending your knees and flexing your hips until your knees are bent at about a 90-degree angle or your heels start to lift off the foot platform. Keep your lower back flat against the support pad. Then extend your knees and return to the starting position.

Muscles developed:
Gluteus maximus, quadriceps, hamstrings

Front   Back

Exercise 11 — Leg Extension (Knee Extension)

Instructions: (a) Adjust the seat so that the pads rest comfortably on top of your lower shins. Loosely grasp the handles. **(b)** Extend your knees until they are almost straight. Return to the starting position.

Knee extensions cause kneecap pain in some people. If you have kneecap pain during this exercise, check with an orthopedic specialist before repeating it.

Front

Muscles developed:
Quadriceps

Exercise 12 — Seated Leg Curl

Instructions: (a) Sit on the seat with your back against the back pad and the leg pad below your calf muscles. **(b)** Flex your knees until your lower and upper legs form a 90 degree angle. Return to the starting position.

Muscles developed:
Hamstrings, gastrocnemius

Back   Back

Exercise 13 — Heel Raise

Instructions: (a) Stand with your head between the pads and one pad on each shoulder. The balls of your feet should be on the platform. Lightly grasp the handles. **(b)** Press down with your toes while lifting your heels. Return to the starting position. Changing the direction your feet are pointing (straight ahead, inward, and outward) will work different portions of your calf muscles.

Muscles developed:
Gastrocnemius, soleus

Back

Note: Abdominal machines and low-back machines are not recommended because of injury risk. Refer to the Free Weights exercise section for appropriate exercises to strengthen the abdominal and low-back muscles. For the rectus abdominus, obliques, and transvere abdominus, perform curl-ups (Exercise 9 in the Free Weights section, p. •••), and for the erector spinae and quadratus lumborum, perform the spine extension and the isometric side bridge (Exercises 10 and 11 in the Free Weights section, p. •••).

Q Will I gain weight if I do resistance exercises?

A Your weight probably will not change significantly as a result of a general fitness program: 1 set of 8–12 repetitions of 8–10 exercises. You will increase muscle mass and lose body fat, so your weight will stay about the same. You may notice a change in how your clothes fit, however, because muscle is denser than fat. Increased muscle mass will help you control body fat. Muscle increases your metabolism, which means you burn more calories every day. If you combine resistance exercises with endurance exercises, you will be on your way to developing a healthier body composition. Concentrate on fat loss rather than weight loss.

Q Do I need more protein in my diet when I train with weights?

A No. Although there is some evidence that power athletes involved in heavy training have a higher-than-normal protein requirement, there is no reason for most people to consume extra protein. Most Americans take in more protein than they need, so even if there is an increased protein need during heavy training, it is probably supplied by the average diet. Consuming a protein-rich snack before or after training may promote muscle hypertrophy.

Q What causes muscle soreness the day or two following a weight training workout?

A The muscle pain you feel a day or two after a heavy weight training workout is caused by injury to the muscle fibers and surrounding connective tissue. Contrary to popular belief, delayed-onset muscle soreness is not caused by lactic acid buildup. Scientists believe that injury to muscle fibers causes inflammation, which in turn causes the release of chemicals that break down part of the muscle tissue and cause pain. After a bout of intense exercise that causes muscle injury and delayed-onset muscle soreness, the muscles produce protective proteins that prevent soreness during future workouts. If you don't work out regularly, you lose these protective proteins and become susceptible to soreness again.

Q Will strength training improve my sports performance?

A Strength developed in the weight room does not automatically increase your power in sports such as skiing, tennis, or cycling. Hitting a forehand in tennis and making a turn on skis are precise skills that require coordination between your nervous system and muscles. For skilled people, movements become reflex—you don't think about them when you do them. Increasing strength can disturb this coordination. Only by simultaneously practicing a sport and improving fitness can you expect to become more powerful in the skill. Practice helps you integrate your new strength with your skills, which makes you more powerful. Consequently, you can hit the ball harder in tennis or make more graceful turns on the ski slopes. (Refer to Chapter 2 for more on the concept of specificity of physical training.)

Q Will I improve faster if I train every day?

A No. Your muscles need time to recover between training sessions. Doing resistance exercises every day will cause you to become overtrained, which will increase your chance of injury and impede your progress. If your strength training program reaches a plateau, try one of these strategies:

- Train less frequently. If you are currently training the same muscle groups three or more times per week, you may not be allowing your muscles to fully recover from intense workouts.

- Change exercises. Using different exercises for the same muscle group may stimulate further strength development.

- Vary the load and number of repetitions. Try increasing or decreasing the loads you are using and changing the number of repetitions accordingly.

- Vary the number of sets. If you have been performing 1 set of each exercise, add sets.

- If you are training alone, find a motivated training partner. A partner can encourage you and assist you with difficult lifts, forcing you to work harder.

Q If I stop training, will my muscles turn to fat?

A No. Fat and muscle are two different kinds of tissue, and one cannot turn into the other. Muscles that aren't used become smaller (atrophy), and body fat may increase if caloric intake exceeds calories burned. Although the result of inactivity may be smaller muscles and more fat, the change is caused by two separate processes.

Q Should I wear a weight belt when I lift?

A Until recently, most experts advised people to wear weight belts. However, several studies have shown that weight belts do not prevent back injuries and may, in fact, increase the risk of injury by encouraging people to lift more weight than they are capable of lifting with good form. Although wearing a belt may allow you to lift more weight in some lifts, you may not get the full benefit of your program because use of a weight belt reduces the effectiveness of the workout on the muscles that help support your spine.

For more Common Questions Answered about strength training, visit the Online Learning Center.

SUMMARY

• Hypertrophy, or increased muscle fiber size, occurs when weight training causes the number of myofibrils to increase; total muscle size thereby increases. Strength also increases through muscle learning. Most women do not develop large muscles from weight training.

• Improvements in muscular strength and endurance lead to enhanced physical performance, protection against injury, improved body composition, better self-image, improved muscle and bone health with aging, and reduced risk of chronic disease.

• Muscular strength can be assessed by determining the amount of weight that can be lifted in one repetition of an exercise; muscular endurance can be assessed by determining the number of repetitions of a particular exercise that can be performed.

• Static (isometric) exercises (contraction without movement) are most useful when a person is recovering from an injury or surgery or needs to overcome weak points in a range of motion.

• Dynamic (isotonic) exercises involve contraction that results in movement. The two most common types are constant resistance (free weights) and variable resistance (many weight machines).

• Free weights and weight machines have pluses and minuses for developing fitness, although machines tend to be safer.

• Lifting heavy weights for only a few repetitions helps develop strength. Lifting lighter weights for more repetitions helps develop muscular endurance.

• A strength training program for general fitness includes at least 1 set of 8–12 repetitions (enough to cause fatigue) of 8–10 exercises, along with warm-up and cool-down periods; the program should be carried out at least 2 days per week.

• Safety guidelines for strength training include using proper technique, using spotters and collars when necessary, and taking care of injuries.

• Supplements or drugs that are promoted as instant or quick "cures" usually don't work and are either dangerous or expensive or both.

FOR FURTHER EXPLORATION

BOOKS

Bailes, J., and J. McCloskey. 2005. *When Winning Costs Too Much: Steroids, Supplements, and Scandal in Today's Sports World.* New York: Taylor Trade. *An overview of issues relating to the use of steroids and other performance aids.*

Delavier, F. 2005. *Strength Training Anatomy,* 2nd ed. Champaign, Ill.: Human Kinetics. *Includes exercises for all major muscle groups as well as full anatomical pictures of the muscular system. Women's* *Strength Training Anatomy, a matching volume for women, was published in 2003.*

Fahey, T. D. 2007. *Basic Weight Training for Men and Women,* 6th ed. New York: McGraw-Hill. *A practical guide to developing training programs, using free weights, tailored to individual needs.*

Goldenberg, L., and P. Twist. 2007. *Strength Ball Training.* Champaign, Ill.: Human Kinetics. *A guide to incorporating exercise balls and medicine balls into a complete weight training program.*

Lethi, A., et al. 2007. *Free-Weight Training.* Berkeley, Calif.: Thunder Bay Press. *A complete guide to training with free weights, with special instructions for using weights with an exercise ball.*

Page, P. A. 2005. *Strength Band Training.* Champaign, Ill.: Human Kinetics. *Describes and illustrates more than 100 resistance band exercises, targeting every major muscle group.*

ORGANIZATIONS AND WEB SITES

American College of Sports Medicine Position Stand: Progression Models in Resistance Training for Healthy Adults. Provides an in-depth look at strategies for setting up a strength training program and making progress based on individual program goals; look for the February 2002 Position Stand.
http://www.acsm-msse.org

Exercise: A Guide from the National Institute on Aging. Provides practical advice on fitness for seniors; includes animated instructions for specific weight training exercises.
http://weboflife.ksc.nasa.gov/exerciseandaging/toc.html

Georgia State University: Strength Training. Provides information about the benefits of strength training and ways to develop a safe and effective program; also includes illustrations of a variety of exercises.
http://www.gsu.edu/~wwwfit/strength.html

Human Anatomy On-line. Provides text, illustrations, and animation about the muscular system, nerve-muscle connections, muscular contraction, and other topics.
http://www.innerbody.com/htm/body.html

Kansas State University: Nutritional Supplements for Athletes. Provides information and links to recent research findings about specific supplements.
http://www.oznet.ksu.edu/nutrition/supplements.htm

National Strength and Conditioning Association. A professional organization that focuses on strength development for fitness and athletic performance.
http://www.nsca-lift.org

Pilates Method Alliance. Provides information about Pilates and about instructor certification; includes a directory of instructors.
http://www.pilatesmethodalliance.com

United States Department of Agriculture, Food and Nutrition Information Center: Dietary Supplements page. Provides information and fact sheets about a wide variety of dietary supplements, their uses, and their effects.
http://fnic.nal.usda.gov/nal_display/index.php?info_center=4&tax_level=1&tax_subject=274

University of California, San Diego/Muscle Physiology Home Page. Provides an introduction to muscle physiology, including information about types of muscle fibers and energy cycles.
http://muscle.ucsd.edu

University of Michigan/Muscles in Action. Interactive descriptions of muscle movements.

http://www.med.umich.edu/lrc/Hypermuscle/Hyper.html

See also the listings in Chapter 2.

SELECTED BIBLIOGRAPHY

Acacio, B. D., et al. 2004. Pharmacokinetics of dehydroepiandrosterone and its metabolites after long-term daily oral administration to healthy young men. *Fertility and Sterility* 81(3): 595–604.

American College of Sports Medicine. 2006. *ACSM's Guidelines for Exercise Testing and Prescription.* Philadelphia: Lippincott Williams and Wilkins.

American College of Sports Medicine. 2006. *ACSM's Resource Manual for Guidelines for Exercise Testing and Prescription,* 5th ed. Philadelphia: Lippincott Williams and Wilkins.

American College of Sports Medicine. 2005. *News Release: Pilates Research Offers New Information on Popular Technique* (http://www.acsm.org/Content/ContentFolders/NewsReleases/2005/PILATES_RESEARCH_OFFERS_NEW_INFORMATION_ON_POPULAR_TECHNIQUE.htm; retrieved November 19, 2007).

American College of Sports Medicine. 2002. Position Stand: Progression models in resistance training for healthy adults. *Medicine and Science in Sports and Exercise* 34(2): 364–380.

Andersen, L. L., et al. 2005. The effect of resistance training combined with timed ingestion of protein on muscle fiber size and muscle strength. *Metabolism* 54: 151–156.

Anton, M. M., et al. 2006. Resistance training increases basal limb blood flow and vascular conductance in aging humans. *Journal of Applied Physiology* 101(5): 1351–1355.

Baar, K. 2006. Training for endurance and strength: Lessons from cell signaling. *Medicine and Science in Sports and Exercise* 38(11): 1939–1944.

Blazevich, A. J., et al. 2007. Lack of human muscle architectural adaptation after short-term strength training. *Muscle and Nerve* 35(1): 78–86.

Brooks, N., et al. 2006. Strength training improves muscle quality and insulin sensitivity in Hispanic older adults with type 2 diabetes. *International Journal of Medical Sciences* 4(1): 19–27.

Brooks, G. A., et al. 2005. *Exercise Physiology: Human Bioenergetics and Its Applications.* New York: McGraw-Hill.

Burt, J., et al. 2007. A comparison of once versus twice per week training on leg press strength in women. *The Journal of Sports Medicine and Physical Fitness* 47(1): 13–17.

Centers for Disease Control and Prevention. 2004. Strength training among adults aged ≥65 years. *Morbidity and Mortality Weekly Report* 53(2): 25–28.

Crews, L. 2005. Mind-body exercise: Yoga and Pilates. *ACSM Fit Society Page,* Spring.

Cribb, P. J., et al. 2007. Effects of whey isolate, creatine, and resistance training on muscle hypertrophy. *Medicine and Science in Sports and Exercise* 39(2): 298–307.

Cribb, P. J., and A. Hayes. 2006. Effects of supplement timing and resistance exercise on skeletal muscle hypertrophy. *Medicine and Science in Sports and Exercise* 38(11): 1918–1925.

Cronin, J., and B. Crewther. 2004. Training volume and strength and power development. *Journal of Science and Medicine in Sport* 7: 144–155.

Earle, R. W., and T. R. Baechle, eds. 2004. *NSCA's Essentials of Personal Training.* Champaign, Ill: Human Kinetics.

Ferguson, T. B., and D. G. Syrotuik. 2006. Effects of creatine monohydrate supplementation on body composition and strength indices in experienced resistance trained women. *Journal of Strength and Conditioning Research* 20(4): 939–946.

Field, A. E., et al. 2005. Exposure to the mass media, body shape concerns, and use of supplements to improve weight and shape among male and female adolescents. *Pediatrics* 116(2): e214–220.

Food and Drug Administration. 2006 Update. *Sales of Supplements Containing Ephedrine Alkaloids (Ephedra) Prohibited* (http://www.fda.gov/oc/initiatives/ephedra/february2004/default.htm; retrieved May 9, 2007).

Food and Drug Administration. 2004. *Questions and Answers: Androstenedione* (http://www.cfsan.fda.gov/~dms/androqa.html).

Get on the bandwagon. 2005. *University of California, Berkeley Wellness Letter,* January.

Glowacki, S. P., et al. 2004. Effects of resistance, endurance, and concurrent exercise on training outcomes in men. *Medicine and Science in Sports and Exercise* 36: 2119–2127.

Guallar-Castillon, P., et al. 2007. Waist circumference as a predictor of disability among older adults. *Obesity* (Silver Spring) 15(1): 233–244.

Hartgens, F., and H. Kuipers. 2004. Effects of androgenic-anabolic steroids in athletes. *Sports Medicine* 34: 513–554.

Haskell, W. L., et al. 2007. Physical activity and public health: updated recommendation for adults from the American College of Sports Medicine and the American Heart Association. *Circulation.* 116(9): 1081–1093.

Ibanez, J., et al. 2005. Twice-weekly progressive resistance training decreases abdominal fat and improves insulin sensitivity in older men with type 2 diabetes. *Diabetes Care* 28: 662–667.

Jurca, R., et al. 2004. Associations of muscle strength and fitness with metabolic syndrome in men. *Medicine and Science in Sports and Exercise* 36: 1301–1307.

Kemmler, W. K., et al. 2006. Predicting maximal strength in trained postmenopausal woman. *Journal of Strength and Conditioning Research* 20(4): 838–842.

Kemmler, W. K., et al. 2004. Effects of single- vs. multiple-set resistance training on maximum strength and body composition in trained postmenopausal women. *Journal of Strength and Conditioning Research* 18: 689–694.

Kraemer, W. J., et al. 2004. Changes in muscle hypertrophy in women with periodized resistance training. *Medicine and Science in Sports and Exercise* 36: 697–708.

Leyk, D., et al. 2007. Hand-grip strength of young men, women and highly trained female athletes. *European Journal of Applied Physiology* 99(4): 415–421.

Liu-Ambrose, T., et al. 2004. Resistance and agility training reduce fall risk in women aged 75 to 85 with low bone mass: A 6-month randomized, controlled trial. *Journal of the American Geriatrics Society* 52: 657–665.

Magkos, F., and S. A. Kavouras. 2004. Caffeine and ephedrine: Physiological, metabolic and performance-enhancing effects. *Sports Medicine* 34: 871–889.

Nader, G. A. 2006. Concurrent strength and endurance training: From molecules to man. *Medicine and Science in Sports and Exercise* 38(11): 1965–1970.

Peterson, J. A. 2005. 10 common mistakes made while strength training. *ACSM's Health & Fitness Journal* 9(2): 44.

Sorace, P., and T. LaFontaine, 2005. Resistance training muscle power: Design programs that work! *ACSM's Health &Fitness Journal* 9(2): 6–12.

Sosnoff, J. J., and K. M. Newell. 2006. Are age-related increases in force variability due to decrements in strength? *Experimental Brain Research* 174(1): 86–94.

Thiblin, I., and A. Petersson. 2005. Pharmacoepidemiology of anabolic androgenic steroids: A review. *Fundamental and Clinical Pharmacology* 19: 27–44.

Tsourlou, T., et al. 2006. The effects of a twenty-four-week aquatic training program on muscular strength performance in healthy elderly women. *Journal of Strength and Conditioning Research* 20(4): 811–818.

Wieser, M., and P. Haber. 2007. The effects of systematic resistance training in the elderly. *International Journal of Sports Medicine* 28(1): 59–65.

Willardson, J. M. 2006. A brief review: Factors affecting the length of the rest interval between resistance exercise sets. *Journal of Strength and Conditioning Research* 20(4): 978–984.

Willardson, J. M., and L. N. Burkett. 2005. A comparison of 3 different rest intervals on the exercise volume completed during a workout. *Journal of Strength and Conditioning Research* 19: 23–26.

LAB 4.1 Assessing Your Current Level of Muscular Strength

For best results, don't do any strenuous weight training within 48 hours of any test. Use great caution when completing 1-RM tests; do not take the maximum bench press test if you have any injuries to your shoulders, elbows, back, hips, or knees. In addition, do not take these tests until you have had at least one month of weight training experience.

The Maximum Bench Press Test

Equipment

The free weights bench press test uses the following equipment:

1. Flat bench (with or without racks)
2. Barbell
3. Assorted weight plates, with collars to hold them in place
4. One or two spotters
5. Weight scale

If a weight machine is preferred, use the following equipment:

1. Universal Gym Dynamic Variable Resistance Machine
2. Weight scale

Preparation

Try a few bench presses with a small amount of weight so you can practice your technique, warm up your muscles, and, if you use free weights, coordinate your movements with those of your spotters. Weigh yourself and record the results.

Body weight: _____ lb

Maximum bench press test.

Instructions

1. Use a weight that is lower than the amount you believe you can lift. For free weights, men should begin with a weight about 2/3 of their body weight; women should begin with the weight of just the bar (45 lb).

2. Lie on the bench with your feet firmly on the floor. If you are using a weight machine, grasp the handles with palms away from you; the tops of the handles should be aligned with the tops of your armpits.

   If you are using free weights, grasp the bar slightly wider than shoulder width with your palms away from you. If you have one spotter, she or he should stand directly behind the bench; if you have two spotters, they should stand to the side, one at each end of the barbell. Signal to the spotter when you are ready to begin the test by saying "1, 2, 3." On "3," the spotter should help you lift the weight to a point over your midchest (nipple line).

3. Push the bars or barbell until your arms are fully extended. Exhale as you lift. If you are using free weights, the weight moves from a low point at the chest straight up. Keep your feet firmly on the floor, don't arch your back, and push the weight evenly with your right and left arms. Don't bounce the weight on your chest.

4. Rest for several minutes, then repeat the lift with a heavier weight. It will probably take several attempts to determine the maximum amount of weight you can lift (1 RM).

   1 RM: _____ lb   Check one: _____ Free weights _____ Universal _____ Other

5. If you used free weights, convert your free weights bench press score to an estimated value for 1 RM on the Universal bench press using the appropriate formula:

   Males: Estimated Universal 1 RM = (1.016 × free weights 1 RM _____ lb) + 18.41 = _____ lb

   Females: Estimated Universal 1 RM = (0.848 × free weights 1 RM _____ lb) + 21.37 = _____ lb

Rating Your Bench Press Result

1. Divide your Universal 1-RM value by your body weight.

    1 RM _____ lb ÷ body weight _____ lb = _____

2. Find this ratio in the table to determine your bench press strength rating. Record the rating here and in the chart at the end of this lab.

    Bench press strength rating: _____

Strength Ratings for the Maximum Bench Press Test

			Pounds Lifted/Body Weight (lb)			
Men	*Very Poor*	*Poor*	*Fair*	*Good*	*Excellent*	*Superior*
Age: Under 20	Below 0.89	0.89–1.05	1.06–1.18	1.19–1.33	1.34–1.75	Above 1.75
20–29	Below 0.88	0.88–0.98	0.99–1.13	1.14–1.31	1.32–1.62	Above 1.62
30–39	Below 0.78	0.78–0.87	0.88–0.97	0.98–1.11	1.12–1.34	Above 1.34
40–49	Below 0.72	0.72–0.79	0.80–0.87	0.88–0.99	1.00–1.19	Above 1.19
50–59	Below 0.63	0.63–0.70	0.71–0.78	0.79–0.89	0.90–1.04	Above 1.04
60 and over	Below 0.57	0.57–0.65	0.66–0.71	0.72–0.81	0.82–0.93	Above 0.93
Women						
Age: Under 20	Below 0.53	0.53–0.57	0.58–0.64	0.65–0.76	0.77–0.87	Above 0.87
20–29	Below 0.51	0.51–0.58	0.59–0.69	0.70–0.79	0.80–1.00	Above 1.00
30–39	Below 0.47	0.47–0.52	0.53–0.59	0.60–0.69	0.70–0.81	Above 0.81
40–49	Below 0.43	0.43–0.49	0.50–0.53	0.54–0.61	0.62–0.76	Above 0.76
50–59	Below 0.39	0.39–0.43	0.44–0.47	0.48–0.54	0.55–0.67	Above 0.67
60 and over	Below 0.38	0.38–0.42	0.43–0.46	0.47–0.53	0.54–0.71	Above 0.71

SOURCE: Based on norms from The Cooper Institute of Aerobic Research, Dallas, Texas; from *The Physical Fitness Specialist Manual*, revised 2002. Used with permission.

Predicting 1 RM from Multiple-Repetition Lifts Using Free Weights

Instead of doing the 1-RM maximum strength bench press test, you can predict your 1 RM from multiple-repetition lifts.

Instructions

1. Choose a weight you think you can bench press five times.
2. Follow the instructions for lifting the weight given in the Maximum Bench Press Test.
3. Do as many repetitions of the bench press as you can. A repetition counts only if done correctly.
4. Refer to the chart on p. 125, or calculate predicted 1 RM using the Brzycki equation:

    1 RM = *weight*/(1.0278 − [0.0278 × *number of repetitions*])

    1 RM = _____ lb × (1.0278 − [0.0278 × _____ repetitions]) = _____

5. Divide your predicted 1-RM value by your body weight.

    1 RM _____ lb ÷ body weight _____ lb = _____

6. Find this ratio in the table above to determine your bench press strength rating. Record the rating here and in the chart at the end of the lab.

    Bench press strength rating: _____

Weight Lifted (lb)	Repetitions											
	1	2	3	4	5	6	7	8	9	10	11	12
66	66	68	70	72	74	77	79	82	85	88	91	95
77	77	79	82	84	87	89	92	96	99	103	107	111
88	88	91	93	96	99	102	106	109	113	117	122	127
99	99	102	105	108	111	115	119	123	127	132	137	143
110	110	113	116	120	124	128	132	137	141	147	152	158
121	121	124	128	132	136	141	145	150	156	161	168	174
132	132	136	140	144	149	153	158	164	170	176	183	190
143	143	147	151	156	161	166	172	178	184	191	198	206
154	154	158	163	168	173	179	185	191	198	205	213	222
165	165	170	175	180	186	192	198	205	212	220	229	238
176	176	181	186	192	198	204	211	219	226	235	244	254
187	187	192	198	204	210	217	224	232	240	249	259	269
198	198	204	210	216	223	230	238	246	255	264	274	285
209	209	215	221	228	235	243	251	259	269	279	289	301
220	220	226	233	240	248	256	264	273	283	293	305	317
231	231	238	245	252	260	268	277	287	297	308	320	333
242	242	249	256	264	272	281	290	300	311	323	335	349
253	253	260	268	276	285	294	304	314	325	337	350	364
264	264	272	280	288	297	307	317	328	340	352	366	380
275	275	283	291	300	309	319	330	341	354	367	381	396
286	286	294	303	312	322	332	343	355	368	381	396	412
297	297	305	314	324	334	345	356	369	382	396	411	428
308	308	317	326	336	347	358	370	382	396	411	427	444

SOURCE: Brzycki, M. 1993. Strength testing—predicting a one-rep max from reps to fatigue. *The Journal of Physical Education, Recreation and Dance* 64: 88–90.

Functional Leg Strength Tests

The following tests assess functional leg strength using squats. Most people do squats improperly, increasing their risk of knee and back pain. Before you add weight-bearing squats to your weight training program, you should determine your functional leg strength, check your ability to squat properly, and give yourself a chance to master squatting movements. The following leg strength tests will help you in each of these areas.

These tests are progressively more difficult, so do not move to the next test until you have scored at least a 3 on the current test. On each test, give yourself a rating of 0, 1, 3, or 5, as described in the instructions that follow the fifth test.

1. Chair Squat

Instructions

1. Sit up straight in a chair with your back resting against the backrest and your arms at your sides. Your feet should be placed more than shoulder-width apart so that you can get them under the body.

2. Begin the motion of rising out of the chair by flexing (bending) at the hips—not the back. Then squat up using a hip hinge movement (no spine movement). Stand without rocking forward, bending your back, or using external support, and keep your head in a neutral position.

3. Return to the sitting position while maintaining a straight back and keeping your weight centered over your feet. Your thighs should abduct (spread) as you sit back in the chair. Use your rear hip and thigh muscles as much as possible as you sit.

Do five repetitions.

Your rating: _____

(See rating instructions that follow.)

2. Single-Leg Step-Up

Instructions

1. Stand facing a bench, with your right foot placed on the middle of the bench, right knee bent at 90 degrees, and arms at your sides.
2. Step up on the bench until your right leg is straight, maximizing the use of the hip muscles.
3. Return to the starting position. Keep your hips stable, back straight, chest up, shoulders back, and head neutral during the entire movement.

Do five repetitions for each leg.

Your rating: _____

(See rating instructions that follow.)

3. Unweighted Squat

Instructions

1. Stand with your feet placed slightly more than shoulder-width apart, toes pointed out slightly, hands on hips or across your chest, head neutral, and back straight. Center your weight over your arches or slightly behind.
2. Squat down, keeping your weight centered over your arches and actively flexing (bending) your hips until your legs break parallel. During the movement, keep your back straight, shoulders back, and chest out, and let your thighs part to the side so that you are "squatting between your legs."
3. Push back up to the starting position, hinging at the hips and not with the spine, maximizing the use of the rear hip and thigh muscles, and maintaining a straight back and neutral head position.

Do five repetitions.

Your rating: _____

(See rating instructions that follow.)

4. Single-Leg Lunge-Squat with Rear-Foot Support

Instructions

1. Stand about 3 feet in front of a bench (with your back to the bench).
2. Place the instep of your left foot on the bench, and put most of your weight on your right leg (your left leg should be bent), with your hands at your sides.
3. Squat on your right leg until your thigh is parallel with the floor. Keep your back straight, chest up, shoulders back, and head neutral.
4. Return to the starting position.

   Do three repetitions for each leg.

   Your rating: _____

   (See rating instructions that follow.)

5. Single-Leg Squat from a Bench

Preparation

This exercise is the most difficult of the functional leg tests. Use spotters if you haven't done this exercise before or if you do not have the leg strength to perform three repetitions easily.

Instructions

1. Stand on the middle of a bench with your weight on your right leg and your arms extended in front of you. During the test, maintain a straight back and keep your weight over the arches of your feet.
2. Squat down on your right leg until your thigh is parallel with the ground, maximizing the use of your rear hip and thigh muscles. Do not rock forward on your toes or bend at the waist, and maintain a neutral head position.
3. Return to the starting position (stand up) by straightening your right hip and knee, maximizing the use of your rear hip and thigh muscles.

   Perform three repetitions for each leg.

   Your rating: _____

   (See rating instructions that follow.)

Rating Your Functional Leg Strength Test Results

5 points: Performed the exercise properly with good back and thigh position, weight centered over the middle or rear of the foot, chest out, and shoulders back; good use of hip muscles on the way down and on the way up, with head in a neutral position throughout the movement; maintained good form during all repetitions; abducted (spread) the thighs on the way down during chair squats and double-leg squats; for single-leg exercises, showed good strength on both sides; for single-leg lunge-squat with rear-foot support, maintained straight back, and knees stayed behind toes.

3 points: Weight was forward on the toes, with some rounding of the back; used thigh muscles excessively, with little use of hip muscles; head and chest were too far forward; showed little abduction of the thighs during double-leg squats; when going down for single-leg exercises, one side was stronger than the other; form deteriorated with repetitions; for single-leg lunge-squat with rear-foot support and single-leg squat from a bench, could not reach parallel (thigh parallel with floor).

1 point: Had difficulty performing the movement, rocking forward and rounding back badly; used thigh muscles excessively, with little use of hip muscles on the way up or on the way down; chest and head were forward; on unweighted squats, had difficulty reaching parallel; and showed little abduction of the thighs; on single-leg exercises, one leg was markedly stronger than the other; could not perform multiple repetitions.

0 points: Could not perform the exercise.

Summary of Results

Maximum bench press test from either the 1-RM test or the multiple-repetition test: Weight pressed: _____ lb Rating: _____

Functional leg strength tests (0–5): Chair squat: _____ Single-leg step-up: _____ Unweighted squat: _____

Single-leg lunge-squat with rear-foot support: _____ Single-leg squat from a bench: _____

Remember that muscular strength is specific: Your ratings may vary considerably for different parts of your body.

Using Your Results

How did you score? Are you surprised by your ratings for muscular strength? Are you satisfied with your current ratings?

If you're not satisfied, set realistic goals for improvement:

Are you satisfied with your current level of muscular strength as evidenced in your daily life—for example, your ability to lift objects, climb stairs, and engage in sports and recreational activities?

If you're not satisfied, set realistic goals for improvement:

What should you do next? Enter the results of this lab in the Preprogram Assessment column in Appendix D. If you've set goals for improvement, begin planning your strength training program by completing the plan in Lab 4.3. After several weeks of your program, complete this lab again and enter the results in the Postprogram Assessment column of Appendix D. How do the results compare?

LAB 4.2 Assessing Your Current Level of Muscular Endurance

For best results, don't do any strenuous weight training within 48 hours of any test. To assess endurance of the abdominal muscles, perform the curl-up test. To assess endurance of muscles in the upper body, perform the push-up test. To assess endurance of the muscles, perform the squat endurance test.

The Curl-Up Test

Equipment

1. Four 6-inch strips of self-stick Velcro or heavy tape
2. Ruler
3. Partner
4. Mat (optional)

Preparation

Affix the strips of Velcro or long strips of tape on the mat or testing surface. Place the strips 3 inches apart.

Instructions

1. Start by lying on your back on the floor or mat, arms straight and by your sides, shoulders relaxed, palms down and on the floor, and fingers straight. Adjust your position so that the longest fingertip of each hand touches the end of the near strip of Velcro or tape. Your knees should be bent about 90 degrees, with your feet about 12–18 inches from your buttocks.

2. To perform a curl-up, flex your spine while sliding your fingers across the floor until the fingertips of each hand reach the second strip of Velcro or tape. Then return to the starting position; the shoulders must be returned to touch the mat between curl-ups, but the head need not touch. Shoulders must remain relaxed throughout the curl-up, and feet and buttocks must stay on the floor. Breathe easily, exhaling during the lift phase of the curl-up; do not hold your breath.

3. Once your partner says "go," perform as many curl-ups as you can at a steady pace with correct form. Your partner counts the curl-ups you perform and calls a stop to the test if she or he notices any incorrect form or drop in your pace.

Number of curl-ups: _____

Rating Your Curl-Up Test Result

Your score is the number of completed curl-ups. Refer to the appropriate portion of the table for a rating of your abdominal muscular endurance. Record your rating below and in the summary at the end of this lab.

Rating: _____

Ratings for the Curl-Up Test

	Number of Curl-Ups					
Men	*Very Poor*	*Poor*	*Average*	*Good*	*Excellent*	*Superior*
Age: 16–19	Below 48	48–57	58–64	65–74	75–93	Above 93
20–29	Below 46	46–54	55–63	64–74	75–93	Above 93
30–39	Below 40	40–47	48–55	56–64	65–81	Above 81
40–49	Below 38	38–45	46–53	54–62	63–79	Above 79
50–59	Below 36	36–43	44–51	52–60	61–77	Above 77
60–69	Below 33	33–40	41–48	49–57	58–74	Above 74
Women						
Age: 16–19	Below 42	42–50	51–58	59–67	68–84	Above 84
20–29	Below 41	41–51	52–57	58–66	67–83	Above 83
30–39	Below 38	38–47	48–56	57–66	67–85	Above 85
40–49	Below 36	36–45	46–54	55–64	65–83	Above 83
50–59	Below 34	34–43	44–52	53–62	63–81	Above 81
60–69	Below 31	31–40	41–49	50–59	60–78	Above 78

SOURCE: Ratings based on norms calculated from data collected by Robert Lualhati on 4545 college students, 16–80 years of age, at Skyline College, San Bruno, California. Used with permission.

The Push-Up Test

Equipment: Mat or towel (optional)

Preparation

In this test, you will perform either standard push-ups or modified push-ups, in which you support yourself with your knees. The Cooper Institute developed the ratings for this test with men performing push-ups and women performing modified push-ups. Biologically, males tend to be stronger than females; the modified technique reduces the need for upper-body strength in a test of muscular endurance. Therefore, for an accurate assessment of upper-body endurance, men should perform standard push-ups and women should perform modified push-ups. However, in using push-ups as part of a strength training program, individuals should choose the technique most appropriate for increasing their level of strength and endurance—regardless of gender.

Instructions

1. *For push-ups:* Start in the push-up position with your body supported by your hands and feet. *For-modified push-ups:* Start in the modified push-up position with your body supported by your hands and knees. *For both positions,* keep your arms and your back straight and your fingers pointed forward.

2. Lower your chest to the floor with your back straight, and then return to the starting position.
3. Perform as many push-ups or modified push-ups as you can without stopping.

   Number of push-ups: _____ or number of modified push-ups: _____

Rating Your Push-Up Test Result

Your score is the number of completed push-ups or modified push-ups. Refer to the appropriate portion of the table for a rating of your upper-body endurance. Record your rating below and in the summary at the end of this lab.

Rating: _____

Ratings for the Push-Up and Modified Push-Up Tests

Men			Number of Push-Ups			
	Very Poor	*Poor*	*Fair*	*Good*	*Excellent*	*Superior*
Age: 18–29	Below 22	22–28	29–36	37–46	47–61	Above 61
30–39	Below 17	17–23	24–29	30–38	39–51	Above 51
40–49	Below 11	11–17	18–23	24–29	30–39	Above 39
50–59	Below 9	9–12	13–18	19–24	25–38	Above 38
60 and over	Below 6	6–9	10–17	18–22	23–27	Above 27

Women			Number of Modified Push-Ups			
	Very Poor	*Poor*	*Fair*	*Good*	*Excellent*	*Superior*
Age: 18–29	Below 17	17–22	23–29	30–35	36–44	Above 44
30–39	Below 11	11–18	19–23	24–30	31–38	Above 38
40–49	Below 6	6–12	13–17	18–23	24–32	Above 32
50–59	Below 6	6–11	12–16	17–20	21–27	Above 27
60 and over	Below 2	2–4	5–11	12–14	15–19	Above 19

SOURCE: Based on norms from The Cooper Institute of Aerobic Research, Dallas, Texas; from *The Physical Fitness Specialist Manual*, revised 2002. Used with permission.

The Squat Endurance Test

Instructions

1. Stand with your feet placed slightly more than shoulder width apart, toes pointed out slightly, hands on hips or across your chest, head neutral, and back straight. Center your weight over your arches or slightly behind.

2. Squat down, keeping your weight centered over your arches, until your thighs are parallel with the floor. Push back up to the starting position, maintaining a straight back and neutral head position.

3. Perform as many squats as you can without stopping.

   Number of squats: _____

Rating Your Squat Endurance Test Result

Your score is the number of completed squats. Refer to the appropriate portion of the table for a rating of your leg muscular endurance. Record your rating below and in the summary at the end of this lab.

Rating: _____

Ratings for the Squat Endurance Test

Men			Number of Squats Performed				
	Very Poor	*Poor*	*Below Average*	*Average*	*Above Average*	*Good*	*Excellent*
Age 18–25	<25	25–30	31–34	35–38	39–43	44–49	>49
26–35	<22	22–28	29–30	31–34	35–39	40–45	>45
36–45	<17	17–22	23–26	27–29	30–34	35–41	>41
46–55	<9	13–17	18–21	22–24	25–38	29–35	>35
56–65	<9	9–12	13–16	17–20	21–24	25–31	>31
65+	<7	7–10	11–14	15–18	19–21	22–28	>28

Women							
	Very Poor	*Poor*	*Below Average*	*Average*	*Above Average*	*Good*	*Excellent*
Age 18–25	<18	18–24	25–28	29–32	33–36	37–43	>43
26–35	<20	13–20	21–24	25–28	29–32	33–39	>39
36–45	<7	7–14	15–18	19–22	23–26	27–33	>33
46–55	<5	5–9	10–13	14–17	18–21	22–27	>27
56–65	<3	3–6	7–9	10–12	13–17	18–24	>24
65+	<2	2–4	5–10	11–13	14–16	17–23	>23

SOURCE: www.topendsports.com/testing/tests/home-squat.htm

Summary of Results

Curl-up test: Number of curl-ups: _____ Rating: _____

Push-up test: Number of push-ups: _____ Rating: _____

Squat endurance test: Number of squats: _____ Rating: _____

Remember that muscular endurance is specific: Your ratings may vary considerably for different parts of your body.

Using Your Results

How did you score? Are you surprised by your ratings for muscular endurance? Are you satisfied with your current ratings?

If you're not satisfied, set realistic goals for improvement:

Are you satisfied with your current level of muscular endurance as evidenced in your daily life—for example, your ability to carry groceries or your books, hike, and do yard work?

If you're not satisfied, set realistic goals for improvement:

What should you do next? Enter the results of this lab in the Preprogram Assessment column in Appendix D. If you've set goals for improvement, begin planning your strength training program by completing the plan in Lab 4.3. After several weeks of your program, complete this lab again and enter the results in the Postprogram Assessment column of Appendix D. How do the results compare?

LAB 4.3 Designing and Monitoring a Strength Training Program

1. *Set goals*. List goals for your strength training program. Your goals can be specific or general, short or long term. In the first section, include specific, measurable goals that you can use to track the progress of your fitness program—for example, raising your upper-body muscular strength rating from fair to good or being able to complete 10 repetitions of a lat pull with 125 pounds of resistance. In the second section, include long-term and more qualitative goals, such as improving self-confidence and reducing your risk for back pain.

Specific Goals: Current Status   Final Goals

_____   _____

_____   _____

_____   _____

Other goals: _____

_____

2. *Choose exercises*. Based on your goals, choose 8–10 exercises to perform during each weight training session. If your goal is general training for wellness, use one of the sample programs in Figure 4.4 (p. 102) and on pp. 111–119. List your exercises and the muscles they develop in your program plan.

3. *Frequency: Choose the number of training sessions per week*. Work out at least 2 nonconsecutive days per week. Indicate the days you will train in your program plan; be sure to include days of rest to allow your body to recover.

4. *Intensity: Choose starting weights*. Experiment with different amounts of weight until you settle on a good starting weight, one that you can lift easily for 10–12 repetitions. As you progress in your program, add more weight. Fill in the starting weight for each exercise in your program plan.

5. *Time: Choose a starting number of sets and repetitions*. Include at least 1 set of 8–12 repetitions of each exercise. (When you add weight, you may have to decrease the number of repetitions slightly until your muscles adapt to the heavier load.) If your program is focusing on strength alone, your sets can contain fewer repetitions using a heavier load. If you are over approximately age 50–60, your sets should contain more repetitions (10–15) using a lighter load. Fill in the starting number of sets and repetitions of each exercise in your program plan.

6. *Monitor your progress*. Use the workout card on the next page to monitor your progress and keep track of exercises, weights, sets, and repetitions.

Program Plan for Weight Training

Exercise	Muscle(s) Developed	Frequency (check ✓)							Intensity: Weight (lb)	Time	
		M	T	W	Th	F	Sa	Su		Repetitions	Sets

WORKOUT CARD FOR _____

Exercise/Date	Wt	Sets	Reps	Wt	Sets	Reps	Wt	Sets	Reps	Wt	Sets	Reps	Wt	Sets	Reps	Wt	Sets	Reps	Wt	Sets	Reps	Wt	Sets	Reps	Wt	Sets	Reps	Wt	Sets	Reps	Wt	Sets	Reps	Wt	Sets	Reps

LOOKING AHEAD >>>>>

AFTER READING THIS CHAPTER, YOU SHOULD BE ABLE TO:

- Describe the potential benefits of flexibility and stretching exercises
- List the factors that affect the flexibility in a joint
- Explain the different types of stretching exercises and how they affect muscles
- Describe the intensity, duration, and frequency of stretching exercises that will develop the most flexibility with the lowest risk of injury
- List safe stretching exercises for major joints
- Describe how low-back pain can be prevented and managed

FLEXIBILITY AND LOW-BACK HEALTH

5

TEST YOUR KNOWLEDGE

1. Stretching exercises should be performed

   a. at the start of a warm-up.
   b. first thing in the morning.
   c. after endurance exercise or strength training.

2. If you injure your back, it's usually best to rest in bed until the pain is completely gone.

True or false?

3. It is better to hold a stretch for a short time than to "bounce" while stretching.

True or false?

ANSWERS

1. c. It's best to do stretching exercises when your muscles are warm. Stretching muscles before exercise may temporarily reduce their explosive strength and interfere with neuromuscular control.

2. FALSE. Prolonged bed rest may actually worsen back pain. Limit bed rest to a day or less, treat pain and inflammation with cold and then heat, and begin moderate physical activity as soon as possible.

3. TRUE. "Bouncing" during stretching can damage your muscles. This type of stretching, called ballistic stretching, should be used only by well-conditioned athletes for specific purposes. A person of average fitness should stretch slowly, holding each stretch for 15–30 seconds.

FIT AND WELL ONLINE LEARNING CENTER www.mhhe.com/fahey

Visit the *Fit and Well* Online Learning Center for resources that will help you get the most out of your course!

- Study and review aids include practice quizzes, glossary flashcards, chapter summaries, learning objectives, PowerPoint presentations, Common Questions Answered, student handouts, crossword puzzles, Internet activities, and links to wellness Web sites.
- Behavior change tools include a daily fitness and nutrition journal, a behavior change workbook, sample behavior change plans, and blank behavior change logs to print and use.
- The Chapter 5 resources also include video clips showing how to do all the flexibility and low-back exercises described and illustrated in the chapter (look for the video icon).

Flexibility—the ability of a joint to move through its normal, full **range of motion**—is important for general fitness and wellness. Flexibility is a highly adaptable physical fitness component. It increases in response to a regular program of stretching exercises and decreases with inactivity. Flexibility is also specific: Good flexibility in one joint doesn't necessarily mean good flexibility in another. Flexibility can be increased through stretching exercises for all major joints.

This chapter describes the factors that affect flexibility and the benefits of maintaining good flexibility. It provides guidelines for assessing your current level of flexibility and putting together a successful stretching program. It also examines the common problem of low-back pain.

TYPES OF FLEXIBILITY

There are two types of flexibility:

- *Static flexibility* is the ability to hold an extended position at one end or point in a joint's range of motion. For example, static flexibility determines how far you can extend your arm across the front of your body or out to the side. Static flexibility depends on your ability to tolerate stretched muscles, the structure of your joints, and the tightness of muscles, tendons, and ligaments.
- *Dynamic flexibility* is the ability to move a joint through its range of motion with little resistance. For example, dynamic flexibility affects your ability to pitch a ball or swing a golf club. Dynamic flexibility depends on static flexibility, but it also involves strength, coordination, and resistance to movement.

Dynamic flexibility is important for daily activities and sports. Because static flexibility is easier to measure and better researched, however, most assessment tests and stretching programs target that type of flexibility.

WHAT DETERMINES FLEXIBILITY?

The flexibility of a joint is affected by its structure, by muscle elasticity and length, and by nervous system regulation. Some factors—joint structure, for example—can't be changed. Other factors, such as the length of resting muscle fibers, can be changed through exercise; these factors should be the focus of a program to develop flexibility.

Joint Structure

The amount of flexibility in a joint is determined in part by the nature and structure of the joint (Figure 5.1). Hinge joints such as those in your fingers and knees allow only limited forward and backward movement; they lock when fully extended. Ball-and-socket joints like the hip enable movement in many different directions and have a greater range of motion. Major joints are surrounded by

FIGURE 5.1 Basic joint structure. A moveable joint is surrounded by a fibrous joint capsule that provides support and stability. The bone surfaces within the joint are lined with cartilage and separated by synovial fluid to cushion the bones and reduce friction as the joint moves. Ligaments can be found both inside and outside the joint capsule and serve to strengthen and reinforce the joint.

joint capsules, semielastic structures that give joints strength and stability but limit movement.

Heredity plays a part in joint structure and flexibility; for example, although everyone has a broad range of motion in the ball-and-socket hip joint, not everyone can do a split. Gender may also play a role. Some studies have found that women on average have greater flexibility in certain joints.

Muscle Elasticity and Length

Soft tissues—including skin, muscles, tendons, and ligaments—also limit the flexibility of a joint. Muscle tissue is the key to developing flexibility because it can be lengthened if it is regularly stretched. The most important component of muscle tissue related to flexibility is the connective tissue that surrounds and envelops every part of muscle tissue, from individual muscle fibers to entire muscles. Connective tissue provides structure, elasticity, and bulk and makes up about 30% of muscle mass. Two principal types of connective tissue are **collagen**—white fibers that provide structure and support—and **elastin**—yellow fibers that are elastic and flexible. Muscles contain both collagen and elastin, closely intertwined, so muscle tissue exhibits the properties of both types of fibers. A recently discovered structural protein in muscles called *titin* also has elastic properties and contributes to flexibility.

When a muscle is stretched, the wavelike elastin fibers straighten; when the stretch is relieved, they rapidly snap back to their resting position. If gently and regularly stretched, connective tissues may lengthen and flexibility may improve. Without regular stretching, the process reverses: These tissues shorten, resulting in decreased flexibility. Regular stretching may contribute to flexibility by lengthening muscle fibers through the addition of contractile units called *sarcomeres.*

The amount of stretch a muscle will tolerate is limited, and as the limits of its flexibility are reached, connective tissue becomes more brittle and may rupture if overstretched. A safe and effective program stretches muscles enough to slightly elongate the tissues but not so much that they are damaged. Research has shown that flexibility is improved best by stretching when muscles are warm (following exercise or the application of heat) and the stretch is applied gradually and conservatively. Sudden, high-stress stretching is less effective and can lead to muscle damage.

Nervous System Regulation

Nerves that send information about the muscular and skeletal systems to the nervous system are called **proprioceptors.** When these nerves detect any change in the position or force of muscles and joints, they send signals to the spine and brain, which in turn send signals back to the muscles to coordinate muscle action in ways that protect muscles and tendons from injury. They help control the speed, strength, and coordination of muscle contractions.

When a muscle is stretched (lengthened), proprioceptors detect the amount and rate of the change in muscle length. The nerves send a signal to the spinal cord, which then sends a signal back to the same muscle, triggering a muscle contraction that resists the change in muscle length. Another signal is sent to the antagonist muscle, causing it to relax, which further facilitates contraction of the stretched muscle. These reflexes occur frequently in active muscles and allow for fine control of muscle length and movement.

Small movements that only slightly stimulate these nerves cause small reflex actions. Rapid, powerful, and sudden changes in muscle length strongly stimulate the receptors and can cause large and powerful reflex muscle contractions. Thus, stretches that involve rapid, bouncy movements can be dangerous and cause injury because each bounce causes a reflex contraction, and so a muscle might be stretching at the same time it is contracting. Performing a gradual stretch and then holding it allows the proprioceptors to adjust to the new muscle length and to reduce the signals sent to the spine, thereby allowing muscles to lengthen and, over time, improving flexibility.

The stretching technique called *proprioceptive neuromuscular facilitation (PNF),* described on p. 140, takes advantage of nerve activity to improve flexibility. For example, contracting a muscle prior to stretching it can help allow the muscle to stretch farther. The advanced strength training technique called plyometrics, described in Chapter 4, also takes advantage of the patterns of nervous system action in stretching and contracting muscles.

Modifying nervous control through movement and specific exercises is the best way to improve the functional range of motion. Stretching regularly trains all of the proprioceptors to allow greater lengthening of the muscles. Proprioceptors adapt very quickly to stretching (or lack of stretching), so frequent training is beneficial for developing flexibility. It is important to note that stretching before exercising can disturb proprioceptors and interfere with motor (movement) control during exercise. This is another good reason to stretch after exercising.

BENEFITS OF FLEXIBILITY AND STRETCHING EXERCISES

Good flexibility provides benefits for the entire musculoskeletal system; it may also prevent injuries and soreness and improve performance in all physical activities.

Joint Health

Good flexibility is essential to good joint health. When the muscles and other tissues that support a joint are tight, the joint is subject to abnormal stresses that can cause joint deterioration. For example, tight thigh muscles cause excessive pressure on the kneecap, leading to pain in the knee joint. Poor joint flexibility can also cause abnormalities in joint lubrication, leading to deterioration of the sensitive cartilage cells lining the joint; pain and further joint injury can result.

Improved flexibility can greatly improve your quality of life, particularly as you get older. People tend to exercise

range of motion   The full motion possible in a joint.

joint capsules   Semielastic structures, composed primarily of connective tissue, that surround major joints.

soft tissues   Tissues of the human body that include skin, fat, linings of internal organs and blood vessels, connective tissues, tendons, ligaments, muscles, and nerves.

collagen   White fibers that provide structure and support in connective tissue.

elastin   Yellow fibers that make connective tissue flexible.

proprioceptor   A nerve that sends information about the muscular and skeletal systems to the nervous system.

QUESTIONS FOR CRITICAL THINKING AND REFLECTION
Have you ever noticed that you are markedly more or less flexible than your friends or classmates? To what do you attribute these differences? Were you aware that you could increase your flexibility with a regular stretching program? Would it be meaningful to you to do so?

less as they age, leading to loss of joint mobility. Aging also decreases the natural elasticity of muscles, tendons, and joints, resulting in stiffness. The problem is often compounded by arthritis. Good joint flexibility may prevent arthritis, and stretching may lessen pain in people who have the condition. Another benefit of good flexibility for older adults is that it increases balance and stability.

Prevention of Low-Back Pain and Injuries

Low-back pain can be related to poor spinal stability, which puts pressure on the nerves leading out from the spinal column. Strength and flexibility in the back, pelvis, and thighs may help prevent this type of back pain. However, few studies have found that trunk flexibility improves back health or reduces the risk of injury (greater spinal mobility may actually increase the risk of low-back problems in some people). Good hip and knee flexibility do protect the spine from excessive motion during the tasks of daily living.

Some studies show that poor flexibility increases the risk for injury. A general stretching program can be effective in reducing the frequency of injuries, as well as their severity. When injuries occur, flexibility exercises can be used in treatment: They reduce symptoms and help restore normal range of motion in affected joints.

Overstretching—stretching muscles to extreme ranges of motion—may decrease the stability of a joint. Although some activities, such as gymnastics and ballet, require extreme joint movements, such flexibility is not recommended for the average person. In fact, extreme flexibility

may increase the risk of injury in activities such as skiing, basketball, and volleyball. As with other types of exercise, moderation is the key to safe training.

Additional Potential Benefits

• **Relief of aches and pains.** Studying or working in one place for a long time can make your muscles tense. Stretching helps relieve tension, so you can go back to work refreshed and effective.

• **Relief of muscle cramps.** Recent research suggests that exercise-related muscle cramps are caused by increased electrical activity within the affected muscle. The best treatment for muscle cramps is gentle stretching, which reduces the electrical activity and allows the muscle to relax.

• **Improved body position and strength for sports (and life).** Good flexibility lets you assume more efficient body positions and exert force through a greater range of motion. For example, swimmers with more flexible shoulders have stronger strokes because they can pull their arms through the water in the optimal position. Some studies also suggest that flexibility training enhances strength development.

• **Maintenance of good posture and balance.** Good flexibility also contributes to body symmetry and good posture. Bad posture can gradually change your body structures. Sitting in a slumped position, for example, can lead to tightness in the muscles in the front of your chest and overstretching and looseness in the upper spine, causing a rounding of the upper back. This condition, called *kyphosis,* is common in older people. It may be prevented by stretching regularly.

• **Relaxation.** Flexibility exercises reduce mental tension, slow your breathing rate, and reduce blood pressure.

ASSESSING FLEXIBILITY

Because flexibility is specific to each joint, there are no tests of general flexibility. The most commonly used flexibility test is the sit-and-reach test, which rates the flexibility of the muscles in the lower back and hamstrings. To assess your flexibility and identify inflexible joints, complete Lab 5.1.

CREATING A SUCCESSFUL PROGRAM TO DEVELOP FLEXIBILITY

A successful program for developing flexibility includes safe exercises executed with the most effective techniques. Your goal should be to attain normal flexibility in the major joints. Extreme flexibility causes joint instability, which can lead to pain in the back, hips, shoulders, and knees. Balanced flexibility (not too much or too little) provides

MOTIVATION BOOSTER

Inspire yourself. List five benefits of flexibility and stretching exercises that are particularly meaningful to you—for example, preventing back pain and relieving neck pain from long hours of computer work. Put the list in a prominent location, and use it as a motivational tool for beginning and maintaining your stretching program.

QUESTIONS FOR CRITICAL THINKING AND REFLECTION

When you think about the health-related components of fitness, how do you rank flexibility? Is it less important to you than cardiorespiratory endurance or muscular strength? If you place a low priority on flexibility and don't include stretching in your program, why do you think this is the case? What influences have shaped your opinions—the media, teachers, coaches, peers? What can you do to increase your motivation and find time to stretch?

Safe Stretching

- Do stretching exercises statically. Stretch to the point of mild discomfort, hold the position for 15–30 seconds, rest for 30–60 seconds, and repeat, trying to stretch a bit farther.

- Do not stretch to the point of pain. Any soreness after a stretching workout should be mild and last no more than 24 hours. If you are sore for a longer period, you stretched too intensely.

- Relax and breathe easily as you stretch. Inhale through the nose and exhale through pursed lips during the stretch. Try to relax the muscles being stretched.

- Perform all exercises on both sides of your body.

- Increase intensity and duration gradually over time. Improved flexibility takes many months to develop.

- Stretch when your muscles are warm. Do gentle warm-up exercises such as easy jogging or calisthenics before doing a stretching routine.

- There are large individual differences in joint flexibility. Don't feel you have to compete with others during stretching workouts.

- Engage in a variety of physical activities to help you develop well-rounded functional physical fitness and allow you to perform all types of training more safely and effectively.

joint stability and facilitates smooth, economical movement patterns. You can achieve balanced flexibility by performing stretching exercises regularly and by using a variety of stretches and stretching techniques.

Applying the FITT Principle

As with the programs described for developing other health-related components of fitness, the acronym FITT can be used to remember key components of a stretching program: Frequency, Intensity, Time, and Type of exercise.

Frequency The ACSM recommends that stretching exercises be performed a minimum of 2–3 days a week, and ideally 5–7 days a week. Doing these exercises often will provide the most benefits. It's best to stretch when your muscles are warm, so try incorporating stretching into your cool-down after cardiorespiratory endurance exercise or weight training.

Never stretch when your muscles are cold; doing so can increase your risk of injury as well as limit the amount of flexibility you can develop. Although stretching before exercise is a time-honored ritual practiced by athletes in many sports, several studies have found that pre-exercise stretching decreases muscle strength and performance and disturbs neuromuscular control. If your workout involves participation in a sport or high-performance activity, you may be better off stretching after your workout; for moderate-intensity activities like walking or cycling, stretching before your workout is unlikely to impair your performance.

Intensity and Time (Duration) For each exercise, slowly stretch your muscles to the point of slight tension or mild discomfort. Hold the stretch for 15–30 seconds. As you hold the stretch, the feeling of slight tension should slowly subside; at that point, try to stretch a bit farther. Throughout the stretch, try to relax and breathe easily. Rest for about 30–60 seconds between each stretch, and do 2–4 repetitions of each stretch. A complete flexibility workout usually takes about 20–30 minutes (Figure 5.2).

Warm-up 5–10 minutes or following an endurance or strength training workout	Stretching exercises for major joints **Sample program**	
	Exercise	*Areas stretched*
	Head turns and tilts	Neck
	Towel stretch	Triceps, shoulders, chest
	Across-the-body and overhead stretches	Shoulders, upper back, back of arm
	Upper-back stretch	Upper back
	Lateral stretch	Trunk muscles
	Step stretch	Hip, front of thigh
	Side lunge	Inner thigh, hip, calf
	Inner thigh stretch	Inner thigh, hip
	Hip and trunk stretch	Trunk, outer thigh, hip, buttocks, lower back
	Modified hurdler stretch	Back of thigh, lower back
	Alternate leg stretcher	Back of thigh, hip, knee, ankle, buttocks
	Lower-leg stretch	Calf, soleus, Achilles tendon

Frequency: 2–3 days per week (minimum); 5–7 days per week (ideal)

Intensity: Stretch to the point of mild discomfort, not pain

Time (duration): All stretches should be held for 15–30 seconds and performed 2–4 times

Type of activity: Stretching exercises that focus on major joints

FIGURE 5.2   The FITT principle for a flexibility program.

WEB Types of Stretching Techniques Stretching techniques vary from simply stretching the muscles during the course of normal activities to sophisticated methods based on patterns of muscle reflexes. Improper stretching can do more harm than good, so it's important to understand the different types of stretching exercises and how they affect the muscles. (See the box "Safe Stretching" for guidelines on creating a safe and effective stretching program.) Four common techniques are static stretches, ballistic stretches, dynamic stretches, and PNF. These techniques can be performed passively or actively.

STATIC STRETCHING In **static stretching**, each muscle is gradually stretched, and the stretch is held for 15–30 seconds. A slow stretch prompts less reaction from proprioceptors, and the muscles can safely stretch farther than usual. Static stretching is the type most often recommended by fitness experts because it's safe and effective.

The key to this technique is to stretch the muscles and joints to the point where a pull is felt, but not to the point of pain. (One note of caution: Excess static stretching can decrease joint stability and increase the risk of injury; this may be a particular concern for women, who naturally have joints that are less stable and more flexible than men.) The sample stretching program presented later in this chapter features static stretching exercises.

BALLISTIC STRETCHING In **ballistic stretching**, the muscles are stretched suddenly in a forceful bouncing movement. For example, touching the toes repeatedly in rapid succession is a ballistic stretch for the hamstrings. A problem with this technique is that the heightened activity of proprioceptors caused by the rapid stretches can continue for some time, possibly causing injuries during any physical activities that follow. Another concern is that triggering strong responses from the nerves can cause a reflex muscle contraction that makes it harder to stretch. For these reasons, ballistic stretching is usually not recommended, especially for people of average fitness.

Ballistic stretching trains the muscle dynamically, so it can be an appropriate stretching technique for some well-trained athletes. For example, tennis players stretch their hamstrings and quadriceps ballistically when they lunge for a ball during a tennis match; because this movement is part of their sport, they might benefit from ballistic training of these muscle groups.

DYNAMIC (FUNCTIONAL) STRETCHING The emphasis in **dynamic stretching** is on functionally based movements. Dynamic stretching is similar to ballistic stretching in that it includes movement, but it differs in that it does not involve rapid bouncing. Instead, dynamic stretching involves moving the joints through the range of motion used in a specific exercise or sport in an exaggerated but controlled manner; movements are fluid rather than jerky. An example of a dynamic stretch is the lunge walk, in which a person takes slow steps with an exaggerated stride length; in each step, a lunge stretch position is reached.

> ### ! MOTIVATION BOOSTER
> **Reward yourself with stretching.** If you have trouble making time for flexibility training, remember that stretching can be relaxing. Make flexibility workouts your reward after a busy day. Warm up for a few minutes, then stretch to reduce physical and mental tension. The immediate benefits may motivate you to stretch regularly.

Slow dynamic stretches can lengthen the muscles in many directions without developing high tension in the tissues; these stretches elongate the tissues and train the neuromuscular system. Because dynamic stretches are based on sports movements or movements used in daily life, they develop functional flexibility that translates well into activities.

Dynamic stretches are more challenging than static stretches; they require balance and coordination and may carry a greater risk of muscle soreness and injury. People just beginning a flexibility program might want to start off with static stretches and try dynamic stretches only after they are comfortable with static stretching techniques and have improved their flexibility. It is also a good idea to seek expert advice on dynamic stretching technique and program development.

Serious athletes may use dynamic stretches as part of their warm-up before a competitive event or a high-intensity training session in order to move their joints through the range of motion required for the activity. Functional flexibility training can also be combined with functional strength training. For example, lunge curls, which combine dynamic lunges with free weights biceps curls, stretch the hip, thigh, and calf muscles; stabilize the core muscles in the trunk; and build strength in the arm muscles. Many activities build functional flexibility and strength at the same time, including yoga, Pilates, taijiquan, Olympic weight lifting, plyometrics, stability training (including Swiss and Bosu ball exercises), medicine ball exercises, and functional training machines (for example, Life Fitness and Cybex).

PROPRIOCEPTIVE NEUROMUSCULAR FACILITATION (PNF) PNF techniques use reflexes initiated by both muscle and joint nerves to cause greater training effects. The most popular PNF stretching technique is the contract-relax stretching method, in which a muscle is contracted before it is stretched. The contraction activates proprioceptors, causing relaxation in the muscle about to be stretched. For example, in a seated stretch of calf muscles, the first step in PNF is to contract the calf muscles. The individual or a partner can provide resistance for an isometric contraction. Following a brief period of relaxation, the next step is to stretch the calf muscles by pulling the tops of the feet toward the body. A duration of 6 seconds for the contraction and 15–30 seconds for the stretch is recommended. PNF appears to be most effective if the individual pushes hard during the isometric contraction.

Another example of a PNF stretch is the contract-relax-contract pattern. In this technique, begin by contracting the muscle to be stretched and then relaxing it. Next, contract the opposing muscle (the antagonist). Finally, stretch the first muscle. For example, using this technique to stretch the hamstrings (the muscles in the back of the thigh) would require the following steps: Contract the hamstrings;

In passive stretching (top), an outside force—such as pressure exerted by another person—helps move the joint and stretch the muscles. In active stretching (bottom), the force to move the joint and stretch the muscles is provided by a contraction of the opposing muscles.

relax the hamstrings; contract the quadriceps (the muscles in the front of the thigh); stretch the hamstrings.

PNF appears to allow more effective stretching and greater increases in flexibility than static stretching, but it tends to cause more muscle stiffness and soreness. It also usually requires a partner and takes more time.

PASSIVE VERSUS ACTIVE STRETCHING Stretches can be done either passively or actively. In **passive stretching**, an outside force or resistance provided by yourself, a partner, gravity, or a weight helps your joints move through their range of motion. For example, a seated stretch of the hamstring and back muscles can be done by reaching the hands toward the feet until a pull is felt in those muscles. You can achieve a greater range of motion (a more intense stretch) using passive stretching. However, because the stretch is not controlled by the muscles themselves, there is a greater risk of injury. Communication between partners in passive stretching is important

to ensure that joints aren't forced outside their normal functional range of motion.

In **active stretching**, a muscle is stretched by a contraction of the opposing muscle (the muscle on the opposite side of the limb). For example, an active seated stretch of the calf muscles occurs when a person actively contracts the muscles on the top of the shin. The contraction of this opposing muscle produces a reflex that relaxes the muscles to be stretched. The muscle can be stretched farther with a low risk of injury.

The only disadvantage of active stretching is that a person may not be able to produce enough stress (enough stretch) to increase flexibility using only the contraction of opposing muscle groups. The safest and most convenient technique is active static stretching, with an occasional passive assist. For example, you might stretch your calves both by contracting the muscles on the top of your shin and by pulling your feet toward you. This way you combine the advantages of active stretching—safety and the relaxation reflex—with those of passive stretching—greater range of motion. People who are just beginning flexibility training may be better off doing active rather than passive stretches. For PNF techniques, it is particularly important to have a knowledgeable partner.

Making Progress

As with any type of training, you will make progress and improve your flexibility if you stick with your program. Judge your progress by noting your body position while stretching. For example, note how far you can lean forward during a modified hurdler stretch. Repeat the assessment tests that appear in Lab 5.1 periodically; be sure to take the test at the same time of day each time. You will likely notice some improvement after only 2–3 weeks of a stretching program; however, attaining significant improvements will take at least 2 months. By then, you can expect flexibility increases of about 10–20% in many joints.

QUESTIONS FOR CRITICAL THINKING AND REFLECTION

Why do you think improper stretching can do more harm than good? How can stretching cause injury? Of all the types of stretching described, which ones do you think would be safest for you? Which ones appeal to you the most?

static stretching   A technique in which a muscle is slowly and gently stretched and then held in the stretched position.

ballistic stretching   A technique in which muscles are stretched by the force generated as a body part is repeatedly bounced, swung, or jerked.

dynamic stretching   A technique in which muscles are stretched by moving joints slowly and fluidly through their range of motion in a controlled manner; also called *functional stretching*.

passive stretching   A technique in which muscles are stretched by force applied by an outside source.

active stretching   A technique in which muscles are stretched by the contraction of the opposing muscles.

Stretches to Avoid

The safe alternatives listed under each stretch are described and illustrated on pp. 143–146 as part of the complete program of safe flexibility exercises presented in this chapter.

Standing Toe Touch

Problem: Puts excessive strain on the spine.

Alternatives: Modified hurdler stretch (Exercise 10), alternate leg stretcher (Exercise 11), and lower-leg stretch (Exercise 12).

Standing Ankle-to-Buttocks Quadriceps Stretch

Problem: Puts excessive strain on the ligaments of the knee.

Alternative: Step stretch (Exercise 6).

Full Squat with Bent Back

Problem: Puts excessive strain on the ankles, knees, and spine.

Alternatives: Alternate leg stretcher (Exercise 11) and lower-leg stretch (Exercise 12).

Prone Arch

Problem: Puts excessive strain on the spine, knees, and shoulders.

Alternatives: Towel stretch (Exercise 2) and step stretch (Exercise 6).

Standing Hamstring Stretch

Problem: Puts excessive strain on the knee and lower back.

Alternatives: Modified hurdler stretch (Exercise 10) and alternate leg stretcher (Exercise 11).

Yoga Plow

Problem: Puts excessive strain on the neck, shoulders, and back.

Alternatives: Head turns and tilts (Exercise 1), across-the-body and overhead stretches (Exercise 3), and upper-back stretch (Exercise 4).

Hurdler Stretch

Problem: Turning out the bent leg can put excessive strain on the ligaments of the knee.

Alternatives: Modified hurdler stretch (Exercise 10).

Neck Circles

Problem: Puts excessive strain on the neck and cervical disks.

Alternatives: Head turns and tilts (Exercise 1).

Note: Prone leg extensions, in which a person lifts both the chest and the legs while lying on the stomach but without grabbing the ankles, should also be avoided; spine extensions (p. 152) provide a safe alternative.

Exercises to Improve Flexibility: A Sample Program

There are hundreds of exercises that can improve flexibility. Your program should include exercises that work all the major joints of the body by stretching their associated muscle groups (refer back to Figure 5.2). The exercises illustrated here are simple to do and pose a minimum risk of injury. Use these exercises to create a well-rounded program for developing flexibility. Be sure to perform each stretch using the proper technique. Hold each position for 15–30 seconds and perform 2–4 repetitions of each exercise. Avoid exercises that put excessive pressure on your joints (see the box "Stretches to Avoid"). Complete Lab 5.2 when you're ready to start your program.

Exercise 1   Head Turns and Tilts

Instructions:

Head turns Turn your head to the right and hold the stretch. Repeat to the left.

Head tilts Tilt your head to the right and hold the stretch. Repeat to the left.

Areas stretched: Neck

Variation: Place your right palm on your right cheek; try to turn your head to the right as you resist with your hand. Repeat on the left side.

Exercise 2   Towel Stretch

Instructions: Roll up a towel and grasp it with both hands, palms down. With your arms straight, slowly lift the towel back over your head as far as possible. The closer together your hands are, the greater the stretch.

Areas stretched: Triceps, shoulders, chest

Variation: Repeat the stretch with your arms down and the towel behind your back. Grasp the towel with your palms forward and thumbs pointing out. Gently raise your arms behind your back.

Exercise 3   Across-the-Body and Overhead Stretches

Instructions: (a) Keeping your back straight, cross your right arm in front of your body and grasp it with your left hand. Stretch your arm, shoulders, and back by gently pulling your arm as close to your body as possible. Hold.
(b) Bend your right arm over your head, placing your right elbow as close to your right ear as possible. Grasp your right elbow with your left hand over your head. Stretch the back of your arm by gently pulling your right elbow back and toward your head. Hold. Repeat both stretches on your left side.

Areas stretched: Shoulders, upper back, back of the arm (triceps)

a

b

Exercise 4 — Upper-Back Stretch

Instructions: Stand with your feet shoulder-width apart, knees slightly bent, and pelvis tucked under. Clasp your hands in front of your body and press your palms forward.

Areas stretched: Upper back

Variation: In the same position, wrap your arms around your body as if you were giving yourself a hug.

Exercise 5 — Lateral Stretch

Instructions: Stand with your feet shoulder-width apart, knees slightly bent, and pelvis tucked under. Raise one arm over your head and bend sideways from the waist. Support your trunk by placing the hand or forearm of your other arm on your thigh or hip for support. Be sure you bend directly sideways and don't move your body below the waist. Repeat on the other side.

Areas stretched: Trunk muscles

Variation: Perform the same exercise in a seated position.

Exercise 6 — Step Stretch

Instructions: Step forward and flex your forward knee, keeping your knee directly above your ankle. Stretch your other leg back so that it is parallel to the floor. Press your hips forward and down to stretch. Your arms can be at your sides, on top of your knee, or on the ground for balance. Repeat on the other side.

Areas stretched: Hip, front of thigh (quadriceps)

Exercise 7 — Side Lunge

Instructions: Stand in a wide straddle with your legs turned out from your hip joints and your hands on your thighs. Lunge to one side by bending one knee and keeping the other leg straight. Keep your knee directly over your ankle; do not bend it more than 90 degrees. Repeat on the other side.

Areas stretched: Inner thigh, hip, calf

Variation: In the same position, lift the heel of the bent knee to provide additional stretch. The exercise may also be performed with your hands on the floor for balance.

Exercise 8 — Inner Thigh Stretch

Instructions: Sit with the soles of your feet together. Push your knees toward the floor using your hands or forearms.

Areas stretched: Inner thigh, hip

Variation: When you first begin to push your knees toward the floor, use your legs to resist the movement. Then relax and press your knees down as far as they will go.

Exercise 9 — Hip and Trunk Stretch

Instructions: Sit with your left leg straight, right leg bent and crossed over the left knee, and right hand on the floor next to your right hip. Turn your trunk as far as possible to the right by pushing against your right leg with your left forearm or elbow. Keep your right foot on the floor. Repeat on the other side.

Areas stretched: Trunk, outer thigh and hip, buttocks, lower back

Exercise 10 — Modified Hurdler Stretch (Seated Single-Leg Hamstring)

Instructions: Sit with your left leg straight and your right leg tucked close to your body. Reach toward your left ankle as far as possible. Repeat for the other leg.

Areas stretched: Back of the thigh (hamstring), lower back

Variation: As you stretch forward, alternately flex and point the foot of your extended leg.

Exercise 11 — Alternate Leg Stretcher

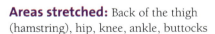

Instructions: Lie flat on your back with both legs straight. **(a)** Grasp your left leg behind the thigh, and pull in to your chest. **(b)** Hold this position, and then extend your left leg toward the ceiling. **(c)** Hold this position, and then bring your left knee back to your chest and pull your toes toward your shin with your left hand. Stretch the back of the leg by attempting to straighten your knee. Repeat for the other leg.

Areas stretched: Back of the thigh (hamstring), hip, knee, ankle, buttocks

Variation: Perform the stretch on both legs at the same time.

a

b

c

Instructions: Stand with one foot about 1–2 feet in front of the other, with both feet pointing forward. **(a)** Keeping your back leg straight, lunge forward by bending your front knee and pushing your rear heel backward. Hold. **(b)** Then pull your back foot in slightly, and bend your back knee. Shift your weight to your back leg. Hold. Repeat on the other side.

Areas stretched: Back of the lower leg (calf, soleus, Achilles tendon)

Variation: Place your hands on a wall and extend one foot back, pressing your heel down to stretch; or stand with the balls of your feet on a step or bench, and allow your heels to drop below the level of your toes.

PREVENTING AND MANAGING LOW-BACK PAIN

More than 85% of Americans experience back pain at some time in their lives. Low-back pain is the second most common ailment in the United States—headache tops the list—and the second most common reason for absences from work and visits to a physician. Low-back pain is estimated to cost as much as $50 billion a year in lost productivity, medical and legal fees, and disability insurance and compensation.

Back pain can result from sudden traumatic injuries, but it is more often the long-term result of weak and inflexible muscles, poor posture, or poor body mechanics during activities like lifting and carrying. Any abnormal strain on the back can result in pain. Most cases of low-back pain clear up within a few weeks or months, but some people have recurrences or suffer from chronic pain.

Function and Structure of the Spine

The spinal column performs many important functions in the body.

- It provides structural support for the body, especially the thorax (upper-body cavity).
- It surrounds and protects the spinal cord.
- It supports much of the body's weight and transmits it to the lower body.
- It serves as an attachment site for a large number of muscles, tendons, and ligaments.
- It allows movement of the neck and back in all directions.

The spinal column is made up of bones called **vertebrae** (Figure 5.3). The spine consists of 7 cervical vertebrae in the neck, 12 thoracic vertebrae in the upper back, and 5 lumbar vertebrae in the lower back. The 9 vertebrae at the base of the spine are fused into two sections and form the sacrum

and the coccyx (tailbone). The spine has four curves: the cervical, thoracic, lumbar, and sacral curves. These curves help bring the body weight supported by the spine in line with the axis of the body.

Although the structure of vertebrae depends on their location on the spine, the different types of vertebrae share

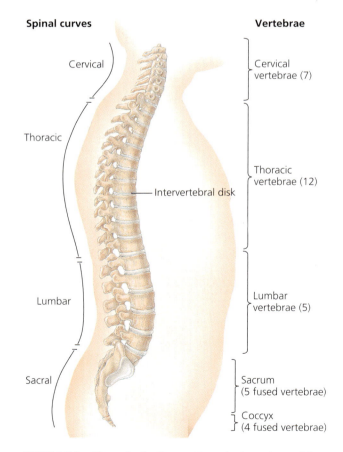

FIGURE 5.3 The spinal column. The spine is made up of five separate regions and has four distinct curves. An intervertebral disk is located between vertebrae.

Spinal cord

Vertebral arch

Intervertebral disk

Vertebral body

Nerve root

FIGURE 5.4 Vertebrae and an intervertebral disk.

common characteristics. Each consists of a body, an arch, and several bony processes (Figure 5.4). The vertebral body is cylindrical, with flattened surfaces where **intervertebral disks** are attached. The vertebral body is designed to carry the stress of body weight and physical activity. The vertebral arch surrounds and protects the spinal cord. The bony processes serve as joints for adjacent vertebrae and attachment sites for muscles and ligaments. **Nerve roots** from the spinal cord pass through notches in the vertebral arch.

Intervertebral disks, which absorb and disperse the stresses placed on the spine, separate vertebrae from each other. Disks are made up of a gel- and water-filled nucleus surrounded by a series of fibrous rings. The liquid nucleus can change shape when it is compressed, allowing the disk to absorb shock. The intervertebral disks also help maintain the spaces between vertebrae where the spinal nerve roots are located.

Core Muscle Fitness

The core muscles include those in the abdomen, pelvic floor, sides of the trunk, back, buttocks, hip, and pelvis. There are 29 of these muscles, attaching to the ribs, hips, spinal column, and other bones in the trunk of the body. As described in Chapter 4, the core muscles stabilize the spine and help transfer force between the upper body and lower body. They stabilize the midsection when you sit, stand, reach, walk, jump, twist, squat, throw, or bend. The muscles on the front, back, and sides of your trunk support your spine when you sit in a chair and fix your midsection as you use your legs to stand up. When hitting a forehand in tennis or batting a softball, most of the force is transferred from the legs and hips, across the core muscles, to the arms. Strong core muscles make movements more forceful and help prevent back pain.

During any dynamic movement, the core muscles work together; some shorten to cause movement, while others contract and hold to provide stability, lengthen to brake the movement, or send signals to the brain about the movements and positions of the muscles and bones (proprioception). When specific core muscles are weak or tired, the

nervous system steps in and uses other muscles. This substitution causes abnormal stresses on the joints, decreases power, and increases the risk of injury. For example, weakness in the transverse abdominis—a muscle deep in the abdomen—creates an unstable spine and can stress muscles and joints in both the upper and lower body.

The best exercises for low-back health are whole-body exercises that force the core muscles to stabilize the spine in many different directions. The low-back exercises presented later in this chapter include several exercises that focus on the core muscles, including the step stretch (lunge), side bridges, and spine extensions. These exercises are generally safe for beginning exercisers and, with physician approval, people with some back pain. More challenging core exercises utilize stability balls or free weights. Stability ball exercises require the core muscles to stabilize the ball (and the body) while performing nearly any type of exercise. Many traditional exercises with free weights can strengthen the core muscles if you do them in a standing position. Weight machines train muscles in isolation, while exercises with free weights done while standing help train the body for real-world movements—an essential principle of core training.

Causes of Back Pain

Back pain can occur at any point along your spine; the lumbar area, because it bears the majority of your weight, is the most common site. Any movement that causes excessive stress on the spinal column can cause injury and pain. The spine is well equipped to bear body weight and the force or stress of body movements along its long axis. However, it is less capable of bearing loads at an angle to its long axis or when the trunk is flexed (bent). You do not have to carry a heavy load or participate in a vigorous contact sport to injure your back. Picking a pencil up from the floor using poor body mechanics—reaching too far out in front of you or bending over with your knees straight, for example—can also result in back pain.

Risk factors associated with low-back pain include age greater than 34 years, degenerative diseases such as arthritis or osteoporosis, a family or personal history of back pain or trauma, a sedentary lifestyle, low job satisfaction, and low socioeconomic status. Smoking increases risk because smoking appears to hasten degenerative changes in the spine. Excess body weight also increases strain on the back, and psychological stress or depression can cause

vertebrae Bony segments composing the spinal column that provide structural support for the body and protect the spinal cord.

intervertebral disk An elastic disk located between adjoining vertebrae, consisting of a gel- and water-filled nucleus surrounded by fibrous rings; serves as a shock absorber for the spinal column.

nerve root The base of each of the 31 pairs of spinal nerves that branch off the spinal cord through spaces between vertebrae.

muscle tension and back pain. Occupations and activities associated with low-back pain are those involving physically hard work, such as frequent lifting, twisting, bending, standing up, or straining in forced positions; those requiring high concentration demands (such as computer programming); and those involving vibrations affecting the entire body (such as truck driving).

Underlying causes of back pain include poor muscle endurance and strength in the core muscles; excess body weight; poor posture or body position when standing, sitting, or sleeping; and poor body mechanics when performing actions like lifting and carrying, or sports movements. Strained muscles, tendons, or ligaments can cause pain and can, over time, lead to injuries to vertebrae, intervertebral disks and surrounding muscles and ligaments.

Stress can cause disks to break down and lose some of their ability to absorb shock. A damaged disk may bulge out between vertebrae and put pressure on a nerve root, a condition commonly referred to as a *slipped disk*. Painful pressure on nerves can also occur if damage to a disk narrows the space between two vertebrae. With age, you lose fluid from the disks, making them more likely to bulge and put pressure on nerve roots. Depending on the amount of pressure on a nerve, symptoms may include numbness in the back, hip, leg, or foot; radiating pain; loss of muscle function; depressed reflexes; and muscle spasm. If the pressure is severe enough, loss of function can be permanent.

Preventing Low-Back Pain

Incorrect posture when standing, sitting, lying, and lifting is responsible for many back injuries. Strategies for maintaining good posture are presented in the box "Good Posture and Low-Back Health." Follow the same guidelines when you engage in sports or recreational activities. Maintain control over your movements, and warm up thoroughly before you exercise. Take special care when lifting weights.

The role of exercise in preventing and treating back pain is still being investigated. However, many experts recommend exercise, especially for people who have already experienced an episode of low-back pain. Regular exercise aimed at increasing muscle endurance and strength in the back and abdomen is often recommended to prevent back pain, as is lifestyle physical activity such as walking. Movement helps lubricate your spinal joints and increases muscle fitness in your trunk and legs. Other lifestyle recommendations for preventing back pain include the following:

- Lose weight, stop smoking, and reduce stress.
- Avoid sitting, standing, or working in the same position for too long. Stand up every hour or half-hour and move around. The cat stretch (p. 151) is a good exercise to perform when you take a break during a long period of sitting.
- Use a supportive seat and a medium-firm mattress. Use lumbar support when driving, particularly for long distances, to prevent muscle fatigue and pain.
- Warm up thoroughly before exercising.
- Progress gradually when attempting to improve strength or fitness.

Managing Acute Back Pain

Sudden back pain usually involves tissue injury. Symptoms may include pain, muscle spasms, stiffness, and inflammation. Many cases of acute back pain go away by themselves within a few days or weeks. You may be able to reduce pain and inflammation by applying cold and then heat (see Chapter 3). Begin with a cold treatment: Apply ice several times a day; once inflammation and spasms subside, you can apply heat using a heating pad or a warm bath. If the pain is bothersome, an over-the-counter, nonsteroidal anti-inflammatory medication such as ibuprofen or naproxen may be helpful; stronger pain medications and muscle relaxants are available by prescription.

Bed rest immediately following the onset of back pain may make you feel better, but it should be of very short duration. Prolonged bed rest—5 days or more—was once thought to be an effective treatment for back pain, but most physicians now advise against it because it may weaken muscles and actually worsen pain. Limit bed rest to one day and begin moderate physical activity as soon as possible. Exercise can increase muscular endurance and flexibility and protect disks from loss of fluid. Three of the back exercises discussed later in the chapter may be particularly helpful following an episode of acute back pain: curl-ups, side bridges, and spine extensions.

See your physician if acute back pain doesn't resolve within a short time. Other warning signals of a more severe problem that requires a professional evaluation include severe pain, numbness, pain that radiates down one or both legs, problems with bladder or bowel control, fever, and rapid weight loss.

Managing Chronic Back Pain

Low-back pain is considered chronic if it persists for more than 3 months. Symptoms vary—some people experience stabbing or shooting pain, and others a steady ache

? **QUESTIONS FOR CRITICAL THINKING AND REFLECTION**

Do you know anyone who suffers from chronic back pain? If so, how has it affected that person's life? How about you—have you ever had back pain? Do you have any of the risk factors listed in the text? If so, what can you do to lower your risk and avoid developing chronic back problems?

Good Posture and Low-Back Health

TAKE CHARGE

Changes in everyday posture and behavior can help prevent and alleviate low-back pain.

- **Lying down.** When resting or sleeping, lie on your side with your knees and hips bent. If you lie on your back place a pillow under your knees. However, do not elevate your knees so much that the curve in your lower spine is flattened. Don't lie on your stomach. Use a medium-firm mattress.

- **Sitting at a computer.** Sit in a slightly reclined position of 100–110 degrees, not an upright 90-degree position. Adjust your chair so your knees are slightly lower than your hips. If your back flattens as you sit, try using a lumbar roll to maintain your back's natural curvature. Place your feet flat on the floor or on a footrest. Place the monitor directly in front of you and adjust it so your eyes are level with the top of the screen; you should be looking slightly downward at the middle of the screen. Adjust the keyboard and mouse so your forearms and wrists are in a neutral position, parallel with the floor.

- **Lifting.** If you need to lower yourself to grasp an object, bend at the knees and hips rather than at the waist. Your feet should be about shoulder-width apart. Lift gradually, keeping your arms straight, by standing up or by pushing with your leg muscles. Keep the object close to your body. Don't twist; if you have to turn with the object, change the position of your feet.

- **Standing.** When you are standing, a straight line should run from the top of your ear through the center of your shoulder, the center of your hip, the back of your kneecap, and the front of your ankle bone. Support your weight mainly on your heels, with one or both knees slightly bent. Try to keep your lower back flat by placing one foot on a stool. Don't let your pelvis tip forward or your back arch. Shift your weight back and forth from foot to foot. Avoid prolonged standing. (To check your posture, stand in a normal way with your back to a wall. Your upper back and buttocks should touch the wall; your heels may be a few inches away. Slide one hand into the space between your lower back and the wall. It should slide in easily but should almost touch both your back and the wall. Adjust your posture as needed, and try to hold this position as you walk away from the wall.)

- **Walking.** Walk with your toes pointed straight ahead. Keep your back flat, head up and centered over your body, and chin in. Swing your arms freely. Don't wear tight or high-heeled shoes. Walking briskly is better for back health than walking slowly.

Yoga for Relaxation and Pain Relief

Certain types of exercise can provide relief from back pain, depending on the pain's underlying cause. Effective exercises stretch the muscles and connective tissue in the hips, stabilize the spine, and strengthen and build endurance in the core muscles of the back and abdomen.

Yoga may be an option for many back pain sufferers because it offers a variety of exercises that target the spine and the core muscles. Yoga is an ancient practice involving slow, gentle movements performed with controlled breathing and focused attention. Yoga practitioners slowly move into a specific posture (called an *asana*) and hold the posture for up to 60 seconds. There are hundreds of asanas, many of which are easy to do and provide good stretches.

Yoga also involves simple breathing exercises that gently stretch the muscles of the upper back while helping the practitioner focus. Yoga experts say that breathing exercises not only encourage relaxation but also clear the mind and can help relieve mild to moderate pain. Yoga enthusiasts end their workouts energized and refreshed but calm and relaxed.

Many medical professionals now recommend yoga for patients with back pain, particularly postures that involve arching and gently stretching the back, such as the cat pose (similar to the cat stretch shown on p. 151) and the child pose (shown here). These are basic asanas that most people can perform repeatedly and hold for a relatively long time.

Because asanas must be performed correctly to be beneficial, qualified instruction is recommended. For those with back pain, physicians advise choosing an instructor who is not only accomplished in yoga but also knowledgeable about back pain and its causes. Such instructors can steer students away from exercises that do more harm than good. It is especially important to choose postures that will benefit the back without worsening the underlying problem. Some asanas can aggravate an injured or painful back if they are performed incorrectly or too aggressively. In fact, a few yoga postures should not be done at all by people with back pain.

If you have back pain, see your physician to determine its cause before beginning any type of exercise program. Even gentle exercise or stretching can be bad for an already injured back, especially if the spinal disks or nerves are involved. For some back conditions, rest or therapy may be better options than exercise, at least in the short term.

---

accompanied by stiffness. Sometimes pain is localized; in other cases, it radiates to another part of the body. Psychological symptoms may also occur. Underlying causes of chronic back pain include injuries, infection, muscle or ligament strains, and disk herniations.

Because symptoms and causes are so varied, different people benefit from different treatment strategies, and researchers have found that many treatments have only limited benefits. Potential treatments include over-the-counter or prescription medications; exercise; physical therapy, massage, yoga, or chiropractic care; acupuncture; percutaneous electrical nerve stimulation (PENS), in which acupuncture-like needles are used to deliver an electrical current; education and advice about posture, exercise, and body mechanics; and surgery (see the box "Yoga for Relaxation and Pain Relief").

Psychological therapy may also be beneficial in some cases. Reducing emotional stress that causes muscle tension can provide direct benefits, and other therapies can help people deal better with chronic pain and its effects on their daily lives. Support groups and expressive writing are strategies that have been found beneficial for people with chronic pain and other conditions.

Exercises for the Prevention and Management of Low-Back Pain

The tests in Labs 5.3 and 5.4 can help you assess low-back muscular endurance and posture. The exercises that follow are designed to help you maintain a healthy back by stretching and strengthening the major muscle groups that affect the back—the abdominal muscles, the muscles along your spine and sides, and the muscles of your hips and thighs. If you have back problems, check with your physician before beginning any exercise program. Perform the exercises slowly and progress very gradually. Stop and consult your physician if any exercise causes back pain. General guidelines for back exercise programs include the following:

• Do low-back exercises at least 3 days per week; many experts recommend that back exercises be done daily.

• Emphasize muscular endurance rather than muscular strength—endurance is more protective.

• Don't do spine exercises involving a full range of motion early in the morning because your disks have a high fluid content early in the day and injuries may occur as a result.

• Engage in regular endurance exercise such as cycling or walking in addition to performing exercises that specifically build muscular endurance and flexibility. Brisk walking with a vigorous arm swing may help relieve back pain. Start with fast walking if your core muscles are weak or you have back pain. After you get in shape, integrate other endurance activities that you enjoy—jogging, cycling, treadmill, elliptical trainer, or stair-climber.

• Be patient and stick with your program. Increased back fitness and pain relief may require as long as 3 months of regular exercise.

LOW-BACK EXERCISES

Exercise 1 — Cat Stretch

Instructions: Begin on all fours with your knees below your hips and your hands below your shoulders. Slowly and deliberately move through a cycle of extension and flexion of your spine. **(a)** Begin by slowly pushing your back up and dropping your head slightly until your spine is extended (rounded). **(b)** Then slowly lower your back and lift your chin slightly until your spine is flexed (relaxed and slightly arched). *Do not press at the ends of the range of motion.* Stop if you feel pain. Do 10 slow, continuous cycles of the movement.

Target: Improved flexibility, relaxation, and reduced stiffness in the spine

Exercise 2 — Step Stretch *(See Exercise 6 in the flexibility program, p. 144.)*

Instructions: Hold each stretch for 15–30 seconds and do 2–4 repetitions on each side.

Target: Improved flexibility, strength, and endurance in the muscles of the hip and the front of the thigh

Exercise 3 — Alternate Leg Stretcher *(See Exercise 11 in the flexibility program, p. 145.)*

Instructions: Hold each stretch for 15–30 seconds and do 2–4 repetitions on each side.

Target: Improved flexibility in the back of the thigh, hip, knee, and buttocks

Exercise 4 — Trunk Twist

Instructions: Lie on your side with top knee bent, lower leg straight, lower arm extended out in front of you on the floor, and upper arm at your side. Push down with your upper knee while you twist your trunk backward. Try to get your shoulders and upper body flat on the floor, turning your head as well. Return to the starting position, and then repeat on the other side. Hold the stretch for 15–30 seconds and do 2–4 repetitions on each side.

Target: Improved flexibility in the lower back and sides

Exercise 5 — Curl-Up

Instructions: Lie on your back with one or both knees bent and arms crossed on your chest or hands under your lower back. Maintain a neutral spine. Tuck your chin in and slowly curl up, one vertebra at a time, as you use your abdominal muscles to lift your head first and then your shoulders. Stop when you can see your knees and hold for 5–10 seconds before returning to the starting position. Do 10 or more repetitions.

Target: Improved strength and endurance in the abdomen

Variation: Add a twist to develop other abdominal muscles. When you have curled up so that your shoulder blades are off the floor, twist your upper body so that one shoulder is higher than the other; reach past your knee with your upper arm. Hold and then return to the starting position. Repeat on the opposite side. Curl-ups can also be done using an exercise ball (see p. 99).

Exercise 6 — Isometric Side Bridge *(See Exercise 11 in the free weights program in Chapter 4, p. 114.)*

Instructions: Hold the bridge position for 10 seconds, breathing normally. Work up to a 60-second hold. Perform one or more repetitions on each side.

Target: Increased strength and endurance in the muscles along the sides of the abdomen

Variation: You can make the exercise more difficult by keeping your legs straight and supporting yourself with your feet and forearm (see Lab 5.3) or with your feet and hand (with elbow straight).

Exercise 7 — Spine Extensions *(See Exercise 10 in the free weights program in Chapter 4, p. 113.)*

Instructions: Hold each position for 10–30 seconds. Begin with one repetition on each side, and work up to several repetitions.

Target: Increased strength and endurance in the back, buttocks, and back of the thighs

Variation: If you have experienced back pain in the past or if this exercise is difficult for you, do the exercise with both hands on the ground rather than with one arm lifted. You can make this exercise more difficult by doing it balancing on an exercise ball. Find a balance point on your chest while lying face down on the ball with one arm and the opposite leg on the ground. Tense your abdominal muscles while reaching and extending with one arm and reaching and extending with the opposite leg. Repeat this exercise using the other arm and leg.

Exercise 8   **Wall Squat (Phantom Chair)**

Instructions: Lean against a wall and bend your knees as though you are sitting in a chair. Support your weight with your legs. Begin by holding the position for 5–10 seconds. Squeeze your gluteal muscles together as you do the exercise. Build up to 1 minute or more. Perform one or more repetitions.

Target: Increased strength and endurance in the lower back, thighs, and abdomen

Exercise 9   **Pelvic Tilt**

Instructions: Lie on your back with knees bent and arms extended to the side. Tilt your pelvis under and try to flatten your lower back against the floor. Tighten your buttock and abdominal muscles while you hold this position for 5–10 seconds. Don't hold your breath. Work up to 10 repetitions of the exercise. Pelvic tilts can also be done standing or leaning against a wall. *Note:* Although this is a popular exercise with many therapists, some experts question the safety of pelvic tilts. Stop if you feel pain in your back at any time during the exercise.

Target: Increased strength and endurance in the abdomen and buttocks

Exercise 10   **Back Bridge**

Instructions: Lie on your back with knees bent and arms extended to the side. Tuck your pelvis under, contract your gluteal muscles, and then lift your tailbone, buttocks, and lower back from the floor. Hold this position for 5–10 seconds with your weight resting on your feet, arms, and shoulders, and then return to the starting position. Work up to 10 repetitions of the exercise.

Target: Increased strength and endurance in the hips and buttocks

Q: Is stretching the same as warming up?

A: No. They are two distinct activities. A warm-up is light exercise that involves moving the joints through the same motions used during the activity; it increases body temperature so your metabolism works better when you're exercising at high intensity. Stretching increases the movement capability of your joints, so you can move more easily with less risk of injury. It is best to stretch at the end of your aerobic or weight training workout, when your muscles are warm. Warmed muscles stretch better than cold ones and are less prone to injury.

Q: How much flexibility do I need?

A: This question is not always easy to answer. If you're involved in a sport such as gymnastics, figure skating, or ballet, you are often required to reach extreme joint motions to achieve success. However, nonathletes do not need to reach these extreme joint positions. In fact, too much flexibility may, in some cases, create joint instability and increase your risk of injury. As with other types of fitness, moderation is the key. You should regularly stretch your major joints and muscle groups but not aspire to reach extreme flexibility.

Q: Can I stretch too far?

A: Yes. As muscle tissue is progressively stretched, it reaches a point where it becomes damaged and may rupture. The greatest danger occurs during passive stretching when a partner is doing the stretching for you. It is critical that your stretching partner not force your joint outside its normal functional range of motion.

Q: Can physical training limit flexibility?

A: Weight training, jogging, or any physical activity will decrease flexibility if the exercises are not performed through a full range of motion. When done properly, weight training increases flexibility. However, because of the limited range of motion used during the running stride, jogging tends to compromise flexibility. It is important for runners to do flexibility exercises for the hamstrings and quadriceps regularly.

Q: Does stretching affect muscular strength?

A: Several recent studies have found that stretching decreases strength, power, and motor control following the stretch. This is one reason some experts suggest that people not stretch as part of their exercise warm-up. It is important to warm up before any workout by engaging in 5–10 minutes of light exercise such as walking or slow jogging. Flexibility training increases muscle strength over time.

For more Common Questions Answered about flexibility and low-back health, visit the Online Learning Center.

TIPS FOR TODAY AND THE FUTURE

To improve and maintain your flexibility, perform stretches that work the major joints at least twice a week.

RIGHT NOW YOU CAN

- Stand up and stretch—do either the upper-back stretch or the across-the-body stretch shown in the chapter.
- Practice the recommended sitting and standing postures suggested in the chapter. If needed, adjust your chair or find something to use as a footrest.

IN THE FUTURE YOU CAN

- Build up your flexibility by incorporating more sophisticated stretching exercises into your routine.
- Increase the frequency of your flexibility workouts to 5 or more days per week.
- Increase the efficiency of your workouts by adding stretching exercises to the cool-down period of your endurance or strength workouts.

SUMMARY

- Flexibility, the ability of joints to move through their full range of motion, is highly adaptable and specific to each joint.

- Range of motion can be limited by joint structure, muscle inelasticity, and proprioceptor activity.

- Developing flexibility depends on stretching the elastic tissues within muscles regularly and gently until they lengthen. Overstretching can make connective tissue brittle and lead to rupture.

- Signals sent between muscle and tendon nerves and the spinal cord can enhance flexibility.

- The benefits of flexibility include preventing abnormal stresses that lead to joint deterioration and possibly reducing the risk of injuries and low-back pain.

- Stretches should be held for 15–30 seconds; perform 2–4 repetitions. Flexibility training should be done a minimum of

2–3 days per week (ideally, 5–7 days per week), preferably following activity, when muscles are warm.

- Static stretching is done slowly and held to the point of mild tension; ballistic stretching consists of bouncing stretches and can lead to injury. Dynamic stretching involves moving joints slowly and fluidly through their range of motion. Proprioceptive neuromuscular facilitation uses muscle receptors in contracting and relaxing a muscle.

- Passive stretching, using an outside force in moving muscles and joints, achieves a greater range of motion (and has a higher injury risk) than active stretching, which uses opposing muscles to initiate a stretch.

- The spinal column consists of vertebrae separated by intervertebral disks. It provides structure and support for the body and protects the spinal cord. The core muscles stabilize the spine and transfer force between the upper and lower body.

- Acute back pain can be treated as a soft tissue injury, with cold treatment followed by application of heat (once swelling subsides); prolonged bed rest is not recommended. A variety of treatments have been suggested for chronic back pain, including regular exercise, physical therapy, acupuncture, education, and psychological therapy.

- In addition to good posture, proper body mechanics, and regular physical activity, a program for preventing low-back pain includes exercises that develop flexibility, strength, and endurance in the muscle groups that affect the lower back.

FOR FURTHER EXPLORATION

BOOKS

Alter, M. J. 2004. *Science of Flexibility,* 3rd ed. Champaign, Ill.: Human Kinetics. *An extremely well-researched book that discusses the scientific basis of stretching exercises and flexibility.*

Anderson, B., and J. Anderson. 2003. *Stretching,* 20th anniv. ed. Bolinas, Calif.: Shelter Publications. *A best-selling exercise book, updated with more than 200 stretches for 60 sports and activities.*

Blahnik, J. 2004. *Full-Body Flexibility.* Champaign, Ill.: Human Kinetics. *Presents a blend of stretching techniques derived from sports training, martial arts, yoga, and Pilates.*

McGill, S. 2006. *Ultimate Back Fitness and Performance, 3rd ed .* Waterloo, Canada: Backfit Pro. *Written by one of the premier researchers in the world on back biomechanics and back pain; describes mechanisms of back pain and exercises and movement patterns for preventing it.*

Nelson, A. G., et al. 2006. *Stretching Anatomy.* Champaign, Ill.: Human Kinetics. *A guide to stretching that features highly detailed illustrations of the muscles that are affected by each exercise.*

ORGANIZATIONS AND WEB SITES

American Academy of Orthopaedic Surgeons. Provides information about a variety of joint problems.
   http://orthoinfo.aaos.org

CUErgo: Cornell University Ergonomics Web Site. Provides information about how to arrange a computer workstation to prevent back pain and repetitive strain injuries, as well as other topics related to ergonomics.
   http://ergo.human.cornell.edu

Exercise: A Guide from the National Institute on Aging. Gives practical advice on fitness for seniors; includes animated instructions for specific flexibility exercises.
   http://weboflife.ksc.nasa.gov/exerciseandaging/toc.html

Georgia State University: Flexibility. Provides information about the benefits of stretching and ways to develop a safe and effective program; includes illustrations of stretches.
   http://www.gsu.edu/~wwwfit/flexibility.html

MedlinePlus Interactive Tutorial: How to Prevent Back Pain. An interactive, illustrated tutorial of the causes and prevention of back pain.
   http://www.nlm.nih.gov/medlineplus/tutorials/
      howtopreventbackpain/htm/index.htm

NIH Back Pain Fact Sheet. Provides basic information on the prevention and treatment of back pain.
   http://www.ninds.nih.gov/disorders/backpain/backpain.htm

Southern California Orthopedic Institute. Provides information on a variety of orthopedic problems, including back injuries; also has illustrations of spinal anatomy.
   http://www.scoi.com

Stretching and Flexibility. Provides information on the physiology of stretching and different types of stretching exercises.
   http://www.ifafitness.com/stretch/index.html

See also the listings for Chapters 2 and 4.

SELECTED BIBLIOGRAPHY

American College of Sports Medicine. 2006. *ACSM's Guidelines for Exercise Testing and Prescription.* Philadelphia: Lippincott Williams and Wilkins.

American College of Sports Medicine. 2006. *ACSM's Resource Manual for Guidelines for Exercise Testing and Prescription,* 5th ed. Philadelphia: Lippincott Williams and Wilkins.

Anton, M. M., et al. 2006. Resistance training increases basal limb blood flow and vascular conductance in aging humans. *Journal of Applied Physiology* 101(5): 1351–1355.

Barnett, A. 2006. Using recovery modalities between training sessions in elite athletes: Does it help? *Sports Medicine* 36(9): 781–796.

Barr, K. P., M. Griggs, and T. Cadby. 2005. Lumbar stabilization: Core concepts and current literature. Part 1. *American Journal of Physical Medicine and Rehabilitation* 84(6): 473–480.

Beach, T. A., et al. 2005. Effects of prolonged sitting on the passive flexion stiffness of the in vivo lumbar spine. *Spine Journal* 5(2): 145–154.

Castellani, J. W., et al. 2006. American College of Sports Medicine position stand: Prevention of cold injuries during exercise. *Medicine and Science in Sports and Exercise* 38(11): 2012–2029.

Davis, D. S., et al. 2005. The effectiveness of three stretching techniques on hamstring flexibility using consistent stretching parameters. *Journal of Strength and Conditioning Research* 19(1): 27–32.

Faigenbaum, A. D., et al. 2006. Dynamic warm-up protocols, with and without a weighted vest, and fitness performance in high school female athletes. *Journal of Athletic Training* 41(4): 357–363.

Fong, D. T., et al. 2007. A systematic review on ankle injury and ankle sprain in sports. *Sports Medicine* (Auckland, New Zealand) 37(1): 73–94.

Friedrich, M., et al. 2005. Long-term effect of a combined exercise and motivational program on the level of disability of patients with chronic low back pain. *Spine* 30(9): 995–1000.

Gajdosik, R. L., et al. 2005. Effects of an eight-week stretching program on the passive-elastic properties and function of the calf muscles of older women. *Clinical Biomechanics* 20(9): 973–983.

Guidetti, L., et al. 2007. Effect of warm up on energy cost and energy sources of a ballet dance exercise. *European Journal of Applied Physiology* 99(3): 275–281.

Hakkinen, A., et al. 2005. Effects of home strength training and stretching versus stretching alone after lumbar disk surgery: A randomized study with a 1-year follow-up. *Archives of Physical Medicine and Rehabilitation* 86(5): 865–870.

Hart, L. 2005. Effect of stretching on sport injury risk: A review. *Clinical Journal of Sports Medicine* 15(2): 113.

Haskell, W. L., et al. 2007. Physical activity and public health: updated recommendation for adults from the American College of Sports Medicine and the American Heart Association. *Circulation.* 116(9): 1081–1093.

Hayden, J. A., M. W. van Tulder, and G. Tomlinson. (2005). Systematic review: Strategies for using exercise therapy to improve outcomes in chronic low back pain. *Annals of Internal Medicine* 142(9): 776–785.

Hurwitz, E. L., H. Morgenstern, and C. Chiao. 2005. Effects of recreational physical activity and back exercises on low back pain and psychological distress: Findings from the UCLA Low Back Pain Study. *American Journal of Public Health* 95(10): 1817–1824.

Kuramoto, A. M. 2006. Therapeutic benefits of Tai Chi exercise: Research review. *Wisconsin Medical Journal* 105(7): 42–46.

Liu-Ambrose, T. Y., et al. 2005. Both resistance and agility training reduce back pain and improve health-related quality of life in older women with low bone mass. *Osteoporosis International,* 9 February [Epub ahead of print].

Malina, R. M. 2006. Weight training in youth-growth, maturation, and safety: An evidence-based review. *Clinical Journal of Sport Medicine* 16(6): 478–487.

Manek, N. J., and A. J. MacGregor. 2005. Epidemiology of back disorders: Prevalence, risk factors, and prognosis. *Current Opinion in Rheumatology* 17(2): 134–140.

Mortimer, M., et al. 2006. Low back pain in a general population. Natural course and influence of physical exercise—a 5-year follow-up of the Musculoskeletal Intervention Center–Norrtalje Study. *Spine* 31(26): 3045–3051.

National Institute of Arthritis and Musculoskeletal and Skin Diseases. 2005. *Back Pain.* NIH Publication No. 05-5285.

Nelson, A. G., et al. 2005. Acute effects of passive muscle stretching on sprint performance. *Journal of Sports Science* 23(5): 449–454.

Newton, R. U., et al. 2006. Determination of functional strength imbalance of the lower extremities. *Journal of Strength and Conditioning Research* 20(4): 971–977.

Nieman, D. C. 2007. *Exercise Testing and Prescription: A Health-Related Approach,* 6th ed. New York: McGraw-Hill.

Park, D. Y., and L. Chou. 2006. Stretching for prevention of Achilles tendon injuries: A review of the literature. *Foot and Ankle International* 27(12): 1086–1095.

Reilly, T., et al. 2006. Thermoregulation in elite athletes. *Current Opinion in Clinical Nutrition and Metabolic Care* 9(6): 666–671.

Shrier, I. 2004. Does stretching improve performance? A systematic and critical review of the literature. *Clinical Journal of Sports Medicine* 14(5): 267–273.

Thacker, S. B., et al. 2004. The impact of stretching on sports injury risk: A systematic review of the literature. *Medicine and Science in Sports and Exercise* 36(3): 371–378.

Topolski, T. D., et al. 2006. The Rapid Assessment of Physical Activity (RAPA) among older adults. *Preventing Chronic Disease* 3(4): A118.

Vibe Fersum, K. 2006. Spinal manipulation and exercise was better than ultrasound and exercise for patients with chronic low back pain. *The Australian Journal of Physiotherapy* 52(4): 306.

Woolstenhulme, M. T., et al. 2006. Ballistic stretching increases flexibility and acute vertical jump height when combined with basketball activity. *Journal of Strength and Conditioning Research* 20(4): 799–803.

LAB 5.1 Assessing Your Current Level of Flexibility

Part I   Sit-and-Reach Test

Equipment

Use a modified Wells and Dillon flexometer or construct your own measuring device using a firm box or two pieces of wood about 30 centimeters (12 inches) high attached at right angles to each other. Attach a metric ruler to measure the extent of reach. With the low numbers of the ruler toward the person being tested, set the 26-centimeter mark of the ruler at the footline of the box. (Individuals who cannot reach as far as the footline will have scores below 26 centimeters; those who can reach past their feet will have scores above 26 centimeters.) Most studies show no relationship between performance on the sit-and-reach test and the incidence of back pain.

Preparation

Warm up your muscles with a low-intensity activity such as walking or easy jogging. Then perform slow stretching movements.

Instructions

1. Remove your shoes and sit facing the flexibility measuring device with your knees fully extended and your feet flat against the device about 10 centimeters (4 inches) apart.

2. Reach as far forward as you can, with palms down, arms evenly stretched, and knees fully extended; hold the position of maximum reach for about 2 seconds.

3. Perform the stretch 2 times, recording the distance of maximum reach to the nearest 0.5 centimeters: _____ cm

Rating Your Flexibility

Find the score in the table below to determine your flexibility rating. Record it here and on the final page of this lab.

Rating: _____

Ratings for Sit-and-Reach Test

	Rating/Score (cm)*				
Men	Needs Improvement	Fair	Good	Very Good	Excellent
Age: 15–19	Below 24	24–28	29–33	34–38	Above 38
20–29	Below 25	25–29	30–33	34–39	Above 39
30–39	Below 23	23–27	28–32	33–37	Above 37
40–49	Below 18	18–23	24–28	29–34	Above 34
50–59	Below 16	16–23	24–27	28–34	Above 34
60–69	Below 15	15–19	20–24	25–32	Above 32
Women					
Age: 15–19	Below 29	29–33	34–37	38–42	Above 42
20–29	Below 28	28–32	33–36	37–40	Above 40
30–39	Below 27	27–31	32–35	36–40	Above 40
40–49	Below 25	25–29	30–33	34–37	Above 37
50–59	Below 25	25–29	30–32	33–38	Above 38
60–69	Below 23	23–26	27–30	31–34	Above 34

*Footline is set at 26 cm.

SOURCE: *The Canadian Physical Activity, Fitness & Lifestyle Approach: CSEP-Health & Fitness Program's Health-Related Appraisal and Counselling Strategy,* 3rd edition, 2003. Reprinted with permission from the Canadian Society for Exercise Physiology.

Part II   Range-of-Motion Assessment

This portion of the lab can be completed by doing visual comparisons or by measuring joint range of motion with a goniometer or other instrument.

Equipment
1. A partner to do visual comparisons or to measure the range of motion of your joints. (You can also use a mirror to perform your own visual comparisons.)
2. For the measurement method, you need a goniometer, flexometer, or other instrument to measure range of motion.

Preparation
Warm up your muscles with some low-intensity activity such as walking or easy jogging.

Instructions
On the following pages, the average range of motion is illustrated and listed quantitatively for some of the major joints. Visually assess the range of motion in your joints, and compare it to that shown in the illustrations. For each joint, note (with a check mark) whether your range of motion is above average, average, or below average and in need of improvement. Average values for range of motion are given in degrees for each joint in the assessment. You can also complete the assessment by measuring your range of motion with a goniometer, flexometer, or other instrument. If you are using this measurement method, identify your rating (above average, average, or below average) and record your range of motion in degrees next to the appropriate category. Although the measurement method is more time-consuming, it allows you to track the progress of your stretching program more precisely and to note changes within the broader ratings categories (below average, above average).

Record your ratings on the following pages and on the chart on the final page of this lab. (Ratings were derived from several published sources.)

Assessment of range of motion using a goniometer.

1. Shoulder Abduction and Adduction

For each position and arm, check one of the following; fill in degrees if using the measurement method.

Shoulder abduction—raise arm up to the side.

Right	Left	
_____	_____	Below average/needs improvement
_____	_____	Average (92–95°)
_____	_____	Above average

Shoulder adduction—move arm down and in front of body.

Right	Left	
_____	_____	Below average/needs improvement
_____	_____	Average (124–127°)
_____	_____	Above average

2. Shoulder Flexion and Extension

For each position and arm, check one of the following; fill in degrees if using the measurement method.

Shoulder flexion—raise arm up in front of the body.

Right   *Left*

_____   _____   Below average/needs improvement

_____   _____   Average (92–95°)

_____   _____   Above average

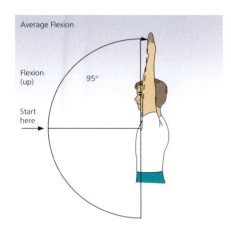

Shoulder extension—move arm down and behind the body.

Right   *Left*

_____   _____   Below average/needs improvement

_____   _____   Average (145–150°)

_____   _____   Above average

3. Trunk/Low-Back Lateral Flexion

Bend directly sideways at your waist. To prevent injury, keep your knees slightly bent, and support your trunk by placing your hand or forearm on your thigh. Check one of the following for each side; fill in degrees if using the measurement method.

Right   *Left*

_____   _____   Below average/needs improvement

_____   _____   Average (36–40°)

_____   _____   Above average

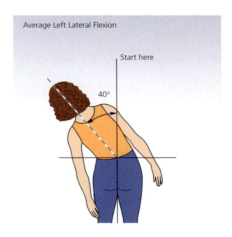

4. Hip Abduction

Raise your leg to the side at the hip. Check one of the following for each leg; fill in degrees if using the measurement method.

Right   *Left*

_____   _____   Below average/needs improvement

_____   _____   Average (40–45°)

_____   _____   Above average

5. Hip Flexion (Bent Knee)

With one leg flat on the floor, bend the other knee and lift the leg up at the hip. Check one of the following for each leg; fill in degrees if using the measurement method.

Right   *Left*

_____   _____   Below average/needs improvement

_____   _____   Average (121–125°)

_____   _____   Above average

6. Hip Flexion (Straight Leg)

With one leg flat on the floor, raise the other leg at the hip, keeping both legs straight. Take care not to put excess strain on your back. Check one of the following for each leg; fill in degrees if using the measurement method.

Right   *Left*

_____   _____   Below average/needs improvement

_____   _____   Average (79–81°)

_____   _____   Above average

7. Ankle Dorsiflexion and Plantar Flexion

For each position and foot, check one of the following; fill in degrees if using the measurement method.

Ankle dorsiflexion—pull your toes toward your shin.

Right   Left

_____ _____ Below average/needs improvement

_____ _____ Average (9–13°)

_____ _____ Above average

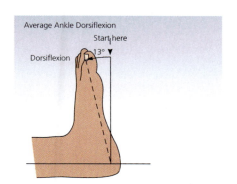

Average Ankle Dorsiflexion

Start here

Dorsiflexion 13°

Plantar flexion—point your toes.

Right   Left

_____ _____ Below average/needs improvement

_____ _____ Average (50–55°)

_____ _____ Above average

Average Ankle Plantar Flexion

Start here

55° Plantar flexion

Rating Your Flexibility

Sit-and-reach test: Score: _____ cm   Rating: _____

Range-of-Motion Assessment

Identify your rating for each joint on each side of the body. If you used the comparison method, put check marks in the appropriate categories; if you measured range of motion, enter the degrees for each joint in the appropriate category.

Joint/Assessment		Right Below Average	Right Average	Right Above Average	Left Below Average	Left Average	Left Above Average
1. Shoulder abduction and adduction	Abduction						
	Adduction						
2. Shoulder flexion and extension	Flexion						
	Extension						
3. Trunk/low-back lateral flexion	Flexion						
4. Hip abduction	Abduction						
5. Hip flexion (bent knee)	Flexion						
6. Hip flexion (straight leg)	Flexion						
7. Ankle dorsiflexion and plantar flexion	Dorsiflexion						
	Plantar flexion						

Using Your Results

How did you score? Are you surprised by your ratings for flexibility? Are you satisfied with your current ratings?

If you're not satisfied, set a realistic goal for improvement:

Are you satisfied with your current level of flexibility as expressed in your daily life—for example, your ability to maintain good posture and move easily and without pain?

If you're not satisfied, set some realistic goals for improvement:

What should you do next? Enter the results of this lab in the Preprogram Assessment column in Appendix D. If you've set goals for improvement, begin planning your flexibility program by completing the plan in Lab 5.2. After several weeks of your program, complete this lab again and enter the results in the Postprogram Assessment column of Appendix D. How do the results compare?

LAB 5.2 Creating a Personalized Program for Developing Flexibility

1. *Goals.* List goals for your flexibility program. On the left, include specific, measurable goals that you can use to track the progress of your fitness program. These goals might be things like raising your sit-and-reach score from fair to good or your bent-leg hip flexion rating from below average to average. On the right, include long-term and more qualitative goals, such as reducing your risk for back pain.

Specific Goals: Current Status

_____
_____
_____

Final Goals

_____
_____
_____

Other goals: _____
_____

2. *Exercises.* The exercises in the program plan below are from the general stretching program presented in Chapter 5. You can add or delete exercises depending on your needs, goals, and preferences. For any exercises you add, fill in the areas of the body affected.

3. *Frequency.* A minimum frequency of 2–3 days per week is recommended; 5–7 days per week is ideal. You may want to do your stretching exercises the same days you plan to do cardiorespiratory endurance exercise or weight training, because muscles stretch better following exercise, when they are warm.

4. *Intensity.* All stretches should be done to the point of mild discomfort, not pain.

5. *Time/duration.* All stretches should be held for 15–30 seconds. (PNF techniques should include a 6-second contraction followed by a 10–30-second assisted stretch.) All stretches should be performed 2–4 times.

Program Plan for Flexibility

Exercise	Areas Stretched	M	T	W	Th	F	Sa	Su
Head turns and tilts	Neck							
Towel stretch	Triceps, shoulders, chest							
Across-the-body and overhead stretches	Shoulders, upper back, back of the arm							
Upper-back stretch	Upper back							
Lateral stretch	Trunk muscles							
Step stretch	Hip, front of thigh							
Side lunge	Inner thigh, hip, calf							
Inner thigh stretch	Inner thigh, hip							
Trunk rotation	Trunk, outer thigh and hip, lower back							
Modified hurdler stretch	Back of the thigh, lower back							
Alternate leg stretcher	Back of the thigh, hip, knee, ankle, buttocks							
Lower-leg stretch	Back of the lower leg							

You can monitor your program using a chart like the one on the next page.

Flexibility Program Chart

Fill in the dates you perform each stretch, the number of seconds you hold each stretch (should be 15–30), and the number of repetitions of each (should be 2–4). For an easy check on the duration of your stretches, count "one thousand one, one thousand two," and so on. You will probably find that over time you'll be able to hold each stretch longer (in addition to being able to stretch farther).

Exercise/Date																						
	Duration																					
	Reps																					
	Duration																					
	Reps																					
	Duration																					
	Reps																					
	Duration																					
	Reps																					
	Duration																					
	Reps																					
	Duration																					
	Reps																					
	Duration																					
	Reps																					
	Duration																					
	Reps																					
	Duration																					
	Reps																					
	Duration																					
	Reps																					
	Duration																					
	Reps																					
	Duration																					
	Reps																					
	Duration																					
	Reps																					
	Duration																					
	Reps																					
	Duration																					
	Reps																					
	Duration																					
	Reps																					
	Duration																					
	Reps																					

LAB 5.3 Assessing Muscular Endurance for Low-Back Health

The three tests in this lab evaluate the muscular endurance of major spine-stabilizing muscles.

Side Bridge Endurance Test

Equipment

1. Stopwatch or clock with a second hand
2. Exercise mat
3. Partner

Preparation

Warm up your muscles with some low-intensity activity such as walking or easy jogging. Practice assuming the side bridge position described below.

Instructions

1. Lie on the mat on your side with your legs extended. Place your top foot in front of your lower foot for support. Lift your hips off the mat so that you are supporting yourself on one elbow and your feet (see photo). Your body should maintain a straight line. Breathe normally; don't hold your breath.

2. Hold the position as long as possible. Your partner should keep track of the time and make sure that you maintain the correct position. Your final score is the total time you are able to hold the side bridge with correct form—from the time you lift your hips until your hips return to the mat.

3. Rest for 5 minutes and then repeat the test on the other side. Record your times here and on the chart at the end of the lab. Right side bridge time: _____ sec   Left side bridge time: _____ sec

Trunk Flexors Endurance Test

Equipment

1. Stopwatch or clock with a second hand
2. Exercise mat or padded exercise table
3. Two helpers
4. Jig angled at 60 degrees from the floor or padded bench (optional)

Preparation

Warm up with some low-intensity activity such as walking or easy jogging.

Instructions

1. To start, assume a sit-up posture with your back supported at an angle of 60 degrees from the floor; support can be provided by a jig, a padded bench, or a spotter (see photos). Your knees and hips should both be flexed at 90 degrees, and your arms should be folded across your chest with your hands placed on the opposite shoulders. Your toes should be secured under a toe strap or held by a partner.

2. Your goal is to hold the starting position (isometric contraction) as long as possible after the support is pulled away. To begin the test, a helper should pull the jig or other support back about 10 centimeters (4 inches). The helper should keep track of the time; if a spotter is acting as your support, she or he should be ready to support your weight as soon as your torso begins to move back. Your final score is the total time you are able to hold the contraction—from the time the support is removed until any part of your back touches the support. Remember to breathe normally throughout the test.

3. Record your time here and on the chart at the end of the lab. Trunk flexors endurance time: _____ sec

Back Extensors Endurance Test

Equipment

1. Stopwatch or clock with a second hand
2. Extension bench with padded ankle support or any padded bench
3. Partner

Preparation

Warm up with some low-intensity activity such as walking or easy jogging.

Instructions

1. Lie face down on the test bench with your upper body extending out over the end of the bench and your pelvis, hips, and knees flat on the bench. Your arms should be folded across your chest with your hands placed on the opposite shoulders. Your feet should be secured under a padded strap or held by a partner.

2. Your goal is to hold your upper body in a straight horizontal line with your lower body as long as possible. Keep your neck straight and neutral; don't raise your head and don't arch your back. Breathe normally. Your partner should keep track of the time and watch your form. Your final score is the total time you are able to hold the horizontal position—from the time you assume the position until your upper body drops from the horizontal position.

3. Record your time here and on the chart below. Back extensors endurance time: _____ sec

Rating Your Test Results for Muscular Endurance for Low-Back Health

The table below shows mean endurance test times for healthy young college students with a mean age of 21 years. Compare your scores with the times shown in the table. (If you are older or have suffered from low-back pain in the past, these ratings are less accurate; however, your time scores can be used as a point of comparison.)

Mean Endurance Times (sec)

	Right side bridge	Left side bridge	Trunk flexors	Back extensors
Men	95	99	136	161
Women	75	78	134	185

SOURCE: From S. M. McGill, 2002, *Low Back Disorders: Evidence-Based Prevention and Rehabilitation*, page 227, table 12.1. © 2002 by Stuart McGill. Reprinted with permission from Human Kinetics (Champaign, IL).

Right side bridge: _____ sec   Rating (above mean, at mean, below mean): _____

Left side bridge: _____ sec   Rating (above mean, at mean, below mean): _____

Trunk flexors: _____ sec   Rating (above mean, at mean, below mean): _____

Back extensors: _____ sec   Rating (above mean, at mean, below mean): _____

Using Your Results

How did you score? Are you surprised by your scores for the low-back tests? Are you satisfied with your current ratings?

If you're not satisfied, set a realistic goal for improvement. The norms in this lab are based on healthy young adults, so a score above the mean may or may not be realistic for you. Instead, you may want to set a specific goal based on time rather than rating; for example, set a goal of improving your time by 10%. Imbalances in muscular endurance have been linked with back problems, so if your rating is significantly lower for one of the three tests, you should focus particular attention on that area of your body.

Goal:

What should you do next? Enter the results of this lab in the Preprogram Assessment column in Appendix D. If you've set a goal for improvement, begin a program of low-back exercises such as that suggested in this chapter. After several weeks of your program, complete this lab again and enter the results in the Postprogram Assessment column of Appendix D. How do the results compare?

LAB 5.4 Posture Evaluation

For each row, have a partner record the point total that corresponds to the illustration that most closely matches your posture. Use a plumb line to help make an accurate assessment of your posture.

5 points	3 points	1 point	Your Score

Head erect (gravity line passes directly through center)	Head twisted or turned to one side slightly	Head twisted or turned to one side markedly	_____

Shoulders level (horizontally)	One shoulder slightly higher than other	One shoulder markedly higher than other	_____

Spine straight	Spine slightly curved laterally	Spine markedly curved laterally	_____

Hips level (horizontally)	One hip slightly higher	One hip markedly higher	_____

Feet pointed straight ahead	Feet pointed out	Feet pointed out markedly; ankles sag in (pronation)	_____

Arches high	Arches lower; feet slightly flat	Arches low; feet markedly flat	_____

LABORATORY ACTIVITIES

5 points	3 points	1 point	Your Score

Neck erect, chin in, head in balance directly above shoulders | Neck slightly forward, chin slightly out | Neck markedly forward, chin markedly out | _____

Chest elevated (breast-bone farthest forward part of body) | Chest slightly depressed | Chest markedly depressed (flat) | _____

Shoulders centered | Shoulders slightly forward | Shoulders markedly forward (shoulder blades protruding in rear) | _____

Upper back normally rounded | Upper back slightly more rounded | Upper back markedly rounded | _____

Trunk erect | Trunk inclined slightly to rear | Trunk inclined markedly to rear | _____

Abdomen flat | Abdomen protruding | Abdomen protruding and sagging | _____

Lower back normally curved | Lower back slightly hollow | Lower back markedly hollow | _____

Total Score (from both pages) (Scores should be between 13 and 65.) _____

If your posture needs improvement, review the information in the box on good posture and low-back health on p. 149. If you scored "1 point" for any item in the evaluation, you may want to consider seeing a physician; professional advice, physical therapy, orthotic devices, or other therapies may help you improve your posture.

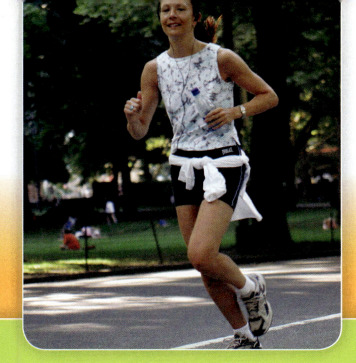

LOOKING AHEAD>>>>>

AFTER READING THIS CHAPTER, YOU SHOULD BE ABLE TO:

- Define fat-free mass, essential fat, and nonessential fat, and describe their functions in the body
- Explain how body composition affects overall health and wellness
- Describe how body mass index, body composition, and body fat distribution are measured and assessed
- Explain how to determine recommended body weight and body fat distribution

BODY COMPOSITION

6

TEST YOUR KNOWLEDGE

1. Exercise helps reduce the risks associated with overweight and obesity even if it doesn't result in improvements in body composition.

True or false?

2. Which of the following is the most significant risk factor for the most common type of diabetes (type 2 diabetes)?

a. smoking
b. low-fiber diet
c. overweight or obesity
d. inactivity

3. In women, excessive exercise and low energy (calorie) intake can cause which of the following?

a. unhealthy reduction in body fat levels
b. amenorrhea (absent menstruation)
c. bone density loss and osteoporosis
d. muscle wasting and fatigue

ANSWERS

1. **TRUE.** Regular physical activity provides protection against the health risks of overweight and obesity. It lowers the risk of death for people who are overweight or obese as well as for those at a normal weight.

2. **c.** All four are risk factors for diabetes, but overweight/obesity is the most significant. It's estimated that 90% of cases of type 2 diabetes could be prevented if people adopted healthy lifestyle behaviors. About 18 million Americans have type 2 diabetes, and more than 6 million of those with diabetes don't know it.

3. **ALL FOUR.** Very low levels of body fat, and the behaviors used to achieve them, have serious health consequences for both men and women.

FIT AND WELL ONLINE LEARNING CENTER www.mhhe.com/fahey

Visit the *Fit and Well* Online Learning Center for resources that will help you get the most out of your course!

- Study and review aids include practice quizzes, glossary flashcards, chapter summaries, learning objectives, PowerPoint presentations, Common Questions Answered, student handouts, crossword puzzles, Internet activities, and links to wellness Web sites.
- Behavior change tools include a daily fitness and nutrition journal, a behavior change workbook, sample behavior change plans, and blank behavior change logs to print and use.

ody composition, the body's relative amounts of fat and fat-free mass, is an important component of fitness for health and wellness. People whose body composition is optimal tend to be healthier, to move more efficiently, and to feel better about themselves. They also have a lower risk of many chronic diseases.

Unfortunately, many people don't succeed in their efforts to obtain a fit and healthy body because they set unrealistic goals and emphasize short-term weight loss rather than the permanent changes in lifestyle that lead to fat loss and a healthy body composition. Successful management of body composition requires the long-term, consistent coordination of many aspects of a wellness program. However, even in the absence of changes in body composition, an active lifestyle can improve wellness (see the box "Body Composition and the Benefits of Physical Activity").

This chapter focuses on defining and measuring body composition. The aspects of lifestyle that affect body composition are discussed in detail in other chapters: physical activity and exercise in Chapters 2–5 and 7, nutrition in Chapter 8, weight management in Chapter 9, and stress management in Chapter 10.

WHAT IS BODY COMPOSITION, AND WHY IS IT IMPORTANT?

The human body can be divided into fat-free mass and body fat. Fat-free mass is composed of all the body's non-fat tissues: bone, water, muscle, connective tissue, organ tissues, and teeth. Body fat includes both essential and nonessential (storage) body fats (Figure 6.1).

• **Essential fat** includes lipids (or fats) incorporated into the nerves, brain, heart, lungs, liver, and mammary glands. These fat deposits, crucial for normal body functioning, make up 3–5% of total body weight in men and 8–12% in women. (The larger percentage in women is

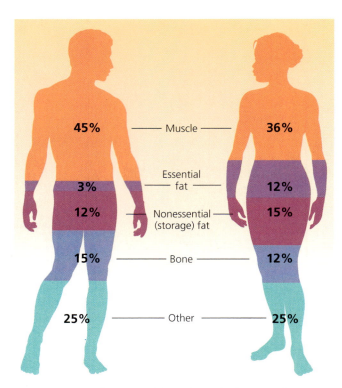

FIGURE 6.1 Body composition of a typical man and woman, 20–24 years old.

SOURCE: Adapted from Brooks, G. A., et al. 2005. *Exercise Physiology: Human Bioenergetics and Its Applications,* 4th ed. New York: McGraw-Hill.

natural and healthy and is due to fat deposits in the breasts, uterus, and other gender-specific sites.)

• **Nonessential (storage) fat** is extra fat or fat reserves stored in the body. Nonessential fat exists primarily within fat cells, or **adipose tissue,** often located just below the skin (subcutaneous fat) and around major organs (visceral fat).

In general, when the amount of fat in the body changes, fat cells increase or decrease in size (rather than in number). The amount of storage fat depends on many factors, including gender, age, heredity, metabolism, diet, and activity level. Excess storage fat is usually the result of consuming more energy (as food) than is expended (in metabolism and physical activity).

Overweight and Obesity Defined

Some of the most commonly used methods of assessing and classifying body composition are described later in this chapter. Some methods are based on body fat, and others on total body weight. Methods based on total body weight are less accurate than those based on body fat, but they are commonly used because body weight is easier to measure than body fat.

In the past, many people relied on height/weight tables (which were based on insurance company mortality statistics) to determine whether they were at a healthy

WEB TERMS

essential fat   The fat in the body necessary for normal body functioning.

nonessential (storage) fat   Extra fat or fat reserves stored in the body.

adipose tissue   Connective tissue in which fat is stored.

percent body fat   The percentage of total body weight that is composed of fat.

overweight   Characterized by a body weight above a recommended range for good health; ranges are set through large-scale population surveys.

obese   Severely overweight, characterized by an excessive accumulation of body fat; overfat. Obesity may also be defined in terms of some measure of total body weight.

Body Composition and the Benefits of Physical Activity

Does physical activity have benefits aside from the help it provides in managing weight and improving body composition? Yes! Physical activity is important for health even if it produces no changes in body composition—that is, even if a person remains overweight or obese. Physical inactivity operates as a risk factor for health problems independently of body composition; conversely, physical activity confers benefits no matter what a person weighs.

Obesity is linked to many serious diseases and physical problems, including cardiovascular disease, diabetes, certain cancers, and premature death. Regular physical activity and exercise block many of the destructive effects of obesity. For example, they improve blood pressure, blood glucose levels, cholesterol levels, and body fat distribution, and they lower the risk of cardiovascular disease, diabetes, and premature death. Although

Relationship among amount of activity, body weight, and risk of premature death.

physical activity and exercise produce these improvements quickly in some people and slowly in others, due to genetic differences, the improvements do occur. Physical activity is particularly

important for the many Americans who have metabolic syndrome or pre-diabetes, both characterized by insulin resistance.

In short, while it is best to have a healthy level of body fat and an active lifestyle, physical activity is important regardless of body composition. Physical activity reduces the risk of health problems and mortality for people of all levels of body fat (see figure).

Which is more important in combating the adverse health effects of obesity—physical activity or physical fitness? Many studies suggest that both are important; the more active and fit you are, the lower your risk of having health problems and dying prematurely. Of the two, however, physical *activity* appears to be more important for health than physical *fitness*. The message: No matter what your current body composition, it helps to get up and move.

SOURCES: Hu, F. B., et al. 2004. Adiposity compared with physical activity in predicting mortality among women. *New England Journal of Medicine* 351(26): 2694–2703. Blair, S. N., Y. Cheng, and J. S. Holder. 2001. Is physical activity or physical fitness more important in defining health benefits? *Medicine and Science in Sports and Exercise* 33(Suppl.): 379–399.

weight. Such tables, however, can be highly inaccurate for some people. Because muscle tissue is denser and heavier than fat, a fit person can easily weigh more than the recommended weight on a height/weight table. For the same reason, an unfit person may weigh less than the table's recommended weight.

When looking at body composition, the most important consideration is the proportion of the body's total weight that is fat—the **percent body fat.** For example, two women may both be 5 feet, 5 inches tall and weigh 130 pounds. But one woman may have only 15% of her body weight as fat, whereas the other woman could have 34% body fat. Although neither woman is overweight by most standards, the second woman is overfat. Too much body fat (not total weight) has a negative effect on health and well-being. Just as the amount of body fat is important, so is its location on your body. Visceral fat is more harmful to health than subcutaneous fat.

Overweight is usually defined as total body weight above the recommended range for good health (as determined by large-scale population surveys). **Obesity** is defined as a more serious degree of overweight. The cutoff point for obesity may be set in terms of percent body fat or in terms of some measure of total body weight.

MOTIVATION BOOSTER

Change the cues in your environment. If you keep unhealthy snacks in your kitchen or desk drawers, replace them with healthier choices. Place your exercise clothes where you can see them. Put motivating notes in visible places around your home.

Prevalence of Overweight and Obesity Among Americans

By any measure, Americans are getting fatter. Since 1960, the average weight among adult men has increased from 166 to 191 pounds; among women, from 140 to 164 pounds. The prevalence of obesity has increased from about 13% in 1960 to about 32% today, and more than 66% of American adults are now overweight (Figure 6.2).

Possible explanations for this increase include more time spent in sedentary work and leisure activities, fewer short trips on foot and more by automobile, fewer daily gym classes for students, more meals eaten outside the home, greater consumption of fast food, increased portion sizes, and increased consumption of soft drinks and convenience foods. According to the

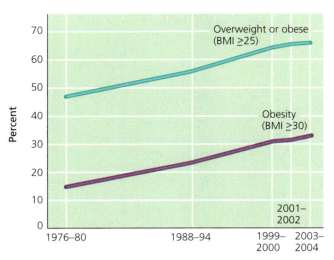

VITAL STATISTICS

FIGURE 6.2   Prevalence of overweight and obesity among American adults age 20–74.

SOURCE: National Center for Health Statistics. 2006. *2003–2004 National Health and Nutrition Examination Survey (NHANES)*. Hyattsville, Md.: National Center for Health Statistics.

USDA, average calorie intake among Americans increased by more than 500 calories per day between 1970 and 2003. Further, the CDC says that nearly 40% of adult Americans are physically inactive and get no exercise at all.

Excess Body Fat and Wellness

As rates of overweight and obesity increase, so do the problems associated with them. Obesity reduces life expectancy by 10–20 years, causes more than 100,000 premature deaths each year, and costs the United States more than $117 billion annually.

Risk of Chronic Disease and Premature Death   Obese people have an overall mortality rate almost twice that of nonobese people, and even mild to moderate overweight is associated with a substantial increase in the risk of heart disease and diabetes. Many overweight and obese people—especially those who are sedentary and eat a poor diet—suffer from a group of symptoms called *metabolic syndrome* (or insulin resistance syndrome). Symptoms include a resistance to the effects of insulin, high blood pressure, high blood glucose levels, abnormal blood fat levels (high triglycerides and low HDLs, or "good" cholesterol), and fat deposits in the abdominal region. Metabolic syndrome increases the risk of heart disease up to three times in men and six times in women. Scientists estimate that nearly 25% of the U.S. population has metabolic syndrome.

Obesity is also associated with increased risk of death from many types of cancer. Other health problems associated with obesity include hypertension, impaired immune function, gallbladder and kidney diseases, skin problems, sleep and breathing disorders, erectile dysfunction, pregnancy complications, back pain, arthritis, and other bone and joint disorders.

Of particular note is the strong association between excess body fat and diabetes mellitus: Obese people are more than three times as likely as nonobese people to develop diabetes, and the incidence of diabetes among Americans has increased dramatically as the rate of obesity has climbed (see the box "Diabetes").

Body Fat Distribution and Health   The distribution of body fat is also an important indicator of health. Men and postmenopausal women tend to store fat in the upper regions of their bodies, particularly in the abdominal area (the "apple shape"). Premenopausal women usually store fat in the hips, buttocks, and thighs (the "pear shape"). Excess fat in the abdominal area increases risk of several diseases, including high blood pressure, diabetes, early-onset heart disease, stroke, certain cancers, and mortality. The reason for this increase in risk is not entirely clear, but it appears that abdominal fat is more easily mobilized and sent into the bloodstream, increasing disease-related blood fat levels.

The risks from body fat distribution are usually assessed by measuring waist circumference. Waist circumference can be used to measure abdominal obesity (an indicator of disease risk) and to monitor changes in body composition over time. More research is needed to determine the precise degree of risk associated with specific values for waist measurement. However, a total waist measurement of more than 40 inches for men and more than 35 inches for women is associated with a significantly increased risk of disease.

Performance of Physical Activities   Too much body fat makes physical activity difficult because moving the body through everyday activities means working harder and using more energy. In general, overfat people are less fit than others and don't have the muscular strength, endurance, and flexibility that make normal activity easy. Because exercise is more difficult, they do less of it, depriving themselves of an effective way to improve body composition.

Emotional Wellness and Self-Image   Obesity can affect psychological as well as physical wellness. Being perceived as fat can be a source of ridicule, ostracism, and sometimes discrimination from others; it can contribute to psychological problems such as depression, anxiety, and low self-esteem.

The popular image of the "ideal" body has changed greatly in the past 50 years, evolving from slightly plump to unhealthily thin. The ideal body—as presented by the media—is an unrealistic goal for most Americans. This is because one's ability to change body composition depends on heredity as well as diet and exercise (see the box "Exercise, Body Image, and Self-Esteem" on p. 174).

Diabetes

Diabetes mellitus is a disease that causes a disruption of normal metabolism. The pancreas, a long, thin organ located behind the stomach, normally secretes the hormone insulin, which stimulates cells to take up glucose (blood sugar) to produce energy. In a person with diabetes, this process is disrupted, causing a buildup of glucose in the bloodstream. Over the long term, diabetes is associated with kidney failure, nerve damage, circulation problems, retinal damage and blindness, and increased rates of heart attack, stroke, and hypertension. The incidence of diabetes among Americans has increased dramatically as the rate of obesity has climbed. Diabetes is currently the sixth leading cause of death in the United States.

Types of Diabetes

About 21 million Americans (7% of the population) have one of two major forms of diabetes. About 5–10% of people with diabetes have the more serious form, known as *type 1 diabetes*. In this type of diabetes, the pancreas produces little or no insulin, so daily doses of insulin are required. (Without insulin, a person with type 1 diabetes can lapse into a coma.) Type 1 diabetes usually strikes before age 30.

The remaining 90–95% of Americans with diabetes have *type 2 diabetes*. This condition can develop slowly, and about a third of affected individuals are unaware of their condition. In type 2 diabetes, the pancreas doesn't produce enough insulin, cells are resistant to insulin, or both. This condition is usually diagnosed in people over age 40, although there has been a tenfold increase in type 2 diabetes in children in the past two decades. About one-third of people with type 2 diabetes must take insulin; others may take medications that increase insulin production or stimulate cells to take up glucose.

A third type of diabetes occurs in about 7% of women during pregnancy. *Gestational diabetes* usually disappears after pregnancy, but over 50% of women who experience it develop type 2 diabetes.

The term *pre-diabetes* describes blood glucose levels that are higher than normal but not high enough for a diagnosis of full-blown diabetes. About 54 million Americans have pre-diabetes, and most people with the condition will develop type 2 diabetes unless they adopt preventive lifestyle measures.

The major factors involved in the development of diabetes are age, obesity, physical inactivity, a family history of diabetes, and lifestyle. Excess body fat reduces cell sensitivity to insulin, and insulin resistance is almost always a precursor of type 2 diabetes. Ethnic background also plays a role. African Americans and Hispanics are 55% more likely than non-Hispanic whites to develop type 2 diabetes; more than 20% of Hispanics over age 65 have diabetes. Native Americans also have a higher-than-average incidence of diabetes. The American Diabetes Association's Web site (http://www.diabetes.org) includes an interactive diabetes risk assessment.

Treatment

There is no cure for diabetes, but it can be successfully managed by keeping blood sugar levels within safe limits through diet, exercise, and, if necessary, medication. Blood sugar levels can be monitored using a home test, and close control of glucose levels can significantly reduce the rate of serious complications. Nearly 90% of people with type 2 diabetes are overweight when diagnosed, and an important step in treatment is to lose weight. Even a small amount of exercise and weight loss can be beneficial. People with diabetes should obtain carbohydrates from whole grains, fruits, vegetables, and low-fat dairy products; carbohydrates and monounsaturated fat together should provide 60–70% of total daily calories. Regular exercise and a healthy diet are often sufficient to control type 2 diabetes.

Prevention

It is estimated that 90% of cases of type 2 diabetes could be prevented if people adopted healthy lifestyle behaviors, including regular physical activity, a moderate diet, and modest weight loss. For people with pre-diabetes, lifestyle measures are more effective than medication for delaying or preventing the development of diabetes. Studies of people with pre-diabetes show that a 5–7% weight loss can lower diabetes onset by nearly 60%. Exercise (endurance and/or strength training) makes cells more sensitive to insulin and helps stabilize blood glucose levels; it also helps keep body fat at healthy levels.

Eating a moderate diet to help control body fat is perhaps the most important dietary recommendation for the prevention of diabetes. However, the composition of the diet may also be important. Studies have linked diets low in fiber and high in sugar, refined carbohydrates, saturated fat, red meat, and high-fat dairy products to increased risk of diabetes; diets rich in whole grains, fruits, vegetables, legumes, fish, and poultry may be protective. Specific foods linked to higher diabetes risk include regular (nondiet) cola beverages, white bread, white rice, french fries, processed meats (bacon, sausage, hot dogs), and sugary desserts.

Warning Signs and Testing

Be alert for the warning signs of diabetes:

- Frequent urination
- Extreme hunger or thirst
- Unexplained weight loss
- Extreme fatigue
- Blurred vision
- Frequent infections
- Cuts and bruises that are slow to heal
- Tingling or numbness in the hands and feet
- Generalized itching, with no rash

The best way to avoid complications is to recognize these symptoms and get early diagnosis and treatment. Type 2 diabetes is often asymptomatic in the early stages, however, and major health organizations now recommend routine screening for people over age 45 and anyone younger who is at high risk, including anyone who is obese.

Screening involves a blood test to check glucose levels after either a period of fasting or the administration of a set dose of glucose. A fasting glucose level of 126 mg/dl or higher indicates diabetes; a level of 100–125 mg/dl indicates pre-diabetes. If you are concerned about your risk for diabetes, talk with your physician about being tested.

Exercise, Body Image, and Self-Esteem

If you gaze into the mirror and wish you could change the way your body looks, consider getting some exercise—not to reshape your contours but to firm up your body image and enhance your self-esteem. In one study, 82 adults completed a 12-week aerobic exercise program (using cycle ergometry) and had 12 months of follow-up. Compared with the control group, the participants not only improved their fitness but also benefited psychologically in tests of mood, anxiety, and self-concept. These same physical and psychological benefits were still significant at the 1-year follow-up.

One reason for the findings may be that people who exercise regularly often gain a sense of mastery and competence that enhances their self-esteem and body image. In addition, exercise contributes to a more toned look, which many adults prefer. Research suggests that physically active people are more comfortable with their bodies and their image than sedentary people are. In one workplace study, 60 employees were asked to complete a 36-session stretching program whose main purpose was to prevent muscle strains at work. At the end of the program, besides the significant increase by all participants in measurements of flexibility, their perceptions of their bodies improved, as did their overall sense of self-worth.

Similar results were obtained in a Norwegian study, in which 219 middle-aged people at risk for heart disease were randomly assigned to one of four groups: diet, diet plus exercise, exercise, and no intervention. The greater the participation of individuals in the exercise component of the program, the higher their scores in perceived competence/self-esteem and coping.

SOURCES: DiLorenzo, T. M., et al. 1999. Long-term effects of aerobic exercise on psychological outcomes. *Preventive Medicine* 28(1): 75–85. Sorensen, M., et al. 1999. The effect of exercise and diet on mental health and quality of life in middle-aged individuals with elevated risk factors for cardiovascular disease. *Journal of Sports Science* 17(5): 369–377. Moore, T. M. 1998. A workplace stretching program. *AAOHN Journal* 46(12): 563–568.

Most people should have the goal of developing a fit, healthy-looking body. The key to achieving this "look" is adopting a balance of proper nutrition and exercise and shedding unrealistic expectations about body composition—expectations that can negatively effect self-image and even lead to eating disorders and other problems.

Problems Associated with Very Low Levels of Body Fat

Though not as prevalent a problem as overweight or obesity, having too little body fat is also dangerous. Essential fat is necessary for the functioning of the body, and health experts generally view too little body fat— less than 8–12% for women and 3–5% for men—as a threat to health and well-being. Extreme leanness is linked with reproductive, circulatory, and immune system disorders and with premature death. Extremely lean people may experience muscle wasting and fatigue. They are also more likely to have eating disorders, which are described in more detail in Chapter 9. For women, an extremely low percentage of body fat is associated with **amenorrhea** and loss of bone mass (see the box "The Female Athlete Triad").

ASSESSING BODY MASS INDEX, BODY COMPOSITION, AND BODY FAT DISTRIBUTION

Like many people, you may weigh yourself from time to time on a scale in your bathroom, at the gym, or at a doctor's office. Although a scale can tell your total weight, it can't reveal whether a fluctuation in weight is due to a change in muscle, body water, or fat. Most importantly, a scale can't differentiate between overweight and overfat.

There are a number of simple, inexpensive ways to estimate healthy body weight and healthy body composition that are more accurate than the bathroom scale. These assessments can provide you with information about the health risks associated with your current body weight and body composition. They can also help you establish reasonable goals and set a starting point for current and future decisions about weight loss and weight gain.

Calculating Body Mass Index

Body mass index (BMI) is a measure of body weight that is useful for classifying the health risks of body weight if you don't have access to more sophisticated methods. Though more accurate than height-weight tables, body

QUESTIONS FOR CRITICAL THINKING AND REFLECTION

How do you view your own body composition? Where do you think you've gotten your ideas about how your body should look and perform? In light of what you've learned in this chapter, do the ideals and images promoted in our culture seem reasonable? Do they seem healthy?

The Female Athlete Triad

While obesity is at epidemic levels in the United States, many girls and women strive for unrealistic thinness in response to pressure from peers and a society obsessed with appearance. This quest for thinness has led to an increasingly common, underreported condition called the **female athlete triad.**

The triad consists of three interrelated disorders: abnormal eating patterns (and excessive exercising), followed by lack of menstrual periods (amenorrhea), followed by decreased bone density (premature osteoporosis). Left untreated, the triad can lead to decreased physical performance, increased incidence of bone fractures, disturbances of heart rhythm and metabolism, and even death.

Abnormal eating is the event from which the other two components of the triad flow. Abnormal eating ranges from moderately restricting food intake, to binge eating and purging (bulimia), to severely restricting food intake (anorexia nervosa). Whether serious or relatively mild, eating disorders prevent women from consuming enough calories to meet their bodies' needs.

Disordered eating, combined with intense exercise and emotional stress, can suppress the hormones that control the

Abnormal eating patterns and excessive exercising

Premature osteoporosis

Amenorrhea

menstrual cycle. If the menstrual cycle stops for three consecutive months, the condition is called amenorrhea. Prolonged amenorrhea can lead to osteoporosis; bone density may erode to the point that a woman in her 20s will have the bone density of a woman in her 60s. Women with osteoporosis have fragile, easily fractured bones. Some researchers have found that even a few missed menstrual periods can decrease bone density.

All physically active women and girls have the potential to develop one or more components of the female athlete triad; for example, it is estimated that 5–20% of women who exercise regularly and vigorously may develop amenorrhea. But the triad is most prevalent among athletes who participate in certain sports: those in which appearance

is highly important, those that emphasize a prepubertal body shape, those that require contour-revealing clothing for competition, those that require endurance, and those that use weight categories for participation. Such sports include gymnastics, figure skating, swimming, distance running, cycling, cross-country skiing, track, volleyball, rowing, horse racing, and cheerleading.

The female athlete triad can be life-threatening, and health professionals are taking it seriously. Typical signs of the eating disorders that trigger the condition are extreme weight loss, dry skin, loss of hair, brittle fingernails, cold hands and feet, low blood pressure and heart rate, swelling around the ankles and hands, and weakening of the bones. Female athletes who have repeated stress fractures may be suffering from the condition. Early intervention is the key to stopping this series of interrelated conditions. Unfortunately, once the condition has progressed, long-term consequences, especially bone loss, are unavoidable. Teenagers may need only to learn about good eating habits; college-age women with a long-standing problem may require intensive psychological counseling.

SOURCES: Beals, K. A., and N. L. Meyer. 2007. Female athlete triad update. *Clinics in Sports Medicine* 26(1): 69–89. Brunet, M. 2005. Female athlete triad. *Clinics in Sports Medicine* 24(3): 623–636. Art: Adapted from Yeager, K. K., et al. 1993. The female athlete triad: Disordered eating, amenorrhea, osteoporosis. *Medicine and Science in Sports and Exercise* 25:775–777. Reprinted by permission of Lippincott Williams and Wilkins.

mass index is also based on the concept that weight should be proportional to height. BMI is a fairly accurate measure of the health risks of body weight for average (nonathletic) people, and it is easy to calculate and rate. Researchers frequently use BMI in conjunction with waist circumference in studies that examine the health risks associated with body weight.

Because BMI doesn't distinguish between fat weight and fat-free weight, however, it can be inaccurate for some groups. For example, athletes who weight train have more muscle mass than average people and may be classified as overweight by the BMI scale; because their "excess" weight is in the form of muscle, however, it is healthy. Further, BMI is not particularly useful for tracking changes in body composition—gains in muscle mass and losses of fat. Women are likely to have more body fat for a given BMI than men. If you are an athlete, a serious weight trainer, or a person of short stature, do not use BMI as your primary means of assessing whether

your current weight is healthy; instead, try one of the methods described in the next section for estimating percent body fat.

BMI is calculated by dividing your body weight (expressed in kilograms) by the square of your height (expressed in meters). The following example is for a

amenorrhea Absent or infrequent menstruation, sometimes related to low levels of body fat and excessive quantity or intensity of exercise.

body mass index (BMI) A measure of relative body weight correlating highly with more direct measures of body fat, calculated by dividing total body weight (in kilograms) by the square of body height (in meters).

female athlete triad A condition consisting of three interrelated disorders: abnormal eating patterns (and excessive exercising) followed by lack of menstrual periods (amenorrhea) and decreased bone density (premature osteoporosis).

TERMS

Table 6.1 Body Mass Index (BMI) Classification and Disease Risk

Classification	BMI (kg/m²)	Obesity Class	Disease Risk Relative to Normal Weight and Waist Circumference*	
			Men ≤ 40 in. (102 cm) Women ≤ 35 in. (88 cm)	> 40 in. (102 cm) > 35 in. (88 cm)
Underweight**	<18.5		—	—
Normal†	18.5–24.9		—	—
Overweight	25.0–29.9		Increased	High
Obesity	30.0–34.9	I	High	Very high
	35.0–39.9	II	Very high	Very high
Extreme obesity	≥40.0	III	Extremely high	Extremely high

*Disease risk for type 2 diabetes, hypertension, and cardiovascular disease. The waist circumference cutoff points for increased risk are 40 inches (102 cm) for men and 35 inches (88 cm) for women.

**Research suggests that a low BMI can be healthy in some cases, as long as it is not the result of smoking, an eating disorder, or an underlying disease process. A BMI of 17.5 or less is sometimes used as a diagnostic criterion for the eating disorder anorexia nervosa.

†Increased waist circumference can also be a marker for increased risk, even in persons of normal weight.

SOURCE: Adapted from National Heart, Lung, and Blood Institute. 1998. *Clinical Guidelines on the Identification, Evaluation, and Treatment of Overweight and Obesity in Adults: The Evidence Report.* Bethesda, Md.: National Institutes of Health.

person who is 5 feet, 3 inches tall (63 inches) and weighs 130 pounds:

1. Divide body weight in pounds by 2.2 to convert weight to kilograms:

   130 ÷ 2.2 = 59.1

2. Multiply height in inches by 0.0254 to convert height to meters:

   63 × 0.0254 = 1.6

3. Multiply the result of step 2 by itself to get the square of the height measurement:

   1.6 × 1.6 = 2.56

4. Divide the result of step 1 by the result of step 3 to determine BMI:

   59.1 ÷ 2.56 = 23

An alternative equation, based on pounds and inches, is

   $BMI = [weight / (height \times height)] \times 703$

Space for your own calculations can be found in Lab 6.1, and a complete BMI chart appears in Lab 6.2.

Under guidelines from the National Institutes of Health (NIH), a person is classified as overweight if he or she has a BMI of 25 or above and obese if he or she has a BMI of 30 or above (Table 6.1). More than 60% of American adults have a BMI of 25 or above. At high values of BMI (over 25), the risk of arthritis, diabetes, hypertension, endometrial cancer, and other disorders increases substantially. The increased risk of type 2 diabetes at even fairly low values of BMI, especially among women, is of particular concern (Figure 6.3).

In classifying the health risks associated with overweight and obesity, the NIH guidelines consider body fat

distribution and other disease risk factors in addition to BMI. As described earlier, excess fat in the abdomen is of greater concern than excess fat in other areas. Methods of assessing body fat distribution are discussed later in the chapter; the NIH guidelines use measurement of waist

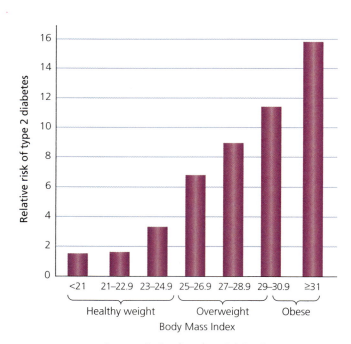

FIGURE 6.3 Body mass index (BMI) and risk of type 2 diabetes in women. The risk of diabetes goes up even for women at the high end of the healthy BMI range, but it is extremely high in overweight and obese women.

SOURCE: Hankinson, S. E., et al. 2001. *Healthy Women, Healthy Lives: A Guide to Preventing Disease from the Landmark Nurses' Health Study.* New York: Simon and Schuster.

circumference (see Table 6.1). At a given level of overweight, people with a large waist circumference and/or additional disease risk factors are at greater risk for health problems. For example, a man with a BMI of 27, a waist circumference of more than 40 inches, and high blood pressure is at greater risk for health problems than another man who has a BMI of 27 but has a smaller waist circumference and no other risk factors.

Thus, optimal BMI for good health depends on many factors; if your BMI is 25 or above, consult a physician for help in determining a healthy BMI for you. Despite its widespread use, BMI does have limitations. Although it is good for large population studies, it is less useful for measuring changes in body composition in individuals.

Estimating Percent Body Fat

Assessing body composition involves estimating percent body fat. The only method for directly measuring the percentage body weight that is fat is autopsy—the dissection and chemical analysis of the body. However, there are indirect techniques that can provide an estimate of percent body fat. One of the most accurate is underwater weighing. Other techniques include skinfold measurements, the Bod Pod, bioelectrical impedance analysis, and dual-energy X-ray absorptiometry.

All of these methods have a margin of error, so it is important not to focus too much on precise values. For example, underwater weighing has a margin of error of about ±3%, meaning that if a person's percent body fat is actually 17%, the test result may be between 14% and 20%. The results of different methods may also vary, so if you plan to track changes in body composition over time, be sure to use the same method each time to perform the assessment. Table 6.2 provides estimated ranges for healthy percent body fat.

Underwater Weighing   In hydrostatic (underwater) weighing, an individual is submerged and weighed under water. The percentages of fat and fat-free weight are calculated from body density. Muscle has a higher density and fat a lower density than water (1.1 grams per cubic centimeter for fat-free mass, 0.91 gram per cubic centimeter for fat, and 1 gram per cubic centimeter for water). Therefore, fat people tend to float and weigh less under water, and lean people tend to sink and weigh more under water. Most university exercise physiology departments or sports medicine laboratories have an underwater weighing facility. If you want an accurate assessment of your body composition, find a place that does underwater weighing.

Skinfold Measurements   Skinfold measurement is a simple, inexpensive, and practical way to assess body composition. Skinfold measurements can be used to

Table 6.2	Percent Body Fat Classification, by Age and Sex		
	Percent Body Fat (%)		
	20–39 Years	40–59 Years	60–79 Years
Women			
Essential*	8–12	8–12	8–12
Low/athletic**	13–20	13–22	13–23
Recommended	21–32	23–33	24–35
Overfat†	33–38	34–39	36–41
Obese†	≥39	≥40	≥42
Men			
Essential*	3–5	3–5	3–5
Low/athletic**	6–7	6–10	6–12
Recommended	8–19	11–21	13–24
Overfat†	20–24	22–27	25–29
Obese†	≥25	≥28	≥30

Note: The cutoffs for recommended, overfat, and obese ranges in this table are based on a study that linked BMI classifications from the National Institutes of Health with predicted percent body fat (measured using dual energy X-ray absorptiometry).

*Essential body fat is necessary for the basic functioning of the body.

**Percent body fat in the low/athletic range may be appropriate for some people as long as it is not the result of illness or disordered eating habits.

†Health risks increase as percent body fat exceeds the recommended range.

SOURCES: Gallagher, D., et al. 2000. Healthy percentage body fat ranges: An approach for developing guidelines based on body mass index. *American Journal of Clinical Nutrition* 72: 694–701. American College of Sports Medicine. 2006. *ACSM's Resource Manual for Guidelines for Exercise Testing and Prescription*, 5th ed. Philadelphia: Lippincott Williams and Wilkins.

assess body composition because equations can link the thickness of skinfolds at various sites to percent body fat calculations from more precise laboratory techniques.

Skinfold assessment typically involves measuring the thickness of skinfolds at several different sites on the body. You can sum up the skinfold values as an indirect measure of body fatness. For example, if you plan to create a fitness (and dietary change) program to improve body composition, you can compare the sum of skinfold values over time as an indicator of your program's progress and of improvements in body composition. You can also plug your skinfold values into equations like those in Lab 6.1 that predict percent body fat. When using these equations, however, it is important to remember that they have a fairly substantial margin of error (±4% if performed by a skilled technician)—so don't focus too much on specific values. The sum represents only a relative measure of body fatness.

Skinfolds are measured with a device called a **caliper,** which is a pair of spring-loaded, calibrated jaws. High-quality calipers are made of metal and have parallel jaw surfaces and constant spring tension. Inexpensive plastic calipers are also available; to ensure accuracy, plastic calipers should be spring-loaded and have metal jaws. Refer to Lab 6.1 for instructions on how to take skinfold measurements.

Taking accurate measurements with calipers requires patience, experience, and considerable practice. It's best to take several measurements at each site (or have several different people take each measurement) to help ensure accuracy. Be sure to take the measurements in the exact location called for in the procedure. Because the amount of water in your body changes during the day, skinfold measurements taken in the morning and evening often differ. If you repeat the measurements in the future to track changes in your body composition, measure skinfolds at approximately the same time of day.

The Bod Pod   The Bod Pod, a small chamber containing computerized sensors, measures body composition by air displacement rather than water displacement; the technical name of the technique is *plethysmography*. It determines the percentage of fat by calculating how much air is displaced by the person sitting inside the chamber. The Bod Pod has an error rate of about ±2–4% in determining percent body fat.

Bioelectrical Impedance Analysis (BIA)   The BIA technique works by sending a small electrical current through the body and measuring the body's resistance to it. Fat-free tissues, where most body water is located, are good conductors of electrical current, whereas fat is not. Thus, the amount of resistance to electrical current is related to the amount of fat-free tissue in the body (the lower the resistance, the greater the fat-free mass) and can be used to estimate percent body fat.

Bioelectrical impedance analysis has an error rate of about ±4–5%. To reduce error, follow the manufacturer's instructions carefully and avoid overhydration or underhydration (more or less body water than normal). Because measurement varies with the type of BIA analyzer, use the same instrument to compare measurements over time.

Advanced Techniques: DEXA and TOBEC   Dual-energy X-ray absorptiometry (DEXA) works by measuring

In underwater weighing (top), percent body fat is calculated from body density; muscle has a higher density than water, so people with more muscle weigh relatively more under water. The Bod Pod (middle) measures air displacement, which can be used to calculate percent body fat. DEXA (bottom) uses high- and low-energy X-ray beams to measure fat and lean tissue.

QUESTIONS FOR CRITICAL THINKING AND REFLECTION

Calculate your BMI using the formula given in the chapter, and compare it with the BMIs of several of your classmates. Do the results surprise you? How well do you think BMI reflects body composition? Why do you think it is such a commonly used measure?

MOTIVATION BOOSTER

Monitor your progress—your way. If changing your body composition is a goal, choose a method of monitoring your progress that works for you. For some people, weighing themselves frequently is discouraging and actually reduces their motivation. In some cases, it even promotes eating disorders. For other people, though, weighing is highly motivating and keeps their program on track. If weighing doesn't work for you, use another measure of progress, such as the amount of physical activity you incorporate into your day. Changing your body composition is a long-term process, so work toward short-term goals and focus on what is motivating for you.

the tissue absorption of high- and low-energy X-ray beams; studies thus far indicate that it has an error rate of about ±2%. Total body electrical conductivity (TOBEC) estimates lean body mass by passing a body through a magnetic field. Some fitness centers and sports medicine research facilities offer these body composition assessment techniques.

Assessing Body Fat Distribution

Researchers have studied many different methods for measuring body fat distribution. Two of the simplest to perform are waist circumference measurement and waist-to-hip ratio calculation. In the first method, you measure your waist circumference; in the second, you divide your waist circumference by your hip circumference. Waist circumference has been found to be a better indicator of abdominal fat than waist-to-hip ratio. More research is needed to determine the precise degree of risk associated with specific values for these two assessments of body fat distribution. However, as noted earlier, a total waist measurement of more than 40 inches (102 cm) for men and 35 inches (88 cm) for women and a waist-to-hip ratio above 0.94 for young men and 0.82 for young women are associated with a significantly increased risk of heart disease and diabetes. Lab 6.1 shows you how to measure your body fat distribution.

SETTING BODY COMPOSITION GOALS

If assessment tests indicate that fat loss would be beneficial for your health, your first step is to establish a goal. You can use the ratings in Table 6.1 or Table 6.2 to choose a target value for BMI or percent body fat (depending on which assessment you completed).

Make sure your goal is realistic and will ensure good health. Genetics limits your capacity to change your body composition, and few people can expect to develop the body of a fashion model or competitive bodybuilder. However, you can improve your body composition through a program of regular exercise and a healthy diet. If your body composition is in or close to the recom-

mended range, you may want to set a lifestyle goal rather than a specific percent body fat or BMI goal. For example, you might set a goal of increasing your daily physical activity from 20 to 60 minutes or beginning a program of weight training, and then let any improvements in body composition occur as a secondary result of your primary target (physical activity). Remember, a lifestyle that includes regular exercise may be more important for health than trying to reach any ideal weight.

If you are significantly overfat or if you have known risk factors for disease (such as high blood pressure or high cholesterol), consult your physician to determine a body composition goal for your individual risk profile. For people who are obese, small losses of body weight (5–15%) over a 6–12 month period can result in significant health improvements.

Once you've established a body composition goal, you can then set a target range for body weight. Although body weight is not an accurate method of assessing body composition, it's a useful method for tracking progress in a program to change body composition. If you're losing a small or moderate amount of weight and exercising, you're probably losing fat while building muscle mass. Lab 6.2 will help you determine a range for recommended body weight.

Using percent body fat or BMI will generate a fairly accurate target body weight for most people. However, it's best not to stick rigidly to a recommended body weight calculated from any formula; individual genetic, cultural, and lifestyle factors are also important. Decide whether the body weight that the formulas generate for you is realistic, meets all your goals, is healthy, *and* is reasonable for you to maintain.

caliper   A pressure-sensitive measuring instrument with two jaws that can be adjusted to determine thickness.

MAKING CHANGES IN BODY COMPOSITION

Chapter 9 includes specific strategies for losing or gaining weight and improving body composition. In general, lifestyle should be your focus—regular physical activity, endurance exercise, strength training, and a moderate energy intake. Making significant cuts in food intake in order to lose weight and body fat is a difficult strategy to maintain; focusing on increased physical activity is a better approach for many people. In studies of people who have lost weight and maintained the loss, physical activity was the key to long-term success.

You can track your progress toward your target body composition by checking your body weight regularly. Also, focus on how much energy you have and how your clothes fit.

To get a more accurate idea of your progress, you should directly reassess your body composition occasionally during your program: Body composition changes as weight changes. Losing a lot of weight usually includes losing some muscle mass no matter how hard a person exercises, partly because carrying less weight requires the muscular system to bear a smaller burden. (Conversely, a large gain in weight without exercise still causes some gain in muscle mass because muscles are working harder to carry the extra weight.)

TIPS FOR TODAY AND THE FUTURE

A wellness lifestyle can lead naturally to a body composition that is healthy and appropriate for you.

RIGHT NOW YOU CAN

- Find out what types of body composition assessment techniques are available at facilities on your campus or in your community.
- Do 15 minutes of physical activity—walk, jog, bike, swim, or climb stairs.
- Drink a glass of water instead of a soda, and include a high-fiber food such as whole-grain bread or cereal, popcorn, apples, berries, or beans in your next snack or meal.

IN THE FUTURE YOU CAN

- Think about your image of the ideal body type for your sex. Consider where your idea comes from, whether you use this image to judge your own body, and whether it is a realistic goal for you. Write down five positive things about your body.
- Be aware of media messages (especially visual images) that make you feel embarrassed or insecure about your body. Remind yourself that these messages are usually designed to sell a product; they should not form the basis of your body image.

SUMMARY

- The human body is composed of fat-free mass (which includes bone, muscle, organ tissues, and connective tissues) and body fat (essential and nonessential).

- Having too much body fat has negative health consequences, especially in terms of cardiovascular disease and diabetes. Distribution of fat is also a significant factor in health.

- A fit and healthy-looking body, with the right body composition for a particular person, develops from habits of proper nutrition and exercise.

- Measuring body weight is not an accurate way to assess body composition because it does not differentiate between muscle weight and fat weight.

- Body mass index (calculated from weight and height measurements) can help classify the health risks associated with overweight. BMI is sometimes inaccurate, however, particularly in muscular people.

- Techniques for estimating percent body fat include underwater weighing, skinfold measurements, the Bod Pod, bioelectrical impedance analysis, DEXA, and TOBEC.

- Body fat distribution can be assessed through waist measurement or the waist-to-hip ratio.

- Recommended body composition and weight can be determined by choosing a target BMI or target body fat percentage. Keep heredity in mind when setting a goal, and focus on positive changes in lifestyle.

FOR FURTHER EXPLORATION

BOOKS

Bray, G. A., and C. A. Bray. 2002. *An Atlas of Obesity and Weight Control.* London: CRC Press. *Provides detailed information about assessment, classification, and treatment of obesity.*

Heyward, V. H. 2006. *Advanced Fitness Assessment and Exercise Prescription,* 5th ed. Champaign, Ill.: Human Kinetics. *Detailed coverage of assessing body composition, fitness, flexibility, and other aspects of fitness.*

Lean, M., et al. 2007. *ABC of Obesity.* Boston: Blackwell Publishing Limited. *Examines the impact of obesity on the average person's life and discusses some of the most current options for preventing and treating obesity.*

Nathan, D. M., and L. Delahanty. 2006. *Beating Diabetes: A Harvard Medical School Book.* New York: McGraw-Hill. *Provides information on identifying and changing lifestyle behaviors that contribute to the development and worsening of diabetes.*

ORGANIZATIONS AND WEB SITES

American Diabetes Association. Provides information, a free newsletter, and referrals to local support groups; the Web site includes an online diabetes risk assessment.
800-342-2383
http://www.diabetes.org

Before training

After training

Skin

Adipose tissue (fat)

Muscle tissue

Effects of exercise on body composition. Endurance exercise and strength training reduce body fat and increase muscle mass.

Q Is spot reducing effective?

A Spot reducing refers to attempts to lose body fat in specific parts of the body by doing exercises for those parts. Danish researchers have shown that fat use increases in adipose tissue surrounding active muscle, but it is not known if short-term fat use helps reduce fat in specific sites. Most studies show that spot-reducing exercises contribute to fat loss only to the extent that they burn calories. The best way to reduce fat in any specific area is to create an overall negative energy balance: Take in less energy (food) than you use up through exercise and metabolism.

Q How does exercise affect body composition?

A Cardiorespiratory endurance exercise burns calories, thereby helping create a negative energy balance. Weight training does not use many calories and therefore is of little use in creating a negative energy balance. However, weight training increases muscle mass, which maintains a high metabolic rate (the body's energy level) and helps improve body composition. To minimize body fat and increase muscle mass,

thereby improving body composition, combine cardiorespiratory endurance exercise and weight training (see figure).

Q Are people who have a desirable body composition physically fit?

A Having a healthy body composition is not necessarily associated with overall fitness. For example, many bodybuilders have very little body fat but have poor cardiorespiratory capacity and flexibility. Some athletes, such as NFL linemen, weigh 300 pounds or more; they have to lose the weight when they retire if they don't want to jeopardize their health. To be fit, you must rate high on all the components of fitness.

Q What is liposuction, and will it help me lose body fat?

A Suction lipectomy, popularly known as liposuction, has become the most popular type of elective surgery in the world. The procedure involves removing limited amounts of fat from specific areas. Typically, no more than 2.5 kilograms (5.5 pounds) of adipose tissue is removed at a time. The

procedure is usually successful if the amount of excess fat is limited and skin elasticity is good. The procedure is most effective if integrated into a program of dietary restriction and exercise. Side effects include infection, dimpling, and wavy skin contours. Liposuction has a death rate of 1 in 5000 patients, primarily from pulmonary thromboembolism (a blood clot in the lungs) or fat embolism (circulatory blockage caused by a dislodged piece of fat). Other serious complications include shock, bleeding, and impaired blood flow to vital organs.

Q What is cellulite, and how do I get rid of it?

A Cellulite is the name commonly given to ripply, wavy fat deposits that collect just under the skin. The "cottage cheese" appearance stems from the breakdown of tissues supporting the fat. These rippling fat deposits are really the same as fat deposited anywhere else in the body. The only way to control them is to create a negative energy balance—burn up more calories than are taken in. There are no creams or lotions that will rub away surface (subcutaneous) fat deposits, and spot reducing is also ineffective. The solution is sensible eating habits and exercise.

For more Common Questions Answered about body composition, visit the Online Learning Center.

Methods of Body Composition Analysis Tutorials. Provides information about body composition assessment techniques, including underwater weighing, BIA, and DEXA.

    http://nutrition.uvm.edu/bodycomp

National Heart, Lung, and Blood Institute. Provides information on the latest federal obesity standards and a BMI calculator.

    http://www.nhlbi.nih.gov/about/oei/index.htm

National Institute of Diabetes and Digestive and Kidney Diseases Weight-Control Information Network. Provides information about adult obesity: how it is defined and assessed, the risk factors associated with it, and its causes.

    877-946-4627

    http://win.niddk.nih.gov

USDA Food and Nutrition Information Center: Weight and Obesity. Provides links to recent reports and studies on the issue of obesity among Americans.

    http://www.nal.usda.gov/fnic/reports/obesity.html

See also the listings for Chapters 2, 8, and 9.

SELECTED BIBLIOGRAPHY

American College of Sports Medicine. 2006. *ACSM's Resource Manual for Guidelines for Exercise Testing and Prescription,* 5th ed. Philadelphia: Lippincott Williams and Wilkins.

Anderson, D. E. 2007. Reliability of air displacement plethysmography. *Journal of Strength and Conditioning Research* 21(1): 169–172.

Bigaard, J., et al. 2005. Waist circumference and body composition in relation to all-cause mortality in middle-aged men and women. *International Journal of Obesity and Related Metabolic Disorders* 29: 778–784.

Centers for Disease Control and Prevention. 2005. *Frequently Asked Questions About Calculating Obesity-Related Risk* (http://www.cdc.gov/pdf/frequently_asked_questions_about_calculating_obesity-related_risk.pdf; retrieved May 21, 2007).

Centers for Disease Control and Prevention. 2005. National Diabetes Fact Sheet (http://www.cdc.gov/diabetes/pubs/general.htm; retrieved May 21, 2007).

Ekelund, U., S. J. Griffin, and N. J. Wareham. 2007. Physical activity and metabolic risk in individuals with a family history of type 2 diabetes. *Diabetes Care* 30(2): 337–342.

Flegal, K.. M., et al. 2007. Cause-specific excess deaths associated with underweight, overweight, and obesity. *Journal of the American Medical Association* 298 (17): 2028–2037.

Frisard, M. I., F. L. Greenway, and J. P. Delany. 2005. Comparison of methods to assess body composition changes during a period of weight loss. *Obesity Research* 13: 845–854.

Gale, C. R., et al. 2007. Grip strength, body composition, and mortality. *International Journal of Epidemiology* 36(1): 228–235.

Green, J. S., et al. 2004. The effects of exercise training on abdominal visceral fat, body composition, and indicators of the metabolic syndrome in postmenopausal women with and without estrogen replacement therapy: The HERITAGE family study. *Metabolism* 53: 1192–1196.

Guida, B., et al. 2007. Bioelectrical impedance analysis and age-related differences of body composition in the elderly. *Nutrition, Metabolism, and Cardiovascular Disease* 17(3): 175–180.

Holten, M. K., et al. 2004. Strength training increases insulin-mediated glucose uptake, GLUT4 content, and insulin signaling in skeletal muscle in patients with type 2 diabetes. *Diabetes* 53(2): 294–305.

Houston, D. K., et al. 2007. The association between weight history and physical performance in the Health, Aging and Body Composition Study. *International Journal of Obesity.* (Epub ahead of print.)

Hussey, J., et al. 2007. Relationship between the intensity of physical activity, cardiorespiratory fitness and body composition in 7–10-year-old Dublin children. *British Journal of Sports Medicine* 41(5): 311–316.

Janiszewski, P. M., and R. Ross. 2007. Physical activity in the treatment of obesity: Beyond body weight reduction. *Applied Physiology, Nutrition, and Metabolism* 32(3): 512–522.

Joyner, M. J. 2005. Muscle strength, body composition, hormones, and aging. *Exercise and Sport Sciences Reviews* 33: 61–62.

Krakauer, J. C., et al. 2004. Body composition profiles derived from dual-energy X-ray absorptiometry, total body scan, and mortality. *Preventive Cardiology* 7: 109–115.

Liu, J., T. J. Wade, and H. Tan. 2007. Cardiovascular risk factors and anthropometric measurements of adolescent body composition: A cross-sectional analysis of the Third National Health and Nutrition Examination Survey. *International Journal of Obesity* 31(1): 59–64.

Malina, R. M. 2007. Body composition in athletes: Assessment and estimated fatness. *Clinics in Sports Medicine* 26(1): 37–68.

Mattsson, S., and B. J. Thomas. 2006. Development of methods for body composition studies. *Physics in Medicine and Biology* 51(13): R203–228.

Ode, J. J., et al. 2007. Body mass index as a predictor of percent fat in college athletes and nonathletes. *Medicine and Science in Sports and Exercise* 39(3): 403–409.

Plank, L. D. 2005. Dual-energy X-ray absorptiometry and body composition. *Current Opinion in Clinical Nutrition and Metabolic Care* 8: 305–309.

Redman, L. M., et al. 2007. Effect of calorie restriction with or without exercise on body composition and fat distribution. *Journal of Clinical Endocrinology and Metabolism* 92(3): 865–872.

Stookey, J. D., L. S. Adair, and B. M. Popkin. 2005. Do protein and energy intakes explain long-term changes in body composition? *Journal of Nutrition, Health and Aging* 9: 5–17.

Varady, K., et al. 2007. Validation of hand-held bioelectrical impedance analysis with magnetic resonance imaging for the assessment of body composition overweight women. *American Journal of Human Biology* 19(3): 429–433.

Wong, S. L., et al. 2004. Cardiorespiratory fitness is associated with lower abdominal fat independent of body mass index. *Medicine and Science in Sports and Exercise* 36(2): 286–291.

Zhu, S., et al. 2005. Lifestyle behaviors associated with lower risk of having the metabolic syndrome. *Metabolism* 53(11): 1503–1511.

LAB 6.1 Assessing Body Mass Index and Body Composition

Body Mass Index

Equipment

1. Weight scale
2. Tape measure or other means of measuring height

Instructions

Measure your height and weight, and record the results. Be sure to record the unit of measurement.

Height: _____ Weight: _____

Calculating BMI (see also the shortcut chart of BMI values in Lab 6.2)

1. Convert your body weight to kilograms by dividing your weight in pounds by 2.2.

   Body weight _____ lb ÷ 2.2 lb/kg = body weight _____ kg

2. Convert your height measurement to meters by multiplying your height in inches by 0.0254.

   Height _____ in. × 0.0254 m/in. = height _____ m

3. Square your height measurement.

   Height _____ m × height _____ m = height _____ m^2

4. BMI equals body weight in kilograms divided by height in meters squared (kg/m^2).

   Body weight _____ kg ÷ height _____ m^2 = BMI _____ kg/m^2
   (from step 1)   (from step 3)

Rating Your BMI

Refer to the table for a rating of your BMI. Record the results below and on the final page of this lab.

Classification	BMI (kg/m^2)
Underweight	<18.5
Normal	18.5–24.9
Overweight	25.0–29.9
Obesity (I)	30.0–34.9
Obesity (II)	35.0–39.9
Extreme obesity (III)	≥40.0

(See complete version of table on p. 176 for additional information.)

BMI _____ kg/m^2

Classification (from table) _____

Skinfold Measurements

Equipment

1. Skinfold calipers
2. Partner to take measurements
3. Marking pen (optional)

1. *Select and locate the correct sites for measurement.* All measurements should be taken on the right side of the body with the subject standing. Skinfolds are normally measured on the natural fold line of the skin, either vertically or at a slight angle. The skinfold measurement sites for males are chest, abdomen, and thigh; for females, triceps, suprailium, and thigh. If the person taking skinfold measurements is inexperienced, it may be helpful to mark the correct sites with a marking pen.

(a) Chest (b) Abdomen (c) Thigh (d) Triceps (e) Suprailium

(a) Chest. Pinch a diagonal fold halfway between the nipple and the shoulder crease. *(b) Abdomen.* Pinch a vertical fold about 1 inch to the right of the umbilicus (navel). *(c) Thigh.* Pinch a vertical fold midway between the top of the hipbone and the kneecap. *(d) Triceps.* Pinch a vertical skinfold on the back of the right arm midway between the shoulder and elbow. The arm should be straight and should hang naturally. *(e) Suprailium.* Pinch a fold at the top front of the right hipbone. The skinfold here is taken slightly diagonally according to the natural fold tendency of the skin.

2. *Measure the appropriate skinfolds.* Pinch a fold of skin between your thumb and forefinger. Pull the fold up so that no muscular tissue is included; don't pinch the skinfold too hard. Hold the calipers perpendicular to the fold and measure the skinfold about 0.25 inch away from your fingers. Allow the tips of the calipers to close on the skinfold and let the reading settle before marking it down. Take readings to the nearest half-millimeter. Continue to repeat the measurements until two consecutive measurements match, releasing and repinching the skinfold between each measurement. Make a note of the final measurement for each site.

Time of day of measurements: _____

Men	**Women**
Chest: _____ mm	Triceps: _____ mm
Abdomen: _____ mm	Suprailium: _____ mm
Thigh: _____ mm	Thigh: _____ mm

Determining Percent Body Fat

Add the measurements of your three skinfolds. Use this sum as a point of comparison for future assessments and/or find the percent body fat that corresponds to your total in the appropriate table. For example, a 19-year-old female with measurements of 16 mm, 19 mm, and 22 mm would have a skinfold sum of 57 mm; according to the table on p. 185, her percent body fat is 22.7.

Sum of three skinfolds: _____ mm   Percent body fat: _____ %

Percent Body Fat Estimate for Women: Sum of Triceps, Suprailium, and Thigh Skinfolds

Sum of Skinfolds (mm)	Age								
	Under 22	23–27	28–32	33–37	38–42	43–47	48–52	53–57	Over 57
23–25	9.7	9.9	10.2	10.4	10.7	10.9	11.2	11.4	11.7
26–28	11.0	11.2	11.5	11.7	12.0	12.3	12.5	12.7	13.0
29–31	12.3	12.5	12.8	13.0	13.3	13.5	13.8	14.0	14.3
32–34	13.6	13.8	14.0	14.3	14.5	14.8	15.0	15.3	15.5
35–37	14.8	15.0	15.3	15.5	15.8	16.0	16.3	16.5	16.8
38–40	16.0	16.3	16.5	16.7	17.0	17.2	17.5	17.7	18.0
41–43	17.2	17.4	17.7	17.9	18.2	18.4	18.7	18.9	19.2
44–46	18.3	18.6	18.8	19.1	19.3	19.6	19.8	20.1	20.3
47–49	19.5	19.7	20.0	20.2	20.5	20.7	21.0	21.2	21.5
50–52	20.6	20.8	21.1	21.3	21.6	21.8	22.1	22.3	22.6
53–55	21.7	21.9	22.1	22.4	22.6	22.9	23.1	23.4	23.6
56–58	22.7	23.0	23.2	23.4	23.7	23.9	24.2	24.4	24.7
59–61	23.7	24.0	24.2	24.5	24.7	25.0	25.2	25.5	25.7
62–64	24.7	25.0	25.2	25.5	25.7	26.0	26.7	26.4	26.7
65–67	25.7	25.9	26.2	26.4	26.7	26.9	27.2	27.4	27.7
68–70	26.6	26.9	27.1	27.4	27.6	27.9	28.1	28.4	28.6
71–73	27.5	27.8	28.0	28.3	28.5	28.8	29.0	29.3	29.5
74–76	28.4	28.7	28.9	29.2	29.4	29.7	29.9	30.2	30.4
77–79	29.3	29.5	29.8	30.0	30.3	30.5	30.8	31.0	31.3
80–82	30.1	30.4	30.6	30.9	31.1	31.4	31.6	31.9	32.1
83–85	30.9	31.2	31.4	31.7	31.9	32.2	32.4	32.7	32.9
86–88	31.7	32.0	32.2	32.5	32.7	32.9	33.2	33.4	33.7
89–91	32.5	32.7	33.0	33.2	33.5	33.7	33.9	34.2	34.4
92–94	33.2	33.4	33.7	33.9	34.2	34.4	34.7	34.9	35.2
95–97	33.9	34.1	34.4	34.6	34.9	35.1	35.4	35.6	35.9
98–100	34.6	34.8	35.1	35.3	35.5	35.8	36.0	36.3	36.5
101–103	35.3	35.4	35.7	35.9	36.2	36.4	36.7	36.9	37.2
104–106	35.8	36.1	36.3	36.6	36.8	37.1	37.3	37.5	37.8
107–109	36.4	36.7	36.9	37.1	37.4	37.6	37.9	38.1	38.4
110–112	37.0	37.2	37.5	37.7	38.0	38.2	38.5	38.7	38.9
113–115	37.5	37.8	38.0	38.2	38.5	38.7	39.0	39.2	39.5
116–118	38.0	38.3	38.5	38.8	39.0	39.3	39.5	39.7	40.0
119–121	38.5	38.7	39.0	39.2	39.5	39.7	40.0	40.2	40.5
122–124	39.0	39.2	39.4	39.7	39.9	40.2	40.4	40.7	40.9
125–127	39.4	39.6	39.9	40.1	40.4	40.6	40.9	41.1	41.4
128–130	39.8	40.0	40.3	40.5	40.8	41.0	41.3	41.5	41.8

SOURCE: Jackson, A. S., and M. L. Pollock. 1985. Practical assessment of body composition. *The Physician and Sportsmedicine* 13(5): 76–90, Tables 6 & 7, pp. 86, 87. Copyright © 2005 The McGraw-Hill Companies. All rights reserved. Reprinted with permission from The McGraw-Hill Companies.

Sum of Skinfolds (mm)	Age								
	Under 22	23–27	28–32	33–37	38–42	43–47	48–52	53–57	Over 57
8–10	1.3	1.8	2.3	2.9	3.4	3.9	4.5	5.0	5.5
11–13	2.2	2.8	3.3	3.9	4.4	4.9	5.5	6.0	6.5
14–16	3.2	3.8	4.3	4.8	5.4	5.9	6.4	7.0	7.5
17–19	4.2	4.7	5.3	5.8	6.3	6.9	7.4	8.0	8.5
20–22	5.1	5.7	6.2	6.8	7.3	7.9	8.4	8.9	9.5
23–25	6.1	6.6	7.2	7.7	8.3	8.8	9.4	9.9	10.5
26–28	7.0	7.6	8.1	8.7	9.2	9.8	10.3	10.9	11.4
29–31	8.0	8.5	9.1	9.6	10.2	10.7	11.3	11.8	12.4
32–34	8.9	9.4	10.0	10.5	11.1	11.6	12.2	12.8	13.3
35–37	9.8	10.4	10.9	11.5	12.0	12.6	13.1	13.7	14.3
38–40	10.7	11.3	11.8	12.4	12.9	13.5	14.1	14.6	15.2
41–43	11.6	12.2	12.7	13.3	13.8	14.4	15.0	15.5	16.1
44–46	12.5	13.1	13.6	14.2	14.7	15.3	15.9	16.4	17.0
47–49	13.4	13.9	14.5	15.1	15.6	16.2	16.8	17.3	17.9
50–52	14.3	14.8	15.4	15.9	16.5	17.1	17.6	18.2	18.8
53–55	15.1	15.7	16.2	16.8	17.4	17.9	18.5	19.1	19.7
56–58	16.0	16.5	17.1	17.7	18.2	18.8	19.4	20.0	20.5
59–61	16.9	17.4	17.9	18.5	19.1	19.7	20.2	20.8	21.4
62–64	17.6	18.2	18.8	19.4	19.9	20.5	21.1	21.7	22.2
65–67	18.5	19.0	19.6	20.2	20.8	21.3	21.9	22.5	23.1
68–70	19.3	19.9	20.4	21.0	21.6	22.2	22.7	23.3	23.9
71–73	20.1	20.7	21.2	21.8	22.4	23.0	23.6	24.1	24.7
74–76	20.9	21.5	22.0	22.6	23.2	23.8	24.4	25.0	25.5
77–79	21.7	22.2	22.8	23.4	24.0	24.6	25.2	25.8	26.3
80–82	22.4	23.0	23.6	24.2	24.8	25.4	25.9	26.5	27.1
83–85	23.2	23.8	24.4	25.0	25.5	26.1	26.7	27.3	27.9
86–88	24.0	24.5	25.1	25.7	26.3	26.9	27.5	28.1	28.7
89–91	24.7	25.3	25.9	26.5	27.1	27.6	28.2	28.8	29.4
92–94	25.4	26.0	26.6	27.2	27.8	28.4	29.0	29.6	30.2
95–97	26.1	26.7	27.3	27.9	28.5	29.1	29.7	30.3	30.9
98–100	26.9	27.4	28.0	28.6	29.2	29.8	30.4	31.0	31.6
101–103	27.5	28.1	28.7	29.3	29.9	30.5	31.1	31.7	32.3
104–106	28.2	28.8	29.4	30.0	30.6	31.2	31.8	32.4	33.0
107–109	28.9	29.5	30.1	30.7	31.3	31.9	32.5	33.1	33.7
110–112	29.6	30.2	30.8	31.4	32.0	32.6	33.2	33.8	34.4
113–115	30.2	30.8	31.4	32.0	32.6	33.2	33.8	34.5	35.1
116–118	30.9	31.5	32.1	32.7	33.3	33.9	34.5	35.1	35.7
119–121	31.5	32.1	32.7	33.3	33.9	34.5	35.1	35.7	36.4
122–124	32.1	32.7	33.3	33.9	34.5	35.1	35.8	36.4	37.0
125–127	32.7	33.3	33.9	34.5	35.1	35.8	36.4	37.0	37.6

LABORATORY ACTIVITIES

Rating Your Body Composition

Refer to the chart to rate your percent body fat. Record it below and in the chart at the end of this lab.

Rating: _____

Percent Body Fat Classification

	Percent Body Fat (%)				Percent Body Fat (%)		
	20–39 Years	*40–59 Years*	*60–79 Years*		*20–39 Years*	*40–59 Years*	*60–79 Years*
Women				**Men**			
Essential*	8–12	8–12	8–12	Essential*	3–5	3–5	3–5
Low/athletic**	13–20	13–22	13–23	Low/athletic**	6–7	6–10	6–12
Recommended	21–32	23–33	24–35	Recommended	8–19	11–21	13–24
Overfat†	33–38	34–39	36–41	Overfat†	20–24	22–27	25–29
Obese†	≥39	≥40	≥42	Obese†	≥25	≥28	≥30

Note: The cutoffs for recommended, overfat, and obese ranges in this table are based on a study that linked body mass index classifications from the National Institutes of Health with predicted percent body fat (measured using dual-energy X-ray absorptiometry).

*Essential body fat is necessary for the basic functioning of the body.

**Percent body fat in the low/athletic range may be appropriate for some people as long as it is not the result of illness or disordered eating habits.

†Health risks increase as percent body fat exceeds the recommended range.

SOURCES: Gallagher, D., et al. 2000. Healthy percentage body fat ranges: An approach for developing guidelines based on body mass index. *American Journal of Clinical Nutrition* 72: 694–701. American College of Sports Medicine. 2006. *ACSM's Resource Manual for Guidelines for Exercise Testing and Prescription,* 5th ed. Philadelphia: Lippincott Williams and Wilkins.

Other Methods of Assessing Percent Body Fat

If you use a different method, record the name of the method and the result below and in the chart at the end of this lab. Find your body composition rating on the chart above.

Method used: _____ Percent body fat: _____ % Rating (from chart above): _____

Waist Circumference and Waist-to-Hip Ratio

Equipment
1. Tape measure
2. Partner to take measurements

Preparation

Wear clothes that will not add significantly to your measurements.

Instructions

Stand with your feet together and your arms at your sides. Raise your arms only high enough to allow for taking the measurements. Your partner should make sure the tape is horizontal around the entire circumference and pulled snugly against your skin. The tape shouldn't be pulled so tight that it causes indentations in your skin. Record measurements to the nearest millimeter or one-sixteenth of an inch.

Waist. Measure at the smallest waist circumference. If you don't have a natural waist, measure at the level of your navel.
Waist measurement: _____

Hip. Measure at the largest hip circumference. Hip measurement: _____

Waist-to-Hip Ratio: You can use any unit of measurement (for example, inches or centimeters) as long as you're consistent. Waist-to-hip ratio equals waist measurement divided by hip measurement.

Waist-to-hip ratio: _____ ÷ _____ = _____
                             (waist measurement)   (hip measurement)

Determining Your Risk

The table below indicates values for waist circumference and waist-to-hip ratio above which the risk of health problems increases significantly. If your measurement or ratio is above either cutoff point, put a check on the appropriate line below and in the chart at the end of this lab.

Waist circumference: _____ (✓ high risk) Waist-to-hip ratio: _____ (✓ high risk)

Body Fat Distribution

Cutoff Points for High Risk

	Waist Circumference	*Waist-to-Hip Ratio*
Men	More than 40 in. (102 cm)	More than 0.94
Women	More than 35 in. (88 cm)	More than 0.82

SOURCES: National Heart, Lung, and Blood Institute. 1998. *Clinical Guidelines on the Identification, Evaluation, and Treatment of Overweight and Obesity in Adults: The Evidence Report.* Bethesda, Md.: National Institutes of Health. Heyward, V. H., and D. R. Wagner. 2004. *Applied Body Composition Assessment,* 2nd ed. Champaign, Ill.: Human Kinetics.

Rating Your Body Composition

Assessment	*Value*	*Classification*
BMI	_____ kg/m^2	_____
Skinfold measurements or alternative method of determining percent body fat Specify method: _____	_____ % body fat	_____
Waist circumference	_____ in. or cm	_____ (✓ high risk)
Waist-to-hip ratio	_____ (ratio)	_____ (✓ high risk)

Using Your Results

How did you score? Are you surprised by your ratings for body composition and body fat distribution? Are your current ratings in the range for good health? Are you satisfied with your current body composition? Why or why not?

If you're not satisfied, set a realistic goal for improvement:

What should you do next? Enter the results of this lab in the Preprogram Assessment column in Appendix D. If you've determined that you need to improve your body composition, set a specific goal by completing Lab 6.2, and then plan your program using the labs in Chapters 8 and 9. You can also refer to the weight management section of the Daily Fitness and Nutrition Journal on the Online Learning Center. After several weeks or months of an exercise and/or dietary change program, complete this lab again and enter the results in the Postprogram Assessment column of Appendix D. How do the results compare?

Name _____   Section _____   Date _____

LAB 6.2 Setting Goals for Target Body Weight

This lab is designed to help you set body weight goals based on a target BMI or percent body fat. If the results of Lab 6.1 indicate that a change in body composition would be beneficial for your health, you may want to complete this lab to help you set goals.

Remember, though, that a wellness lifestyle—including a balanced diet and regular exercise—is more important for your health than achieving any specific body weight, BMI, or percent body fat. You may want to set goals for improving your diet and increasing physical activity and let your body composition change as a result. If so, use the labs in Chapters 3, 4, 8, and 9 as your guides.

Equipment

Calculator (or pencil and paper for calculations)

Preparation

Determine percent body fat and/or calculate BMI as described in Lab 6.1. Keep track of height and weight as measured for these calculations.

Height: _____   Weight: _____

Instructions: Target Body Weight from Target BMI

Use the chart below to find the target body weight that corresponds to your target BMI. Find your height in the left column, and then move across the appropriate row until you find the weight that corresponds to your target BMI. Remember, BMI is only an indirect measurement of body composition. It is possible to improve body composition without any significant change in weight. For example, a weight training program may result in increased muscle mass and decreased fat mass without any change in overall weight. For this reason, you may want to set alternative or additional goals, such as improving the fit of your clothes or decreasing your waist measurement.

	<18.5 Underweight		18.5–24.9 Normal						25–29.9 Overweight					30–34.9 Obesity (Class I)					35–39.9 Obesity (Class II)					≥40 Extreme Obesity
BMI	17	18	19	20	21	22	23	24	25	26	27	28	29	30	31	32	33	34	35	36	37	38	39	40
Height												Body Weight (pounds)												
4' 10"	81	86	91	96	101	105	110	115	120	124	129	134	139	144	148	153	158	163	168	172	177	182	187	192
4' 11"	84	89	94	99	104	109	114	119	124	129	134	139	144	149	154	159	163	168	173	178	183	188	193	198
5'	87	92	97	102	108	113	118	123	128	133	138	143	149	154	159	164	169	174	179	184	190	195	200	205
5' 1"	90	95	101	106	111	117	122	127	132	138	143	148	154	159	164	169	175	180	185	191	196	201	207	212
5' 2"	93	98	104	109	115	120	126	131	137	142	148	153	159	164	170	175	181	186	191	197	202	208	213	219
5' 3"	96	102	107	113	119	124	130	136	141	147	153	158	164	169	175	181	186	192	198	203	209	215	220	226
5' 4"	99	105	111	117	122	128	134	140	146	152	157	163	169	175	181	187	192	198	204	210	216	222	227	233
5' 5"	102	108	114	120	126	132	138	144	150	156	162	168	174	180	186	192	198	204	210	216	222	229	235	241
5' 6"	105	112	118	124	130	136	143	149	155	161	167	174	180	186	192	198	205	211	217	223	229	236	242	248
5' 7"	109	115	121	128	134	141	147	153	160	166	173	179	185	192	198	204	211	217	224	230	236	243	249	256
5' 8"	112	118	125	132	138	145	151	158	165	171	178	184	191	197	204	211	217	224	230	237	244	250	257	263
5' 9"	115	122	129	136	142	149	156	163	169	176	183	190	197	203	210	217	224	230	237	244	251	258	264	271
5' 10"	119	126	133	139	146	153	160	167	174	181	188	195	202	209	216	223	230	237	244	251	258	265	272	279
5' 11"	122	129	136	143	151	158	165	172	179	187	194	201	208	215	222	230	237	244	251	258	265	273	280	287
6'	125	133	140	148	155	162	170	177	184	192	199	207	214	221	229	236	243	251	258	266	273	280	288	295
6' 1"	129	137	144	152	159	167	174	182	190	197	205	212	220	228	235	243	250	258	265	273	281	288	296	303
6' 2"	132	140	148	156	164	171	179	187	195	203	210	218	226	234	242	249	257	265	273	281	288	296	304	312
6' 3"	136	144	152	160	168	176	184	192	200	208	216	224	232	240	248	256	264	272	280	288	296	304	312	320
6' 4"	140	148	156	164	173	181	189	197	206	214	222	230	238	247	255	263	271	280	288	296	304	312	321	329

SOURCE: Ratings from the National Heart, Lung, and Blood Institute. 1998. *Clinical Guidelines on the Identification, Evaluation, and Treatment of Overweight and Obesity in Adults.* Bethesda, Md.: National Institutes of Health.

Current BMI: _____ Target BMI: _____ Target body weight (from chart): _____

Alternative/additional goals: _____

_____

Note: You can calculate target body weight from target BMI more precisely by using the following formula: (1) convert your height measurement to meters, (2) square your height measurement, (3) multiply this number by your target BMI to get your target weight in kilograms, and (4) convert your target weight from kilograms to pounds:

1. Height _____ in. × 0.0254 m/in. = height _____ m

2. Height _____ m × height _____ m = _____ m^2

3. Target BMI _____ × height _____ m^2 = target weight _____ kg

4. Target weight _____ kg × 2.2 lb/kg = target weight _____ lb

Instructions: Target Body Weight from Target Body Fat Percentages

Use the formula below to determine the target body weight that corresponds to your target percent body fat.

Current percent body fat: _____ Target percent body fat: _____

Formula	*Example: 180-lb male, current percent body fat of 24%, goal of 21%*
1. To determine the fat weight in your body, multiply your current weight by percent body fat (determined through skinfold measurements and expressed as a decimal).	180 lb × 0.24 = 43.2 lb
2. Subtract the fat weight from your current weight to get your current fat-free weight.	180 lb − 43.2 lb = 136.8 lb
3. Subtract your target percent body fat from 1 to get target percent fat-free weight.	1 − 0.21 = 0.79
4. To get your target body weight, divide your fat-free weight by your target percent fat-free weight.	136.8 lb ÷ 0.79 = 173 lb

Note: Weight can be expressed in either pounds or kilograms, as long as the unit of measurement is used consistently.

1. Current body weight _____ × percent body fat _____ = fat weight _____

2. Current body weight _____ − fat weight _____ = fat-free weight _____

3. 1 − target percent body fat _____ = target percent fat-free weight _____

4. Fat-free weight _____ ÷ target percent fat-free weight _____ = target body weight _____

Setting a Goal

Based on these calculations and other factors (including heredity, individual preference, and current health status), select a target weight or range of weights for yourself.

Target body weight: _____

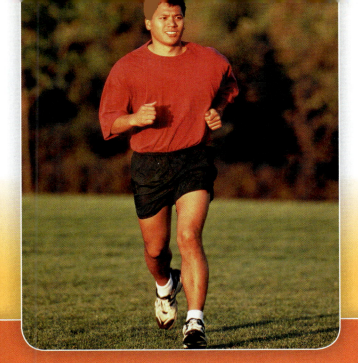

**AFTER READING THIS CHAPTER,
YOU SHOULD BE ABLE TO:**

- Explain the steps for putting together a successful personal fitness program
- Describe strategies that can help you maintain a fitness program over the long term
- Tailor a fitness program to accommodate special health concerns and different life stages

PUTTING TOGETHER

A COMPLETE FITNESS PROGRAM

7

TEST YOUR KNOWLEDGE

1. **Which exercise will allow you to burn the greatest number of calories per pound, if performed vigorously?**

    a. aerobic dance
    b. swimming
    c. bicycling

2. **Falling asleep in a boring class means a person needs more sleep.**

    True or false?

3. **Exercise is not recommended for people with asthma or diabetes.**

    True or false?

ANSWERS

1. **b.** Of the three activities, swimming has the potential to burn 0.088 calories per pound of body weight, per minute of activity, when performed vigorously.

2. **TRUE.** A fully rested person may become bored during an uninteresting or monotonous event but will not fall asleep. Daytime sleepiness is a sign of inadequate sleep, which negatively affects health and athletic performance.

3. **FALSE.** Although special precautions may be needed, people with many types of chronic conditions can exercise safely and enjoy significant health benefits. Regular exercise reduces the risks of acute asthma attacks and improves insulin sensitivity.

FIT AND WELL ONLINE LEARNING CENTER www.mhhe.com/fahey

Visit the *Fit and Well* Online Learning Center for resources that will help you get the most out of your course!

- Study and review aids include practice quizzes, glossary flashcards, chapter summaries, learning objectives, PowerPoint presentations, Common Questions Answered, student handouts, crossword puzzles, Internet activities, and links to wellness Web sites.
- Behavior change tools include a daily fitness and nutrition journal, a behavior change workbook, sample behavior change plans, and blank behavior change logs to print and use.

Understanding the physiological basis and wellness benefits of health-related physical fitness, as explained in Chapters 1–6, is the first step toward creating a well-rounded exercise program. The next challenge is to combine activities into a program that develops all the fitness components and maintains motivation. This chapter presents a step-by-step procedure for creating and maintaining a well-rounded program. At the end of this chapter, you'll find sample programs based on popular activities. The structure these programs provide can be helpful if you're beginning an exercise program for the first time.

DEVELOPING A PERSONAL FITNESS PLAN

If you're ready to create a complete fitness program based on the activities you enjoy most, begin by preparing the program plan and contract in Lab 7.1. By carefully developing your plan and signing a contract, you'll increase your chances of success. The step-by-step procedure outlined here will guide you through the steps of Lab 7.1 to create an exercise program that's right for you. Refer to Figure 7.1 for a sample personal fitness program plan and contract.

If you'd like additional help in setting up your program, choose one of the sample programs at the end of this chapter. Sample programs are provided for walking/jogging/running, cycling, swimming, and calisthenics circuit training; they include detailed instructions for starting a program and developing and maintaining fitness.

1. Set Goals

Ask yourself, "What do I want from my fitness program?" Develop different types of goals—general and specific, long term and short term. General or long-term goals might include things like lowering your risk for chronic disease, improving posture, having more energy, and improving the fit of your clothes.

It's a good idea to also develop some specific, short-term goals based on measurable factors. Specific goals might be:

- Raising $\dot{V}O_{2max}$ by 10%.
- Reducing the time it takes you to jog 2 miles from 22 minutes to 19 minutes.
- Increasing the number of push-ups you can do from 15 to 25.
- Lowering your BMI from 26 to 24.5.

Having specific goals will allow you to track your progress and enjoy the measurable changes brought about by your fitness program. Finally, break your specific goals

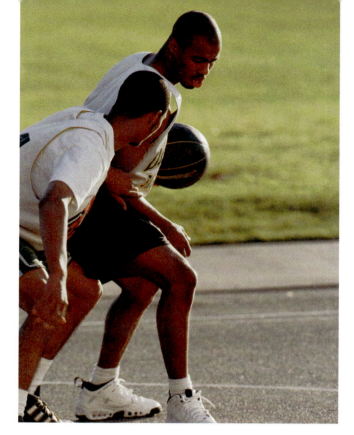

An overall fitness program includes activities to develop all the components of physical fitness.

into several smaller steps (mini-goals), such as those shown in Figure 7.1.

Physical fitness assessment tests are essential to determining your goals. They help you decide which types of exercise you should emphasize, and they help you understand the relative difficulty of attaining specific goals. If you have health problems, such as high blood pressure, heart disease, obesity, or serious joint or muscle disabilities, see your physician before taking assessment tests. Measure your progress by taking these tests about every 3 months.

You'll find it easier to stick with your program if you choose goals that are both important to you and realistic. Remember that heredity, your current fitness level, and other individual factors influence the amount and rate of improvement and the ultimate level of fitness you can expect to reach through physical training. Fitness improves most quickly during the first 6 months of an exercise program. After that, gains come more slowly and usually require a higher-intensity program. Don't expect to improve indefinitely: Improve your fitness to a reasonable target level, and then train consistently to maintain it. Sometimes you may lose fitness—due to illness, injury, missed workouts, or a vacation—so you must begin again at a lower level. Developing fitness is a dynamic process that involves gains and losses. Even if you lose ground occasionally, stay with your program, and you'll be able to achieve your goals.

A. I [Tracie Kaufman] am contracting with myself to follow a physical
        (name)
    fitness program to work toward the following goals:

Specific or short-term goals

1. Improving cardiorespiratory fitness by raising my $\dot{V}O_{2max}$ from 34 to 37 ml/kg/min
2. Improving upper body muscular strength and endurance rating from fair to good
3. Improving body composition (from 28% to 25% body fat)
4. Improving my tennis game (hitting 20 playable shots in a row against the ball machine)

General or long-term goals

1. Developing a more positive attitude about myself
2. Improving the fit of my clothes
3. Building and maintaining bone mass to reduce my risk of osteoporosis
4. Increasing my life expectancy and reducing my risk for diabetes and heart disease

B. **My program plan is as follows:**

Activities	Components (Check X) CRE	MS	ME	F	BC	Time	Frequency (Check X) M	Tu	W	Th	F	S	S	Intensity*
Swimming	X	X	X	X	X	35min	X		X		X			140–170 bpm
Tennis		X	X	X	X	90min					X			RPE= 13–16
Weight training		X	X	X	X	30min		X		X		X		see Lab 4–3
Stretching				X		25min	X		X		X	X		—

*List your target heart rate range or an RPE value if appropriate.

C. My program will begin on [Sept. ▲▼] [21 ▲▼] My program includes the following schedule
    of mini-goals. For each step in my program, I will give myself the reward listed.

Completing 2 full weeks of program (mini-goal 1)	Oct. ▲▼ 5 ▲▼	movie with friends (reward)
$\dot{V}O_{2max}$ of 35 ml/kg/min (mini-goal 2)	Nov. ▲▼ 2 ▲▼	new CD (reward)
Completing 10 full weeks of program (mini-goal 3)	Nov. ▲▼ 30 ▲▼	new sweater (reward)
Percent body fat of 27% (mini-goal 4)	Dec. ▲▼ 22 ▲▼	weekend away (reward)
$\dot{V}O_{2max}$ of 36 ml/kg/min (mini-goal)	Jan. ▲▼ 18 ▲▼	new CD (reward)

D. My program will include the addition of physical activity to my daily routine (such
    as climbing stairs or walking to class):

1. Walking to and from campus job
2. Taking the stairs to dorm room instead of elevator
3. Bicycling to the library instead of driving
4. Doing one active chore a day
5.

E. I will use the following tools to monitor my program and my progress toward
    my goals:

    I'll use a chart that lists the number of laps and minutes I swim and the
    charts for strength and flexibility from Labs 4-3 & 5-2.

I sign this contract as an indication of my personal commitment to reach my goal.

_____ *Tracie Kaufman* _____   Sep. ▲▼ 10 ▲▼
        (your signature)

I have recruited a helper who will witness my contract and

[swim with me three days per week]
(list any way your helper will participate in your program)

_____ *Russell Walker* _____   Sep. ▲▼ 10 ▲▼
        (witness's signature)

FIGURE 7.1   A sample personal fitness program plan and contract.

Table 7.1   A Summary of Sports and Fitness Activities

This table classifies sports and activities as high (H), moderate (M), or low (L) in terms of their ability to develop each of the five components of physical fitness: cardiorespiratory endurance (CRE), muscular strength (MS), muscular endurance (ME), flexibility (F), and body composition (BC). The skill level needed to obtain fitness benefits is noted: Low (L) means little or no skill is required to obtain fitness benefits; moderate (M) means average skill is needed to obtain fitness benefits; and high (H) means much skill is required to obtain fitness benefits. The fitness prerequisite, or conditioning needs of a beginner, is also noted: Low (L) means no fitness prerequisite is required, moderate (M) means some preconditioning is required, and high (H) means substantial fitness is required. The last two columns list the calorie cost of each activity when performed moderately and vigorously. To determine how many calories you burn, multiply the value in the appropriate column by your body weight and then by the number of minutes you exercise. Work up to using 300 or more calories per workout.

Sports and Activities	Components					Skill Level	Fitness Prerequisite	Approximate Calorie Cost (cal/lb/min)	
	CRE	MS*	ME*	F*	BC			Moderate	Vigorous
Aerobic dance	H	M	H	H	H	L	L	.046	.062
Backpacking	H	M	H	M	H	L	M	.032	.078
Badminton, skilled, singles	H	M	M	M	H	M	M	—	.071
Ballet (floor combinations)	M	M	H	H	M	M	L	—	.058
Ballroom dancing	M	L	M	L	M	M	L	.034	.049
Baseball (pitcher and catcher)	M	M	H	M	M	H	M	.039	—
Basketball, half court	H	M	H	M	H	M	M	.045	.071
Bicycling	H	M	H	M	H	M	L	.049	.071
Bowling	L	L	L	L	L	L	L	—	—
Calisthenic circuit training	H	M	H	M	H	L	L	—	.060
Canoeing and kayaking (flat water)	M	M	H	M	M	M	M	.045	—
Cheerleading	M	M	M	M	M	M	L	.033	.049
Elliptical exercise	H	M	H	M	H	L	L	.049	.070
Fencing	M	M	H	H	M	M	L	.032	.078
Field hockey	H	M	H	M	H	M	M	.052	.078
Folk and square dancing	M	L	M	L	M	L	L	.039	.049
Football, touch	M	M	M	M	M	M	M	.049	.078
Frisbee, ultimate	H	M	H	M	H	M	M	.049	.078
Golf (riding cart)	L	L	L	M	L	L	L	—	—
Handball, skilled, singles	H	M	H	M	H	M	M	—	.078
Hiking	H	M	H	L	H	L	M	.051	.073
Hockey, ice and roller	H	M	H	M	H	M	M	.052	.078
Horseback riding	M	M	M	L	M	M	M	.052	.065
Interval circuit training	H	H	H	M	H	L	L	—	.062
Jogging and running	H	M	H	L	H	L	L	.060	.104
Judo	M	H	H	M	M	M	L	.049	.090
Karate	H	M	H	H	H	L	M	.049	.090

*Ratings are for the muscle groups involved.

2. Select Activities

If you have already chosen activities and created separate program plans for different fitness components in Chapters 3–5, you can put those plans together into a single program. It's usually best to include exercises to develop each of the health-related components of fitness.

- Cardiorespiratory endurance is developed by activities such as walking, cycling, and aerobic dance that involve continuous rhythmic movements of large-muscle groups like those in the legs (see Chapter 3).
- Muscular strength and endurance are developed by training against resistance (see Chapter 4).
- Flexibility is developed by stretching the major muscle groups (see Chapter 5).
- Healthy body composition can be developed by combining a sensible diet and a program of regular exercise, including cardiorespiratory endurance exercise to burn calories and resistance training to build muscle mass (see Chapter 6).

Table 7.1 rates many popular activities for their ability to develop each of the health-related components of fitness. Check the ratings of the activities you're considering to make sure the program you put together will develop all fitness components and help you achieve your goals. One strategy is to select one activity for each component of

Table 7.1   A Summary of Sports and Fitness Activities *(continued)*

Sports and Activities	Components					Skill Level	Fitness Prerequisite	Approximate Calorie Cost (cal/lb/min)	
	CRE	MS*	ME*	F*	BC			Moderate	Vigorous
Lacrosse	H	M	H	M	H	H	M	.052	.078
Modern dance (moving combinations)	M	M	H	H	M	L	L	—	.058
Orienteering	H	M	H	L	H	L	M	.049	.078
Outdoor fitness trails	H	M	H	M	H	L	L	—	.060
Popular dancing	M	L	M	M	M	M	L	—	.049
Racquetball, skilled, singles	H	M	M	M	H	M	M	.049	.078
Rock climbing	M	H	H	H	H	H	H	.033	.033
Rope skipping	H	M	H	L	H	M	M	.071	.095
Rowing	H	H	H	H	H	L	L	.032	.097
Rugby	H	M	H	M	H	M	M	.052	.097
Sailing	L	L	M	L	L	M	L	—	—
Skating, ice, roller, and in-line	M	M	M	M	M	H	M	.049	.095
Skiing, alpine	M	H	H	M	M	H	M	.039	.078
Skiing, cross-country	H	M	H	M	H	M	M	.049	.104
Soccer	H	M	H	M	H	M	M	.052	.097
Squash, skilled, singles	H	M	M	M	H	M	M	.049	.078
Stretching	L	L	L	H	L	L	L	—	—
Surfing (including swimming)	M	M	M	M	M	H	M	—	.078
Swimming	H	M	H	M	H	M	L	.032	.088
Synchronized swimming	M	M	H	H	M	H	M	.032	.052
Table tennis	M	L	M	M	M	M	L	—	.045
Tennis, skilled, singles	H	M	M	M	H	M	M	—	.071
Volleyball	M	L	M	M	M	M	L	—	.065
Walking	H	L	M	L	H	L	L	.029	.048
Water polo	H	M	H	M	H	H	M	—	.078
Water skiing	M	M	H	M	M	H	M	.039	.055
Weight training	L	H	H	H	M	L	L	—	—
Wrestling	H	H	H	H	H	H	H	.065	.094
Yoga	L	L	M	H	L	H	L	—	—

*Ratings are for the muscle groups involved.

SOURCE: Kusinitz, I., and M. Fine, *Physical Fitness for Practically Everybody*, Consumer Reports® 1983. Consumers Union of the U.S., Inc., Yonkers, NY 10703-1057, a nonprofit organization. Reprinted with permission for educational purposes only. No commercial use or reproduction permitted. www.ConsumerReports.org®.

fitness—bicycling, weight training, and stretching, for example. Another strategy applies the principle of cross-training, using several different activities to develop a particular fitness component—aerobics classes, swimming, and volleyball for cardiorespiratory endurance, for example. Cross-training is discussed in the next section.

If you select activities that support your commitment rather than activities that turn exercise into a chore, the right program will be its own incentive for continuing. Consider the following factors in making your choices.

• **Fun and interest.** Your fitness program is much more likely to be successful if you choose activities that you enjoy doing. Start by considering any activities you currently engage in and enjoy. Often you can modify your current activities to fit your fitness program. It is a good idea to try a new activity for a while before committing to it.

• **Your current skill and fitness level.** Although many activities are appropriate for beginners, some sports and activities require a moderate level of skill to obtain fitness benefits. For example, a beginning tennis player will probably not be able to sustain rallies long enough to develop cardiorespiratory endurance. Refer to the skill level column in Table 7.1 to determine the level of skill needed for full participation in the activities you're considering. If your current skill level doesn't meet the requirement, you may want to begin your program with a different activity. For example, a beginning tennis player may be better off adhering to a walking program while improving his or her tennis game—or practicing with a ball machine to guarantee steady activity. To build skill for a particular

Choosing Home Exercise Equipment

A home gym can be as simple as a stability ball or as complex as a computerized weight training machine. Regardless, it's best to make sure that your equipment is appropriate for your current needs and will continue to challenge you as your fitness increases. Most importantly, your home exercise equipment should be safe.

Before buying any piece of exercise equipment, consider the following:

- **Your fitness goals.** Make sure the device will help you work on your targeted fitness components. Remember, however, that no single device can "do it all," even though some manufacturers and sellers make such claims. Machines are typically designed for either cardiorespiratory or strength training.

- **Your motivation to use the device.** If you aren't sure whether you'll use the equipment regularly, don't buy it. Instead, try using one regularly at a gym for a few weeks. A try-out period can help you decide whether the device is right for you.

- **Quality.** Look for product reviews in magazines and online. The Federal Trade Commission provides good general advice on shopping for exercise equipment (www.ftc.gov). A personal

trainer may be able to give you recommendations, especially if he or she is not involved in selling equipment. Do not buy a device unless you are sure it is well made. Using low-quality equipment increases your risk of injury.

- **Your space requirements.** Will a treadmill take up your entire living room? Make sure you have enough space to accommodate the device. If necessary, look for equipment that folds up or breaks down to occupy less space between uses.

The most popular types of home equipment for aerobic exercise are treadmills, stationary bikes, cross-country ski machines, stair climbers, and elliptical trainers. When trying out such devices, make sure they support your weight without giving. They should accommodate your full range of motion and should operate smoothly and quietly.

Shop for equipment at a store that specializes in selling such devices. The store should have a highly trained staff and should be able to repair your equipment if it breaks (a real problem with mechanized devices such as treadmills). The staff should be able to tell you all about the equipment's features and warranty.

---

activity, consider taking a class or getting some instruction from a coach or fellow participant.

Your current fitness level may also limit the activities that are appropriate for your program. For example, if you have been inactive, a walking program would be more appropriate than a jogging program. Activities in which participants control the intensity of effort—walking, cycling, and swimming, for example—are more appropriate for a beginning fitness program than sports and activities that are primarily "other paced"—soccer, basketball, and tennis, for example. Refer to the fitness prerequisite column of Table 7.1 to determine the minimum level of fitness required for participation in the activities you're considering. However, staying active is the most important thing. If you like to play tennis but don't like to take walks or jog, then play tennis.

- **Time and convenience.** Unless exercise fits easily into your daily schedule, you are unlikely to maintain your program over the long term. As you consider activities, think about whether a special location or facility is required. Can you participate in the activity close to your

residence, school, or job? Are the necessary facilities open and available at times convenient to you (see Lab 7.2)? Do you need a partner or a team to play? Can you participate in the activity year-round, or will you need to find an alternative during the summer or winter? Would a home treadmill make you more likely to exercise regularly?

- **Cost.** Some sports and activities require equipment, fees, or some type of membership investment. If you are on a tight budget, limit your choices to activities that are inexpensive or free. Investigate the facilities on your campus, which you may be able to use at little or no cost. Many activities require no equipment beyond an appropriate pair of shoes (see the box "Choosing Exercise Footwear," in Chapter 3 for more information). For tips on evaluating exercise equipment, see the box "Choosing Home Exercise Equipment."

- **Special health needs.** If you have special exercise needs due to a particular health problem, choose activities that will conform to your needs and enhance your ability to cope. If necessary, consult your physician about how best to tailor an exercise program to your particular needs and goals. Guidelines and safety tips for exercisers with common chronic conditions are provided later in the chapter.

QUESTIONS FOR CRITICAL THINKING AND REFLECTION

Consider the list of physical activities and sports in Table 7.1. For which ones do you have the necessary fitness prerequisite (rated low, moderate, or high)? Given your current fitness and skill level, which ones could you reasonably incorporate into your exercise program?

3. Set a Target Frequency, Intensity, and Time (Duration) for Each Activity

The next step is to apply the FITT principle and set a starting frequency, intensity, and time (duration) for each type of activity you've chosen (see the summary in Figure 7.2 and the sample in Figure 7.1). Refer to the calculations and plans you completed in Chapters 3–5.

	Cardiorespiratory endurance training	Strength training	Flexibility training
Frequency	3–5 days per week	At least 2 days per week	2–3 days per week (minimum); 5–7 days per week (ideal)
Intensity	55/65–90% of maximum heart rate	Sufficient resistance to fatigue muscles	Stretch to the point of tension
Time	20–60 minutes in sessions lasting 10 minutes or more	8–12 repetitions of each exercise, 1 or more sets	2–4 repetitions of each exercise, held for 15–30 seconds
Type	Continuous rhythmic activities using large muscle groups	Resistance exercises for all major muscle groups	Stretching exercises for all major joints

FIGURE 7.2   A summary of the FITT principle for the health-related components of fitness.

Cardiorespiratory Endurance Exercise   An appropriate frequency for cardiorespiratory endurance exercise is 3–5 times per week. For intensity, note your target heart rate zone or RPE value. Your target total workout time (duration) should be about 20–60 minutes, depending on the intensity of the activity (shorter durations are appropriate for high-intensity activities, longer durations for activities of more moderate intensity). You can exercise in a single session or in multiple sessions of 10 or more minutes.

One way to check whether the total duration you've set is appropriate is to use the **calorie costs** given in Table 7.1. Your goal should be to work up to burning about 300 calories per workout; beginners should start with a calorie cost of about 100–150 calories per workout. Calculate the calorie cost of your activities by multiplying the appropriate factor from Table 7.1 by your body weight and the duration of your workout. For example, walking at a moderate pace burns about 0.029 calorie per minute per pound of body weight. A person weighing 150 pounds could begin her exercise program by walking for 30 minutes, burning about 130 calories. Once her fitness improves, she might choose to start cycling for her cardiorespiratory endurance workouts. Cycling at a moderate pace has a higher calorie cost than walking (0.049 calorie per minute per pound), and if she cycled for 40 minutes, she would burn the target 300 calories during her workout.

Muscular Strength and Endurance Training   A frequency of at least 2 nonconsecutive days per week for strength training is recommended. As described in Chapter 4, a general fitness strength training program includes 1 or more sets of 8–12 repetitions of 8–10 exercises that work all major muscle groups. For intensity, choose a weight that is heavy enough to fatigue your muscles but not so heavy that you cannot complete the full number of repetitions with proper form.

Flexibility Training   Stretches should be performed when muscles are warm at least 2–3 days per week (5–7 days per week is ideal). Stretches should be performed for all major muscle groups. For each exercise, stretch to the point of slight tension or mild discomfort, and hold the stretch for 15–30 seconds; do 2–4 repetitions of each exercise.

4. Set Up a System of Mini-Goals and Rewards

To keep your program on track, set up a system of goals and rewards. Break your specific goals into several steps, and set a target date for each step. For example, if one of the goals of an 18-year-old male student's program is to improve upper-body strength and endurance, he could use the push-up test in Lab 4.2 to set intermediate goals. If he can currently perform 15 push-ups (for a rating of "very poor"), he might set intermediate goals of 17, 20, 25, and 30 push-ups (for a final rating of "fair"). By allowing several weeks between mini-goals and specifying rewards,

---

MOTIVATION BOOSTER

Add music. To add variety and enjoyment to your workouts and to boost your motivation, try exercising to music. Researchers have found that working out to music can boost mood and even keep people working out longer and harder without feeling like they are expending extra effort. Just make sure that music provides a safe distraction and doesn't increase your risk of injury; for example, don't wear headphones while walking, jogging, or cycling on the street.

---

calorie cost   The amount of energy used to perform a particular activity, usually expressed in calories per minute per pound of body weight.

he'll be able to track his progress and reward himself as he moves toward his final goal. Reaching a series of small goals is more satisfying than working toward a single, more challenging, goal that may take months to achieve. Realistic goals, broken into achievable mini-goals, can boost your chances of success. For more on choosing appropriate rewards, see Chapter 1 and Activity 4 in the Behavior Change Workbook at the end of the text.

5. Include Lifestyle Physical Activity in Your Program

As described in Chapter 2, daily physical activity is an important part of a fit and well lifestyle. As part of your fitness program plan, specify ways to be more active during your daily routine. You may find it helpful to first use your health journal to track your activities for several days. Review the records in your journal, identify routine opportunities to be more active, and add these to your program plan in Lab 7.1.

6. Develop Tools for Monitoring Your Progress

A record that tracks your daily progress will help remind you of your ongoing commitment to your program and give you a sense of accomplishment. Figure 7.3 shows you how to create a general program log and record the activity type, frequency, and times (durations). Or, if you wish, complete specific activity logs like those in Labs 3.2, 4.3, and 5.2 in addition to, or instead of, a general log. Post your log in a place where you'll see it often as a reminder and as an incentive for improvement. If you have specific, measurable goals, you can also graph your weekly or monthly progress toward your goal (Figure 7.4). To monitor the overall progress of your fitness program, you may choose to reassess your cardiorespiratory endurance, muscular strength and endurance, flexibility, and body composition every 3 months or so during the improvement phase of your program. Because the results of different fitness tests vary, be sure to compare results for the same assessments over time.

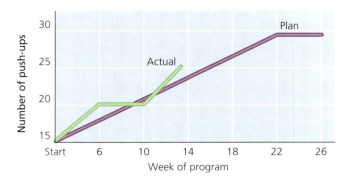

FIGURE 7.4 A sample program progress chart.

7. Make a Commitment

Your final step in planning your program is to make a commitment by signing a contract. Find a witness for your contract—preferably one who will be actively involved in your program. Keep your contract in a visible spot to remind you of your commitment.

PUTTING YOUR PLAN INTO ACTION

Once you've developed a detailed plan and signed your contract, you are ready to begin your fitness program. Refer to the specific training suggestions provided in Chapters 2–5 for advice on beginning and maintaining your program. Many people find it easier to plan a program than to put their plan into action and stick with it over time. For that reason, adherence to healthy lifestyle programs has become an important area of study for psychologists and health researchers. The guidelines below and in the next section reflect research into strategies that help people succeed in sticking with an exercise program.

- **Start slowly and increase fitness gradually.** Overzealous exercising can result in discouraging discomforts and injuries. Your program is meant to last a lifetime. The important first step is to break your established pattern of inactivity. Be patient and realistic. Once your body has adjusted to your starting level of exercise, slowly increase

Name   Tracie Kaufman

Enter time, distance, or another factor (such as heart rate or perceived exertion) to track your progress.

Activity/Date	M	Tu	W	Th	F	S	S	Weekly Total	M	Tu	W	Th	F	S	S	Weekly Total
1 Swimming	800 yd		725 yd		800 yd			2325 yd	800 yd		800 yd		850 yd			2450 yd
2 Tennis					90 min			90 min							95 min	95 min
3 Weight Training		X		X		X				X		X			X	
4 Stretching	X		X		X	X			X			X	X	X	X	

FIGURE 7.3 A sample program log.

the amount of overload. Small increases are the key—achieving a large number of small improvements will eventually result in substantial gains in fitness. It's usually best to increase duration and frequency before increasing intensity.

• **Find an exercise buddy.** The social side of exercise is an important factor for many regular exercisers. Working out with a friend will make exercise more enjoyable and increase your chances of sticking with your program. Find an exercise partner who shares your goals and general fitness level.

• **Ask for support from others.** You have a much greater chance of exercising consistently if you have the support of important people in your life, such as parents, spouse, partner, and friends. Talk with them about your program, and let them know the importance of exercise and wellness in your life. Exercise is not a frivolous pursuit you follow after your work is finished. Rather, it is a critical component of your day (just like sleeping and eating). Good communication will help others become more supportive of and enthusiastic about the time you spend on your wellness program.

• **Vary your activities.** You can make your program more fun over the long term if you participate in a variety of activities that you enjoy. You can also add interest using strategies such as varying the routes you take when walking, running, biking, or in-line skating; finding a new tennis or racquetball partner; changing your music for aerobic dance; or switching to a new volleyball or basketball court.

Varying your activities, a strategy known as cross-training, has other benefits. It can help you develop balanced, total-body fitness. For example, by alternating running with swimming, you build both upper- and lower-body strength. Cross-training can thus prepare you for a wider range of activities and physical challenges. It can also reduce the risk of injury and overtraining because the same muscles, bones, and joints are not continuously subjected to the stresses of the same activity. Cross-training can be done either by choosing different activities on different days or by alternating activities within a single workout.

• **Cycle the duration and intensity of your workouts.** Olympic athletes use a technique called periodization of training, meaning that they vary the duration and intensity of their workouts. Sometimes they exercise very intensely; other times they train lightly or rest. You can use the same technique to improve fitness more quickly and make your training program more varied and enjoyable. For example, if your program consists of walking, weight training, and stretching, pick one day a week for each activity to train a little harder or longer than you normally do. If you usually walk 2 miles in 16 minutes per mile, increase the pace to 15 minutes per mile once a week. If you lift weights twice a week, train more intensely during one of the workouts by using more resistance or performing multiple sets.

• **Adapt to changing environments and schedules.** Most people are creatures of habit and have trouble adjusting to change. Don't use bad weather or a new job as an excuse to give up your exercise program. If you walk in the summer, put on a warm coat and walk in the winter. If you can't go out because of darkness, join a gym and walk on a treadmill.

• **Expect fluctuations and lapses.** On some days, your progress will be excellent, but on others, you'll barely be able to drag yourself through your scheduled activities. Don't let off-days or lapses discourage you or make you feel guilty. Instead, feel a renewed commitment to your fitness program (see the box "Getting Your Fitness Program Back on Track").

• **Choose other healthy lifestyle behaviors.** Exercise provides huge benefits for your health, but other behaviors are also important. Choose a nutritious diet, and avoid harmful habits like smoking and overconsumption of alcohol. Don't skimp on sleep, which has a mutually beneficial relationship with exercise. Physical activity improves sleep, and adequate sleep can improve physical performance (see the box "Sleep").

EXERCISE GUIDELINES FOR PEOPLE WITH SPECIAL HEALTH CONCERNS

Regular, appropriate exercise is safe and beneficial for many people with chronic conditions or other special health concerns. In fact, for many people with special health concerns, the risks associated with *not* exercising are far greater than those associated with a moderate program of regular exercise.

QUESTIONS FOR CRITICAL THINKING AND REFLECTION

How do you typically deal with setbacks? For example, if you have trouble getting motivated to study for exams, what strategies do you use to get back on track? Could those strategies work for keeping your fitness program moving forward? If so, how?

MOTIVATION BOOSTER

Track improvements. In addition to tracking the basic progress of your fitness program, you may find that directly monitoring some of your program's benefits can help keep you motivated and on track. For example, try tracking your energy level. Develop a point scale (1–10 or 1–20), record a value for your energy level each day, and graph the results. Most people find that increasing physical activity quickly boosts their energy level.

Getting Your Fitness Program Back on Track

Lapses are a normal part of any behavior change program. The important point is to move on and avoid becoming discouraged. Try again and keep trying. Know that continued effort will lead to success.

• Don't judge yourself too harshly. Some people make faster gains in fitness than others. Focus on the improvements you've already made from your program and how good you feel after exercise—both physically and mentally.

• Visualize what it will be like to reach your goals. Keep these images in mind as an incentive to stick with your program.

• Use your exercise journal to identify thoughts and behaviors that are causing noncompliance. Devise strategies to combat these problematic patterns. If needed, make additional changes in your environment or find more social support. For example, call a friend to walk with you, or keep exercise clothes in your car or backpack.

• Make changes in your plan and reward system to help renew your enthusiasm for and commitment to your program. Try changing fitness activities or your exercise schedule. Build in more opportunities to reward yourself.

• Plan ahead for difficult situations. Think about what circumstances might make it tough to keep up your fitness routine. Develop strategies to increase your chances of sticking with your program. For example, figure out ways to continue your program during vacation, travel, bad weather, and so on.

• If you're in a bad mood or just don't feel like exercising, remind yourself that physical activity is probably the one thing you can do that will make you feel better. Even if you can only do half your scheduled workout, you'll boost your energy, improve your mood, and help keep your program on track.

The fitness recommendations for the general population presented in this text can serve as a general guideline for any exercise program. For people with special health concerns, however, certain precautions and monitoring may be required. Anyone with special health concerns should consult a physician before beginning an exercise program. The following sections list guidelines and cautions for some common conditions.

Arthritis

• Begin an exercise program as early as possible in the course of the disease.

• Warm up thoroughly before each workout to loosen stiff muscles and lower the risk of injury.

• For cardiorespiratory endurance exercise, avoid high-impact activities that may damage arthritic joints; consider swimming, water walking, or another type of exercise in a warm pool.

• Strength train the whole body; pay special attention to muscles that support and protect affected joints (for example, build quadriceps, hamstring, and calf strength for the knee). Start with small loads and build intensity gradually.

• Perform flexibility exercises daily to maintain joint mobility.

Asthma

• Exercise regularly. Acute attacks are more likely if you exercise only occasionally.

• Carry medication during workouts and avoid exercising alone. Use your inhaler as recommended by your physician.

• Warm up and cool down slowly to reduce the risk of acute attacks.

• When starting an exercise program, choose self-paced endurance activities, especially those involving **interval training** (short bouts of exercise followed by a rest period). Increase the intensity of cardiorespiratory endurance exercise gradually.

• Educate yourself about circumstances that may trigger an asthma attack, and act accordingly. For example, cold, dry air can trigger or worsen an attack. Pollen, dust, and polluted air can also trigger an attack. To avoid attacks in dry air, drink water before, during, and after a workout to moisten your airways. In cold weather, cover your mouth with a mask or scarf to warm and humidify the air you breathe. Also, avoid outdoor activities during pollen season or when the air is polluted or dusty.

Diabetes

• Don't begin an exercise program unless your diabetes is under control and you have discussed exercise safety with your physician. Because people with diabetes have an increased risk for heart disease, an exercise stress test may be recommended.

• Don't exercise alone. Wear a bracelet identifying yourself as having diabetes.

• If you take insulin or another medication, adjust the timing and amount of each dose as needed. Work with your physician and check your blood sugar levels regularly so you can learn to balance your energy intake and output and your medication dosage.

Sleep

The majority of Americans suffer from chronic sleep deprivation. Most of us get between one-half and two fewer hours of sleep each night than we need in order to be fully alert during the day.

Many people view sleep as a luxury or a waste of time, but sleep is absolutely essential for life and health.

- When deprived of sleep for many days, humans and other animals become ill and even die.
- Less extreme sleep deprivation over a long time makes people more vulnerable to a variety of illnesses, including CVD, diabetes, high blood pressure, and psychological disorders.
- Sleep deprivation has been linked to weight gain.
- Inadequate sleep depresses the immune system, making people more vulnerable to infection.
- Lack of sleep affects learning, memory, and attention span, all critical to academic performance.
- Athletes who don't get enough sleep cannot perform at their peak because fatigue slows reaction time and reduces endurance.

Drowsiness is a factor in at least 100,000 auto crashes each year; it impairs driving ability as much as alcohol use. Many of us think that no matter how tired we may be, we can force ourselves to be alert, but we can't. People who are sleep deprived may think they are wide awake but often fall asleep at the wheel for brief periods without even realizing it.

College students are particularly vulnerable to sleep deprivation and poor quality of sleep. Most students lead hectic lives as they juggle studies, work, socializing, and family obligations. Students who live in dormitories are often awakened by nighttime noise. Partying, especially if alcohol and other drugs are used, further disrupts sleep. Financial necessity dictates that many students work part-time or even full-time. There are only so many hours in the day, and many working students find it nearly impossible to get enough sleep to function well in school or at work. To make matters worse, teens and young adults actually need more sleep than older individuals—more than 9 hours of sleep a night—to be well rested.

How do you know if you're getting enough sleep? If you need an alarm to get yourself up every morning, rather than awakening naturally at the appropriate time, chances are you are significantly sleep deprived. Another clue is if you fall asleep within just a few minutes of getting into bed, or if you fall asleep during the day when you don't intend to, such as during lectures or while reading or watching TV.

Sleep you need but don't get is referred to as "sleep debt." Whenever you get less sleep than your body requires, you add to your sleep debt. Week after week, sleep debt can build, leaving you chronically groggy.

If you have a large sleep debt, sleeping in a few extra hours on the weekends won't solve the problem, although it can help a bit. The real solution is to make sleep a priority in your daily life. Remember that the time you spend sleeping will pay for itself in increased productivity. For example, if you go to bed one hour earlier instead of trying to study when you're half awake, you are likely to get the work done in a fraction of the time when you're more alert the next day.

- To prevent abnormally rapid absorption of injected insulin, inject it over a muscle that won't be exercised, and wait at least an hour before exercising.
- Check blood sugar levels before, during, and after exercise, and adjust your diet or insulin dosage as needed. Have high-carbohydrate foods on hand during a workout. Avoid exercise if your blood sugar level is above 250 mg/dl, and ingest carbohydrates prior to exercise if your blood sugar level is below 100 mg/dl.
- Don't lift heavy weights. Straining can damage blood vessels. Instead, perform a higher number of repetitions (15–20) using a lighter load.
- If you have poor circulation or numbness in your extremities, check your skin regularly for blisters and abrasions, especially on your feet. Avoid high-impact activities and wear comfortable shoes.
- For maximum benefit and minimum risk, choose low-to-moderate-intensity activities.

Heart Disease and Hypertension

- Check with your physician about exercise safety before increasing your activity level.
- Exercise at moderate rather than high intensity. Keep your heart rate below the level at which abnormalities appear on an exercise stress test.
- Warm up and cool down gradually, with sessions lasting at least 10 minutes each.
- Monitor your heart rate during exercise, and stop if you experience dizziness or chest pain.
- If your physician has prescribed it, carry nitroglycerin with you during exercise. If you are taking beta-blockers for hypertension, use RPE rather than heart

interval training A training technique that alternates exercise intervals with rest intervals or intense exercise intervals with low-to-moderate intervals.

TERMS

WEB

WELLNESS CONNECTION

rate to monitor exercise intensity (beta-blockers reduce heart rate). Exercise at an RPE level of "fairly light" to "somewhat hard"; your breathing should be unlabored, and you should be able to talk.

- Don't hold your breath when exercising. Doing so can cause sudden, steep increases in blood pressure. Take special care during weight training; don't lift heavy loads. Exhale during the exertion phase of lifts.

- Increase exercise frequency, intensity, and time very gradually.

Obesity

- For maximum benefit and minimum risk, begin by choosing low-to-moderate-intensity activities. Increase intensity slowly as your fitness improves. Studies of overweight people show that exercising at moderate-to-high intensities causes more fat loss than training at low intensities.

- Follow the 2005 Dietary Guidelines recommending that people who want to lose weight or maintain lost weight exercise moderately 60 minutes or more every day. To get the benefit of 60 minutes of exercise, you can exercise all at once or divide your total activity time into sessions of 10, 20, or 30 minutes.

- Choose non- or low-weight-bearing activities such as swimming, water exercises, cycling, or walking. Low-impact activities are less likely to lead to joint problems or injuries.

- Stay alert for symptoms of heat-related problems during exercise (see Chapter 3). Obese people are vulnerable to heat intolerance.

Low-impact activities like walking are a good choice for people who are overweight because they can provide a good workout and are less likely than high-impact activities to cause joint problems or injuries.

- Ease into an exercise program and increase overload gradually. Increase time and frequency of exercise before increasing intensity.

- Include strength training in your fitness program to build or maintain muscle mass.

- Try to include as much lifestyle physical activity in your daily routine as possible.

Osteoporosis

- For cardiorespiratory endurance activities, exercise at the maximum intensity that causes no significant discomfort. If possible, choose low-impact weight-bearing activities to help safely maintain bone density (see Chapter 8 for more strategies for building and maintaining bone density).

- To prevent fractures, avoid any activity or movement that stresses the back or carries a risk of falling.

- Include weight training in your exercise program to improve strength and balance and reduce the risk of falls and fractures. Avoid lifting heavy loads.

MOTIVATION BOOSTER

Join with others. If you have a special health concern and have hesitated to become more active, one helpful strategy is to take a class or join an exercise group specifically designed for your condition. Many health centers and support groups sponsor specially tailored activity programs. Such a class can provide you with both expert advice and exercise partners who share your concerns and goals.

QUESTIONS FOR CRITICAL THINKING AND REFLECTION

Do you have a special physical condition that poses an obstacle to exercising, such as asthma? How have you dealt with this condition in the past? If the condition has prevented you from exercising, how might you deal with it so you can exercise regularly? If necessary, consult with your physician to find ways to exercise despite impediments.

Exercise guidelines for people with disabilities are discussed in Chapter 2 and for people with low-back pain in Chapter 5.

EXERCISE GUIDELINES FOR LIFE STAGES

A fitness program may also need to be adjusted to accommodate the requirements of different life stages.

Children and Adolescents

Lack of physical activity has led to alarming increases in overweight and obesity in children and adolescents. If you have children or are in a position to influence children, keep these guidelines in mind:

- Provide opportunities for children and adolescents to exercise every day. Minimize sedentary activities, such as watching television. Children and adolescents should aim for at least 60 minutes of moderate activity most, but preferably all, days.

- During family outings, choose dynamic activities. For example, go for a walk or park away from a mall and then walk to the stores.

- For children younger than 12, emphasize skill development and fitness rather than excellence in competitive sports. For adolescents, combine participation and training in lifetime sports with traditional, competitive sports.

- Make sure children are developmentally capable of participating in an activity. For example, catching skills are difficult for young children because their nervous system is not developed enough to fully master the skill. When teaching a child to catch a ball, start with a large ball and throw it from a short range. Gradually increase the complexity of the skill once the child has mastered the simpler skill.

- Make sure children get plenty of water when exercising in the heat. Make sure they are dressed properly when exercising in the cold.

Pregnant Women

Exercise is important during pregnancy, but women should be cautious because some types of exercise can pose increased risk to the mother and the unborn child. The following guidelines are consistent with the recommendations of the American College of Obstetrics and Gynecology:

- See your physician about possible modifications needed for your particular pregnancy.

- Continue mild-to-moderate exercise routines at least three times a week. (For most women, this means maintaining an exercise heart rate of 100–160 beats per minute.) Avoid exercising vigorously or to exhaustion, especially in the third trimester. Monitor exercise intensity by assessing how you feel rather than by monitoring your heart rate; RPE levels of 11–13 are appropriate.

- Favor non- or low-weight-bearing exercises such as swimming or cycling over weight-bearing exercises, which can carry increased risk of injury.

- Avoid exercise in a supine position—lying on your back—after the first trimester. This position restricts blood flow to the uterus. Also avoid prolonged periods of motionless standing.

- Avoid exercise that could cause loss of balance, especially in the third trimester, and exercise that might injure the abdomen, stress the joints, or carry a risk of falling (such as contact sports, vigorous racquet sports, skiing, and in-line skating).

- Avoid activities involving extremes in barometric pressure, such as diving and mountain climbing.

- Especially during the first trimester, drink plenty of fluids and exercise in well-ventilated areas to avoid heat stress.

- Do 3–5 sets of 10 Kegel exercises daily. These exercises involve tightening the muscles of the pelvic floor for 5–15 seconds. Kegel exercises are thought to help prevent incontinence (involuntary loss of urine) and speed recovery after giving birth.

- After giving birth, resume prepregnancy exercise routines gradually, based on how you feel.

Older Adults

Older people readily adapt to endurance exercise and strength training. Exercise principles are the same as for younger people, but some specific guidelines apply:

- Include the three basic types of exercise—resistance, endurance, and flexibility.

- For strength training, follow ACSM recommendations that older adults use a lighter weight and perform more (10–15) repetitions than young adults.

- Drink plenty of water and avoid exercising in excessively hot or cold environments. Wear clothes that speed heat loss in warm environments and that prevent heat loss in cold environments.

- Warm up slowly and carefully. Increase intensity and duration of exercise gradually.

- Cool down slowly, continuing very light exercise until the heart rate is below 100.

- To help prevent soft tissue pain, do static stretching after a normal workout.

Sample fitness programs begin on p. 206.

Q Should I exercise every day?

A Some daily exercise is beneficial, and health experts recommend that you engage in at least 30 minutes of moderate physical activity at least 5 days per week. Back experts suggest that you also do back pain prevention exercises daily. However, if you train intensely every day without giving yourself a rest, you will likely get injured or become overtrained. When strength training, for example, rest at least 48 hours between workouts before exercising the same muscle group. For cardio-respiratory endurance exercise, rest or exercise lightly the day after an intense or lengthy workout. Balancing the proper amount of rest and exercise will help you feel better and improve your fitness faster.

Q If exercise is so good for my health, why hasn't my physician ever mentioned to me?

A A recent study by the American College of Sports Medicine (ACSM) suggests that most people would benefit from getting a physician's advice about exercising. According to the study, 65% of patients said they would be more interested in exercising if their physicians suggested it. About 40% of physicians said they talk to their patients about exercise.

To encourage physicians and patients to talk more often about exercise and its benefits, the ACSM and the American Medical Association (AMA) have launched the Exercise is Medicine program. The program advises physicians to give more guidance to patients about exercise and suggests that everyone try to exercise at least 5 days each week. For more information on the program, visit www.exerciseismedicine.org.

For more Common Questions Answered about developing and maintaining a fitness program, visit the *Online Learning Center.*

TIPS FOR TODAY AND THE FUTURE

A complete fitness program includes activities to build and maintain cardiorespiratory endurance, muscular strength and endurance, and flexibility.

RIGHT NOW YOU CAN

- Get a journal to track your daily physical activity and exercise routine.
- Put away your remote control devices—every bit of physical activity can benefit your health.
- Set up your next workout with your training partner.
- Plan to go to bed 15 minutes earlier than usual.

IN THE FUTURE YOU CAN

- Create a schedule that incorporates your workouts into your daily routine. Each week, update the schedule for the upcoming week.
- Learn more about the importance of sleep to good health. If you consistently have trouble sleeping, consult with your physician about seeing a sleep specialist or undergoing a sleep evaluation.

SUMMARY

- Steps for putting together a complete fitness program include (1) setting realistic goals, (2) selecting activities to develop all the health-related components of fitness, (3) setting a target frequency, intensity, and time (duration) for each activity, (4) setting up a system of mini-goals and rewards, (5) making lifestyle physical activity a part of the daily routine, (6) developing tools for monitoring progress, and (7) making a commitment.

- In selecting activities, consider fun and interest, your current skill and fitness levels, time and convenience, cost, and any special health concerns.

- Keys to beginning and maintaining a successful program include starting slowly, increasing intensity and duration gradually, finding a buddy, varying the activities and intensity of the program, and expecting fluctuations and lapses.

- Regular exercise is appropriate and beneficial for people with special health concerns or in particular stages of life; program modifications may be necessary for safety.

FOR FURTHER EXPLORATION

BOOKS, ORGANIZATIONS, AND WEB SITES

American Academy of Orthopaedic Surgeons. Provides information about injuries, treatment, and rehabilitation along with exercise guidelines for people with bone, muscle, and joint pain.
http://www.aaos.org

American College of Obstetricians and Gynecologists. Provides guidelines for promoting a healthy pregnancy and postpartum recovery, including exercise during pregnancy.
http://www.acog.org

American Diabetes Association. Promotes diabetes education, research, and advocacy; includes guidelines for diet and exercise for people with diabetes.
http://www.diabetes.org

American Heart Association. Includes information on fitness for kids as well as diet, exercise, fitness, and weight management for adults.

http://www.heart.org

For additional listings, see Chapters 2–6.

SELECTED BIBLIOGRAPHY

American College of Obstetrics and Gynecology Committee on Obstetric Practice. 2006. *Women's Health: Exercise and Fitness* (http://www.acog.org/publications/patient_education/bp045.cfm; retrieved May 25, 2007).

American College of Sports Medicine. 2006. *ACSM's Guidelines for Exercise Testing and Prescription,* 7th ed. Philadelphia: Lippincott Williams and Wilkins.

American College of Sports Medicine. 2006. *ACSM's Resource Manual for Guidelines for Exercise Testing and Prescription,* 5th ed. Philadelphia: Lippincott Williams and Wilkins.

Bianchi, C., et al. 2007. Treating the metabolic syndrome. *Expert Review of Cardiovascular Therapy* 5(3): 491–506.

Brunet, S., et al. 2005. For the patient: Exercise is important to preventing and controlling type 2 diabetes. *Ethnicity and Disease* 15: 353–354.

Centers for Disease Control and Prevention. 2007. Prevalence of actions to control high blood pressure—20 states, 2005. *Morbidity and Mortality Weekly Report* 56(17): 420–423.

Hogan, M. 2005. Physical and cognitive activity and exercise for older adults: A review. *International Journal of Aging and Human Development* 60: 95–126.

Hu, G., et al. 2007. Epidemiological studies of exercise in diabetes prevention. *Applied Physiology, Nutrition and Metabolism* 32(3): 583–595.

Lee, S., et al. 2005. Exercise without weight loss is an effective strategy for obesity reduction in obese individuals with and without type 2 diabetes. *Journal of Applied Physiology* 99: 1220–1225.

Morris, S. N., and N. R. Johnson. 2005. Exercise during pregnancy: A critical appraisal of the literature. *Journal of Reproductive Medicine* 50: 181–188.

National Sleep Foundation. 2007. *2007 Sleep in America Poll: Summary of Findings.* Washington, D.C.: WBA Market Research.

Nelson, T. F., et al. 2007. Disparities in Overweight and Obesity Among U.S. College Students. *American Journal of Health Behavior* 31(4): 363–373.

Riebe, D., et al. 2005. Long-term maintenance of exercise and healthy eating behaviors in overweight adults. *Preventive Medicine* 40: 769–778.

Vorona, R. D., et al. 2005. Overweight and obese patients in a primary care population report less sleep than patients with a normal body mass index. *Archives of Internal Medicine* 165(1): 25–30.

SAMPLE PROGRAMS FOR POPULAR ACTIVITIES

Sample programs based on four different types of cardiorespiratory activities—walking/jogging/running, bicycling, swimming, and calisthenics circuit training—are presented below. Each sample program includes regular cardiorespiratory endurance exercise, resistance training, and stretching. To choose a sample program, first compare your fitness goals with the benefits of the different types of endurance exercise featured in the sample programs (see Table 7.1). Identify the programs that meet your fitness needs. Next, read through the descriptions of the programs you're considering, and decide which will work best for you based on your present routine, the potential for enjoyment, and adaptability to your lifestyle. If you choose one of these programs, complete the personal fitness program plan in Lab 7.1, the same as if you had created a program from scratch.

No program will produce enormous changes in your fitness level in the first few weeks. Give your program a fair chance. Follow the specifics of the program for 3–4 weeks. Then, if the exercise program doesn't seem suitable, make adjustments to adapt it to your particular needs. But retain the basic elements of the program that make it effective for developing fitness.

GENERAL GUIDELINES

The following guidelines can help make the activity programs more effective for you.

- **Frequency and time.** To experience training effects, exercise for 20–60 minutes at least three times a week.

- **Intensity.** To work effectively for cardiorespiratory endurance training or to improve body composition, raise your heart rate into its target zone. Monitor your pulse or use rates of perceived exertion to monitor your intensity.

  If you've been sedentary, begin very slowly. Give your muscles a chance to adjust to their increased workload. It's probably best to keep your heart rate below target until your body has had time to adjust to new demands. At first you may not need to work very hard to keep your heart rate in its target zone, but as your cardiorespiratory endurance improves, you will probably need to increase intensity.

- **Interval training.** Some of the sample programs involve continuous activity. Others rely on interval training, which calls for alternating a relief interval with exercise (walking after jogging, for example, or coasting after biking uphill). Interval training is an effective way to achieve progressive overload: When your heart rate gets too high, slow down to lower your pulse rate until you're at the low end of your target zone. Interval training can also prolong the total time you spend in exercise and delay the onset of fatigue.

- **Resistance training and stretching guidelines.** For the resistance training and stretching parts of the program, remember the general guidelines for safe and effective exercise. For resistance training, follow these guidelines:

- Train at least 2 nonconsecutive days per week.

- Perform 1 or more sets of 8–12 repetitions of 8–10 exercises.

- Include exercises that work all the major muscle groups: neck, shoulders, chest, arms, upper and lower back, abdomen, thighs, and calves.

For stretching, follow these guidelines:

- Stretch at least 2–3 days per week (ideally, 5–7 days per week), when muscles are warm.

- Stretch to the point of mild discomfort, not pain, and hold the stretch for 15–30 seconds.

- Perform each stretch 2–4 times.

- Stretch all the major muscle groups.

- **Warm-up and cool-down.** Begin each exercise session with a 10-minute warm-up. Begin your activity at a slow pace, and work up gradually to your target heart rate. Always slow down gradually at the end of your exercise session to bring your system back to its normal state. It's a good idea to do stretching exercises to increase your flexibility after cardiorespiratory exercise or strength training because your muscles will be warm and ready to stretch.

- **Record keeping.** After each exercise session, record your daily distance or time on a progress chart.

WALKING/JOGGING/RUNNING SAMPLE PROGRAM

Walking, jogging, and running are the most popular forms of training for people who want to improve cardiorespiratory endurance; they also improve body composition and muscular endurance of the legs. It's not always easy to distinguish among these three endurance activities. For clarity and consistency, we'll consider walking to be any on-foot exercise of less than 5 miles per hour, jogging any pace between 5 and 7.5 miles per hour, and running any pace faster than that. Table 1 divides walking, jogging, and running into nine categories, with rates of speed (in both miles per hour and minutes per mile) and calorie costs for each.

The faster your pace or the longer you exercise, the more calories you burn. The greater the number of calories burned, the higher the potential training effects of these activities. Tables 2 and 3 contain sample walking/jogging programs by time and distance.

Equipment and Technique

These activities require no special skills, expensive equipment, or unusual facilities. Comfortable clothing, well-fitted walking or running shoes, and a stopwatch or ordinary watch with a second hand are all you need.

This table gives the calorie costs of walking, jogging, and running for slow, moderate, and fast paces. Calculations for calorie costs are approximate and assume a level terrain. A hilly terrain would result in higher calorie costs. To get an estimate of the number of calories you burn, multiply your weight by the calories per minute per pound for the speed at which you're doing the activity, and then multiply that by the number of minutes you exercise.

Activity	Speed		Calories per Minute per Pound
	Miles per Hour	Minutes: Seconds per Mile	
Walking			
Slow	2.0	30:00	.020
	2.5	24:00	.023
Moderate	3.0	20:00	.026
	3.5	17:08	.029
Fast	4.0	15:00	.037
	4.5	13:20	.048
Jogging			
Slow	5.0	12:00	.060
	5.5	11:00	.074
Moderate	6.0	10:00	.081
	6.5	9:00	.088
Fast	7.0	8:35	.092
	7.5	8:00	.099
Running			
Slow	8.5	7:00	.111
Moderate	9.0	6:40	.116
Fast	10.0	6:00	.129
	11.0	5:30	.141

SOURCE: Kusinitz, I., and M. Fine, *Physical Fitness for Practically Everybody,* Consumer Reports®, 1983. Consumers Union of the U.S., Inc., Yonkers, NY 10703-1057, a nonprofit organization. Reprinted with permission for educational purposes only. No commercial use or reproduction permitted. www.ConsumerReports.org®.

Developing Cardiorespiratory Endurance

The four variations of the basic walking/jogging/running sample program that follow are designed to help you regulate the intensity, duration, and frequency of your program. Use the following guidelines to choose the variation that is right for you.

• *Variation 1: Walking (starting).* Choose this program if you have medical restrictions, are recovering from illness or surgery, tire easily after short walks, are obese, or have a sedentary lifestyle, and if you want to prepare for the advanced walking program to improve cardiorespiratory endurance, body composition, and muscular endurance.

• *Variation 2: Advanced walking.* Choose this program if you already can walk comfortably for 30 minutes and if you want to develop and maintain cardiorespiratory fitness, a lean body, and muscular endurance.

• *Variation 3: Preparing for a jogging/running program.* Choose this program if you already can walk comfortably for 30 minutes and if you want to prepare for the jogging/running program to improve cardiorespiratory endurance, body composition, and muscular endurance.

• *Variation 4: Jogging/running.* Choose this program if you already can jog comfortably without muscular discomfort, if you already can jog for 15 minutes without stopping or 30 minutes with brief walking intervals within your target heart rate range, and if you want to develop and maintain a high level of cardiorespiratory fitness, a lean body, and muscular endurance.

Variation 1: Walking (Starting)

FIT—frequency, intensity, and time: Walk at first for 15 minutes at a pace that keeps your heart rate below your target zone. Gradually increase to 30-minute sessions. The distance you travel will probably be 1–2 miles. At the beginning, walk every other day. You can gradually increase to daily walking if you want to burn more calories (helpful if you want to change body composition).

Calorie cost: Work up to using 90–135 calories in each session (see Table 1). To increase calorie costs to the target level, walk for a longer time or for a longer distance rather than sharply increasing speed.

At the beginning: Start at whatever level is most comfortable. Maintain a normal, easy pace, and stop to rest as often as you need to. Never prolong a walk past the point of comfort. When walking with a friend (a good motivation), let a comfortable conversation be your guide to pace.

As you progress: Once your muscles have become adjusted to the exercise program, increase the duration of your sessions— but by no more than 10% each week. Increase your intensity only enough to keep your heart rate just below your target. When you're able to walk 1.5 miles in 30 minutes, using 90– 135 calories per session, you should consider moving on to Variation 2 or 3. Don't be discouraged by a lack of immediate progress, and don't try to speed things up by overdoing. Remember that pace and heart rate can vary with the terrain, the weather, and other factors.

Variation 2: Advanced Walking

FIT—frequency, intensity, and time: Start at a pace at the lower end of your target heart rate zone, and begin soon afterward to increase your pace. This might boost your heart rate into the upper levels of your target zone, which is fine for brief periods. But don't overdo the intervals of fast walking. Slow down after a short time to drop your pulse rate. Vary your pattern to allow for intervals of slow, medium, and fast walking. Walk at first for 30 minutes and gradually increase your walking time until eventually you reach 60 minutes, all the while maintaining your target heart rate. The distance you walk will probably be 2–4 miles. Walk at least every other day.

WALKING/JOGGING PROGRESSION BY TIME

This table is based on a walking interval of 3.75 miles per hour, measured in seconds, and a jogging interval of 5.5 miles per hour, measured in minutes:seconds. The combination of the two intervals equals a single set. In the Number of Sets column, the higher figure represents the maximum number of sets to be completed.

	Walk Interval (sec)	Jog Interval (min:sec)	Number of Sets	Total Distance (mi)	Total Time (min:sec)
Stage 1	:60	:30	10–15	1.0–1.7	15:00–22:30
Stage 2	:60	:60	8–13	1.2–2.0	16:00–26:00
Stage 3	:60	2:00	5–19	1.3–2.3	15:00–27:00
Stage 4	:60	3:00	5–7	1.6–2.4	16:00–28:00
Stage 5	:60	4:00	3–6	1.5–2.7	15:00–30:00

SOURCE: Kusinitz, I., and M. Fine, *Physical Fitness for Practically Everybody*, Consumer Reports®, 1983. Consumers Union of the U.S., Inc., Yonkers, NY 10703-1057, a nonprofit organization. Reprinted with permission for educational purposes only. No commercial use or reproduction permitted. www.ConsumerReports.org®.

WALKING/JOGGING PROGRESSION BY DISTANCE

This table is based on a walking interval of 3.75 miles per hour, measured in yards, and a jogging interval of 5.5 miles per hour, also measured in yards. The combination of the two intervals equals a single set. (One lap around a typical track is 440 yards.)

	Walk Interval (yd)	Jog Interval (yd)	Number of Sets	Total Distance (mi)	Total Time (min:sec)
Stage 1	110	55	11–21	1.0–2.0	15:00–28:12
Stage 2	110	110	16	2.0	26:56
Stage 3	110	220	11	2.0	26:02
Stage 4	110	330	8	2.0	24:24
Stage 5	110	440	7	2.2	26:05
Stage 6	110	440	8	2.5	29:49

SOURCE: Kusinitz, I., and M. Fine, *Physical Fitness for Practically Everybody*, Consumer Reports®, 1983. Consumers Union of the U.S., Inc., Yonkers, NY 10703-1057, a nonprofit organization. Reprinted with permission for educational purposes only. No commercial use or reproduction permitted. www.ConsumerReports.org®.

Calorie cost: Work up to using about 200–350 calories in each session (see Table 1).

At the beginning: Begin by walking somewhat faster than you did in Variation 1. Check your pulse to make sure you keep your heart rate within your target zone. Slow down when necessary to lower your heart rate when going up hills or when extending the duration of your walks.

As you progress: As your heart rate adjusts to the increased workload, gradually increase your pace and your total walking time. Gradually lengthen the intervals of fast walking and shorten the relief intervals of slow walking, always maintaining target heart rate. Eventually, you will reach the fitness level you would like to maintain. To maintain that level of fitness, continue to burn the same amount of calories in each session.

Vary your program by changing the pace and distance walked or by walking routes with different terrains and views. Gauge your progress toward whatever calorie goal you've set by using Table 1.

Variation 3: Preparing for a Jogging/Running Program

FIT—frequency, intensity, and time: Start by walking at a moderate pace (3–4 miles per hour or 15–20 minutes per mile). Staying within your target heart rate zone, begin to add brief intervals of slow jogging (5–6 miles per hour or 10–12 minutes per mile). Keep the walking intervals constant at 60 seconds or at 110 yards, but gradually increase the jogging intervals until eventually you jog 4 minutes for each minute of walking. You'll probably cover between 1.5 and 2.5 miles. Each exercise session should last 15–30 minutes. Exercise every other day. If your goals include changing body composition and you want to exercise more frequently, walk on days you're not jogging.

Calorie cost: Work up to using 200–350 calories in each session (see Table 1).

At the beginning: Start slowly. Until your muscles adjust to jogging, you may need to exercise at less than your target heart rate. At the outset, expect to do two to four times as much walking as jogging, and even more if you're relatively inexperienced. Be guided by how comfortable you feel—and by your heart rate—in setting the pace for your progress. Follow the guidelines presented in Chapter 3 for exercising in hot or cold weather. Drink enough liquids to stay adequately hydrated, particularly in hot weather. In addition, use the proper running technique, described below.

• Run with your back straight and your head up. Look straight ahead, not at your feet. Shift your pelvis forward and tuck your buttocks in.

• Hold your arms slightly away from your body. Your elbows should be bent so that your forearms are parallel to the ground. You may cup your hands, but do not clench your fists. Allow your arms to swing loosely and rhythmically with each stride.

• Let your heel hit the ground first in each stride. Then roll forward onto the ball of your foot and push off for the next stride. If you find this difficult, you can try a more flat-footed style, but don't land on the balls of your feet.

• Keep your steps short by allowing your foot to strike the ground in line with your knee. Keep your knees bent at all times.

• Breathe deeply through your mouth. Try to use your abdominal muscles rather than just your chest muscles to take deep breaths.

• Stay relaxed.

As you progress: Adjust your ratio of walking to jogging to keep within your target heart rate zone as much as possible. When you have progressed to the point at which most of your 30-minute session is spent jogging, consider moving on to Variation 4. To find a walking/jogging progression that suits you, refer to Tables 2 and 3 (one uses time, the other distance). Which one you choose will depend, to some extent, on where you work out. If you have access to a track or can use a measured distance with easily visible landmarks to indicate yardage covered, you may find it convenient to use distance as your organizing principle. If you'll be using parks, streets, or woods, time intervals (measured with a watch) would probably work better. The progressions in Tables 2 and 3 are not meant to be rigid; they are guidelines to help you develop your own rate of progress. Let your progress be guided by your heart rate, and increase your intensity and duration only to achieve your target zone.

Variation 4: Jogging/Running

FIT—frequency, intensity, and time: The key is to exercise within your target heart rate zone. Most people who sustain a continuous jog/run program will find that they can stay within their target heart rate zone with a speed of 5.5–7.5 miles per hour (8–11 minutes per mile). Start by jogging steadily for 15 minutes. Gradually increase your jog/run session to a regular 30–60 minutes (or about 2.5–7 miles). Exercise at least every other day. Increasing frequency by doing other activities on alternate days will place less stress on the weight-bearing parts of your lower body than will a daily program of jogging/running.

Calorie cost: Use about 300–750 calories in each session (see Table 1).

At the beginning: The greater number of calories you burn per minute makes this program less time-consuming for altering body composition than the three other variations in the walking/jogging/running program.

As you progress: If you choose this variation, you probably already have a moderate-to-high level of cardiorespiratory fitness. To stay within your target heart rate zone, increase your distance or both pace and distance as needed. Add variety to your workouts by varying your route, intensity, and duration. Alternate short runs with long runs. If you run for 60 minutes one day, try running for 30 minutes the next session. Or try doing sets that alternate hard and easy intervals—even walking, if you feel like it. You can also try a road race now and then, but be careful not to do too much too soon.

Developing Muscular Strength and Endurance and Flexibility

Walking, jogging, and running provide muscular endurance workouts for your lower body; they also develop muscular strength of the lower body to a lesser degree. If you'd like to increase your running speed and performance, you might want to focus your program on lower-body exercises. (Don't neglect upper-body strength, however; it is important for overall wellness.) For flexibility, pay special attention to the hamstrings and quadriceps, which are not worked through their complete range of motion during walking or jogging.

BICYCLING SAMPLE PROGRAM

Bicycling can also lead to large gains in physical fitness. For many people, cycling is a pleasant and economical alternative to driving and a convenient way to build fitness.

Equipment and Technique

Cycling has its own special array of equipment, including headgear, lighting, safety pennants, and special shoes. The

bike is the most expensive item, ranging from about $100 to well over $1000. Avoid making a large investment until you're sure you'll use your bike regularly. While investigating what the marketplace has to offer, rent or borrow a bike. Consider your intended use of the bike. Most cyclists who are interested primarily in fitness are best served by a sturdy 10-speed rather than a mountain bike or sport bike. Stationary cycles are good for rainy days and areas that have harsh winters.

Clothing for bike riding shouldn't be restrictive or binding, nor should it be so loose-fitting or so long that it might get caught in the chain. Clothing worn on the upper body should be comfortable but not so loose that it catches the wind and slows you down. Always wear a helmet to help prevent injury in case of a fall or crash. Wearing glasses or goggles can protect the eyes from dirt, small objects, and irritation from wind.

To avoid saddle soreness and injury, choose a soft or padded saddle, and adjust it to a height that allows your legs to almost reach full extension while pedaling. Make certain the saddle doesn't put too much pressure on sensitive areas. Wear a pair of well-padded gloves if your hands tend to become numb while riding or if you begin to develop blisters or calluses. To prevent backache and neck strain, warm up thoroughly and periodically shift the position of your hands on the handlebars and your body in the saddle. Keep your arms relaxed and don't lock your elbows. To protect your knees from strain, pedal with your feet pointed straight ahead or very slightly inward, and don't pedal in high gear for long periods.

Bike riding requires a number of precise skills that practice makes automatic. If you've never ridden before, consider taking a course. In fact, many courses are not just for beginners. They'll help you develop skills in braking, shifting, and handling emergencies, as well as teach you ways of caring for and repairing your bike. For safe cycling, follow these rules:

- Always wear a helmet.

- Keep on the correct side of the road. Bicycling against traffic is usually illegal and always dangerous.

- Obey all traffic signs and signals.

- On public roads, ride in single file, except in low-traffic areas (if the law permits). Ride in a straight line; don't swerve or weave in traffic.

- Be alert; anticipate the movements of other traffic and pedestrians. Listen for approaching traffic that is out of your line of vision.

- Slow down at street crossings. Check both ways before crossing.

- Use hand signals—the same as for automobile drivers—if you intend to stop or turn. Use audible signals to warn those in your path.

- Maintain full control. Avoid anything that interferes with your vision. Don't jeopardize your ability to steer by carrying anything (including people) on the handlebars.

- Keep your bicycle in good shape. Brakes, gears, saddle, wheels, and tires should always be in good condition.

- See and be seen. Use a headlight at night and equip your bike with rear reflectors. Use side reflectors on pedals, front and rear. Wear light-colored clothing or use reflective tape at night; wear bright colors or use fluorescent tape by day.

- Be courteous to other road users. Anticipate the worst and practice preventive cycling.

- Use a rear-view mirror.

Developing Cardiorespiratory Endurance

Cycling is an excellent way to develop and maintain cardiorespiratory endurance and a healthy body composition.

FIT—frequency, intensity, and time: If you've been inactive for a long time, begin your cycling program at a heart rate that is 10–20% below your target zone. Beginning cyclists should pedal at about 80–100 revolutions per minute; adjust the gear so that you can pedal at that rate easily. Your bicycle may display different types of useful information, including speed, distance traveled, heart rate, altitude, and revolutions per minute, and it may provide a cadence signal to help you maintain your pace. Once you feel at home on your bike, try 1 mile at a comfortable speed, and then stop and check your heart rate. Increase your speed gradually until you can cycle at 12–15 miles per hour (4–5 minutes per mile), a speed fast enough to bring most new cyclists' heart rate into their target zone. Allow your pulse rate to be your guide: More highly fit individuals may need to ride faster to achieve their target heart rate. Cycling for at least 20 minutes three times a week will improve your fitness.

Calorie cost: Use Table 4 to determine the number of calories you burn during each outing. You can increase the number of calories burned by cycling faster or for a longer time (it's usually better to increase distance than to add speed).

At the beginning: It may require several outings to get the muscles and joints of your legs and hips adjusted to this new activity. Begin each outing with a 10-minute warm-up. When your muscles are warm, stretch your hamstrings and your back and neck muscles. Until you become a skilled cyclist, select routes with the fewest hazards and avoid heavy automobile traffic.

As you progress: Interval training is also effective with bicycling. Simply increase your speed for periods of 4–8 minutes or for specific distances, such as 1–2 miles. Then coast for 2–3 minutes. Alternate the speed intervals and slow intervals for a total of 20–60 minutes, depending on your level of fitness. Hilly terrain is also a form of interval training.

Developing Muscular Strength and Endurance and Flexibility

Bicycling develops a high level of endurance and a moderate level of strength in the muscles of the lower body. If one of your goals is to increase your cycling speed and performance, be sure to include exercises for the quadriceps, hamstrings, and buttocks muscles in your strength training program. For flexibility, pay special attention to the hamstrings and quadriceps, which are not worked through their complete range of motion during bike riding, and to the muscles in your lower back, shoulders, and neck.

CALORIE COSTS FOR BICYCLING

This table gives the approximate calorie costs per pound of body weight for cycling from 5 to 60 minutes for distances of .50 mile up to 15 miles on a level terrain. To use the table, find on the horizontal line the time most closely approximating the number of minutes you cycle. Next, locate on the vertical column the approximate distance in miles you cover. The figure at the intersection represents an estimate of the calories used per minute per pound of body weight. Multiply this figure by your body weight. Then multiply the product of these two figures by the number of minutes you cycle to get the total number of calories burned. For example, assuming you weigh 154 pounds and cycle 6 miles in 40 minutes, you would burn 260 calories: $154 \times .042$ (calories per pound, from table) $= 6.5 \times 40$ (minutes) $= 260$ calories burned.

Distance (mi)	Time (min)											
	5	10	15	20	25	30	35	40	45	50	55	60
.50	.032											
1.00	.062	.032										
1.50		.042	.032									
2.00		.062	.039	.032								
3.00			.062	.042	.036	.032						
4.00				.062	.044	.039	.035	.032				
5.00				.097	.062	.045	.041	.037	.035	.032		
6.00					.088	.062	.047	.042	.039	.036	.034	.032
7.00						.081	.062	.049	.043	.040	.038	.036
8.00							.078	.062	.050	.044	.041	.039
9.00								.076	.062	.051	.045	.042
10.00								.097	.074	.062	.051	.045
11.00									.093	.073	.062	.052
12.00										.088	.072	.062
13.00											.084	.071
14.00												.081
15.00												.097

SOURCE: Kusinitz, I., and M. Fine, *Physical Fitness for Practically Everybody*, Consumer Reports®, 1983. Consumers Union of the U.S., Inc., Yonkers, NY 10703-1057, a nonprofit organization. Reprinted with permission for educational purposes only. No commercial use or reproduction permitted. www.ConsumerReports.org®.

SWIMMING SAMPLE PROGRAM

Swimming is excellent for developing all-around fitness. Because water supports the body weight of the swimmer, swimming places less stress than weight-bearing activities on joints, ligaments, and tendons and tends to cause fewer injuries.

Equipment and Safety Guidelines

Aside from having access to a swimming pool, the only equipment required for a swimming program is a swimsuit and a pair of swimming goggles (that fit and do not leak) to protect the eyes from irritation in chlorinated pools. Following these few simple rules can help keep you safe and healthy during your swimming sessions:

- Swim only in a pool with a qualified lifeguard on duty.

- Always walk carefully on wet surfaces.

- Dry your ears well after swimming. If you experience the symptoms of swimmer's ear (itching, discharge, or even a partial hearing loss), consult your physician. If you swim while recovering from swimmer's ear, protect your ears with a few drops of lanolin on a wad of lamb's wool.

- To avoid back pain, try not to arch your back excessively when you swim.

- Be courteous to others in the pool.

If you swim in a setting other than a pool with a lifeguard, remember the following important rules:

- Don't swim beyond your skill and endurance limits.

- Avoid being chilled: don't swim in water colder than 70°F.

- Never drink alcohol before going swimming.

- Never swim alone.

Developing Cardiorespiratory Endurance

Any one or any combination of common swimming strokes— front crawl stroke, breaststroke, backstroke, butterfly stroke, sidestroke, or elementary backstroke—can help develop and maintain cardiorespiratory fitness. (Swimming may not be as helpful as walking, jogging, or cycling for body fat loss.)

FIT—frequency, intensity, and time: Because swimming is not a weight-bearing activity and is not done in an upright position, it elicits a lower heart rate per minute. Therefore, you'll need to adjust your target heart rate zone. To calculate your target heart rate for swimming, use this formula:

Maximum swimming heart rate (MSHR) = 205 − age
Target heart rate zone = 65 − 90% of MSHR

For example, a 19-year-old would calculate her target heart rate zone for swimming as follows:

MSHR = 205 − 19 = 186 bpm
65% intensity 0.65 × 186 = 121 bpm
90% intensity 0.90 × 186 = 167 bpm

Base your duration of swimming on your intensity and target calorie costs. Swim at least three times a week.

Calorie cost: Calories burned while swimming are the result of the pace: how far you swim and how fast (Table 5). Work up to using at least 300 calories per session.

At the beginning: If you are an inexperienced swimmer, invest in the time and money for instruction. You'll make more rapid gains in fitness if you learn correct swimming technique. If you've been sedentary and haven't done any swimming for a long time, begin your program with 2–3 weeks, three times a week, of leisurely swimming at a pace that keeps your heart rate 10–20% below your target zone. Start swimming laps of the width of the pool if you can't swim the length. To keep your heart rate below target, take rest intervals as needed. Swim one lap, then rest 15–90 seconds as needed. Start with 10 minutes of swim/rest intervals and work up to 20 minutes. How long it takes will depend on your swimming skills and muscular fitness.

As you progress: Gradually increase the duration, or the intensity, or both duration and intensity of your swimming to raise your heart rate to a comfortable level within your target zone. Gradually increase your swimming intervals and decrease your rest intervals as you progress. Once you can swim the length of the pool at a pace that keeps your heart rate on target, continue swim/rest intervals for 20 minutes. Your rest intervals should be 30–45 seconds. You may find it helpful to get out of the pool during your rest intervals and walk until you've lowered your heart rate. Next, swim two laps of the pool length per swim interval and continue swim/rest intervals for 30 minutes. For the 30-second rest interval, walk (or rest) until you've lowered your heart rate. Gradually increase the number of laps you swim consecutively and the total duration of your session until you reach your target calorie expenditure and fitness level. But take care not to swim at too fast a pace: It can raise your heart rate too high and limit your ability to sustain your swimming. Alternating strokes can rest your muscles and help prolong your swimming time. A variety of strokes will also let you work more muscle groups. You can also vary your program by incorporat-

SAMPLE PROGRAM TABLE 5
CALORIE COSTS FOR SWIMMING

To use this table, find on the top horizontal row the distance in yards that most closely approximates the distance you swim. Next, locate on the appropriate vertical column (below the distance in yards) the time it takes you to swim the distance. Then locate in the first column on the left the approximate number of calories burned per minute per pound for the time and distance. To find the total number of calories burned, multiply your weight by the calories per minute per pound. Then multiply the product of these two numbers by the time it takes you to swim the distance (minutes:seconds). For example, assuming you weigh 130 pounds and swim 500 yards in 20 minutes, you would burn 106 calories: 130 × .041 (calories per pound, from table) = 5.33 × 20 (minutes) = 106 calories burned.

Calories per Minute per Pound	Distance (yd)					
	25	100	150	250	500	750
.033	1:15	5:00	7:30	12:30	25:00	30:30
.041	1:00	4:00	6:00	10:00	20:00	30:00
.049	0:50	3:20	5:00	8:20	18:40	25:00
.057	0:43	2:52	4:18	7:10	17:20	21:30
.065	0:37.5	2:30	3:45	6:15	10:00	
.073	0:33	2:13	3:20	5:30	8:50	
.081	0:30	2:00	3:00	5:00	8:00	
.090	0:27	1:48	2:42	4:30	7:12	
.097	0:25	1:40	2:30	4:10	6:30	

SOURCE: Kusinitz, I., and M. Fine, *Physical Fitness for Practically Everybody*, Consumer Reports®, 1983. Consumers Union of the U.S., Inc., Yonkers, NY 10703-1057, a nonprofit organization. Reprinted with permission for educational purposes only. No commercial use or reproduction permitted. www.ConsumerReports.org®.

ing kick boards, pull-buoys, hand paddles, or fins into some of your workouts.

Developing Muscular Strength and Endurance and Flexibility

The swimming program outlined in this section will result in moderate gains in strength and large gains in endurance in the muscles used during the strokes you've chosen. To improve your swimming performance, include exercises that work key muscles. For example, if you swim primarily front crawl, include exercises to increase strength in your shoulders, arms, and upper back. (Training the muscles you use during swimming can also help prevent injuries.) For flexibility, pay special attention to the muscles you use during swimming, particularly the shoulders and back.

CALISTHENICS CIRCUIT-TRAINING SAMPLE PROGRAM

Calisthenics are rhythmic exercises that typically develop muscular strength, muscular endurance, and flexibility. Because cal-

isthenic exercises require little or no equipment, they can be performed at home or while traveling. As commonly practiced, such exercises do not constitute a well-rounded fitness program because they do not develop cardiorespiratory endurance. However, a calisthenics program based on circuit training can be the basis of a complete fitness program.

Circuit training is a system of organizing a series of exercises that are performed consecutively. Exercises for different muscle groups follow one another, providing a well-rounded workout and helping to delay the onset of fatigue. When you have performed all the exercises in this model program, you will have completed one circuit; a workout consists of three trips around the circuit. By performing the exercises continuously and not resting between exercises or circuits, you can develop the cardiorespiratory endurance component of fitness. In addition, some of the individual exercises, such as jumping jacks or running in place, develop cardiorespiratory endurance.

Equipment

To time your exercises (which is required only once, when you create your work description), you need a clock or watch with a second hand. If you plan to perform calisthenics regularly, it's a good idea to get a pair of cross-training athletic shoes. Choose an exercise area that is well ventilated and comfortable, with enough room for you to do the exercises without interference. You may want to perform the floor exercises (such as curl-ups) on an exercise mat or a nonskid rug.

Technique

To perform a complete calisthenics cross-training circuit, you need to be able to perform the following exercises smoothly.

- *Arm circles.* Stand with your feet shoulder-width apart and your knees slightly bent. Maintain good posture to protect the lower back. Hold your arms out to the side at shoulder height with palms up. Rotate your arms forward in a circular motion. Keep your shoulders down. Halfway through the time limit or work description, reverse the direction of your circles.

- *Jumping jacks.* Start with your feet together and your hands at your sides. Jump into a straddle position and clap your hands over your head. Then jump back to the starting position and lower your arms to your sides. Always land with your knees slightly bent. Land on the balls of your feet and then press your heels down. If you prefer a low-impact movement, step to the side into the straddle position and then step back into the starting position; alternate legs.

- *Push-ups.* Depending on your level of muscular strength and endurance, you can perform either standard push-ups or modified push-ups. For standard push-ups, begin with your body supported by your hands and feet; for modified push-ups, begin with your body supported by your hands and knees. Lower your chest to the floor with your back straight and your fingers pointed forward. Return to the starting position. (See Lab 4.2, p. 130.)

- *Squats.* Stand with feet shoulder-width apart and toes pointed slightly outward. Keeping your head up and lower back straight, squat down until your thighs are approximately parallel with the floor. Don't let your knees extend out in front of your toes. Hold this position for about 2 seconds.

Return to the starting position. (See Lab 4.1, p. 126, and Lab 4.2, p. 131.)

- *Curls-ups.* Lie on your back on the floor with your arms folded across your chest, knees bent, and feet on the floor. Curl your trunk up and forward by raising your head and shoulders from the ground. Lower to the starting position. (See Lab 4.2, p. 129.)

Alternative instructions (performing curl-ups this way provides better protection for the back during the exercise): Lie on your back on a mat with one knee bent and foot flat on the floor. Place your hands under your lower back and maintain a neutral spine (don't flatten your back to the mat). Curl up as far as possible by contracting the rectus abdominis muscle ("6-pack muscle") rather than your neck and shoulder muscles. As fitness improves, do the exercise with arms folded on your chest. Eventually, place your hands lightly on your forehead, but do not pull on your head and neck.

- *Side leg raises.* Lie on your right side, with your right arm extended flat along the floor in front of your body. Bend your right knee, keeping your knee and thigh in line with your torso. Place your left hand on the floor in front of your chest for balance. Keeping your left leg straight, foot flexed, and toes and knee facing forward (not up), lift your leg 1–2 feet off the floor. Then lower it to the starting position. Do half of your total repetitions on this side, and then do the same number of repetitions on the other side.

- *Heel raises.* Stand with your feet shoulder-width apart and your toes pointed slightly outward. Press down with your toes while lifting your heels. Return to the starting position. Do not bounce. (See Exercise 8 in the free weights portion of the Weight Training Exercises in Chapter 4, p. 113.)

- *Upper-back flies.* Stand with your feet 1½–2 times shoulder-width apart and your knees slightly bent. Keeping your back straight, lean forward at the hips until your torso is diagonal to the floor. Let your arms hang forward, with elbows slightly bent and hands fisted. Leading with your elbows, open your arms to the side and pull your shoulder blades together. Return to the starting position. Lift your arms smoothly and with resistance; do not bounce or swing them.

- *Lunges.* Begin with your feet shoulder-width apart and your hands at your sides or resting on your shoulders. Step forward onto your right foot until your right thigh is almost parallel to the floor. Your right knee should be directly above your right ankle and should not push out in front of your toes. Bend your left knee and drop it directly below your torso in line with your left ankle; your lower left leg should be about parallel to the floor. (See Exercise 6 in the Flexibility Exercises in Chapter 5, p. 144.) Return to the starting position, using the gluteal muscles to push off the floor. Contract the abdominals to relieve pressure on your knees and lower back. Alternate legs. (*Note:* Do not perform lunges if you have knee problems.)

- *Back bridges.* Lie on your back with knees bent and arms extended to the side. Tuck your pelvis under and then lift your tailbone, buttocks, and lower back from the floor. Hold for 5–10 seconds, with your weight resting on your feet, arms, and shoulders. Return to the starting position. (See Exercise 10 in the Low Back Exercises in Chapter 5, p. 153.)

- *Spine extension.* Start on your hands and knees, with your knees below your hips and your hands below your shoulders. Simultaneously raise and straighten your right arm and left leg until they are in line with your spine. Hold this position for 30 seconds. Do not raise either the arm or the leg above spine level (that is, don't arch your back). Return to the starting position and immediately repeat the movement with the left arm and right leg. Do not raise your arms and legs excessively or increase the low back curve by tilting the pelvis. (See Exercise 10 in the free weights portion of the Weight Training Exercises in Chapter 4, p. 114.)

- *Side bridges.* Lie on your side with your knees bent and your top arm lying alongside your body. Lift your hips so that your weight is supported by your forearm and knees. (See Exercise 11 in the free weights portion of the Weight Training Exercises in Chapter 4, p. 115). Hold the position for 10 seconds, breathing normally. Repeat on the other side. As you increase fitness, make the exercise more difficult by doing it with straight legs and supporting yourself with your feet and forearm or with your feet and hand (arm extended, elbow straight). (See Lab 5.3, p. 165.) Hold your spine straight—don't let it sag during the exercise.

- *Running in place.* Run with your knees lifted and land with the ball of your foot first. Follow through by pressing your heel to the floor. If you prefer a low-impact movement, march in place, lifting your knees high. (When you count repetitions of running or marching, count alternate steps.)

Developing Cardiorespiratory Endurance

Calisthenics can help develop cardiorespiratory fitness provided the intensity is moderate to intense. Maximize the cardiorespiratory benefits by moving rapidly between exercises and doing each movement vigorously.

FIT—frequency, intensity, and time: Do the workout 3–5 days per week. Exercise intensely enough to raise your heart rate into the target zone: 65–90% of maximum heart rate or an RPE of 12–18. (If you have been inactive for a long time, start out at a heart rate that is 10–20% below your target zone.) Exercise at an intensity that allows you to comfortably carry on a conversation. Begin by doing the calisthenics circuit one time. As you gain fitness, build up gradually until you can complete 3 circuits (see "As you progress," p. 215).

Calorie cost: To estimate the number of calories you burn, first determine the amount of time it takes to complete a circuit, multiply the calories per minute per pound (.060) by your weight, then multiply that figure by the number of minutes you need to complete one circuit of exercises. For example, assuming you weigh 145 pounds and complete a circuit in 15 minutes, you would burn 131 calories per circuit: 145 × .060 (calories per pound for vigorous training) = 8.7 × 15 (minutes) = 131 calories burned. To burn more calories, increase your repetitions, work faster, and/or work longer.

At the beginning: Before doing your first full calisthenic workout, you need to set up a work description—the number of repetitions of each exercise you will perform in each circuit. To do this, determine the maximum number of repetitions of each exercise you can perform in the time listed in the following table.

For example, count the maximum number of arm circles you can do in 30 seconds, and record that number in the "Max" column. Rest fully between exercises to obtain true maximums. Once you have filled in the "Max" column, write half of this number in the "Work Description" column labeled "1/2 Max." Once you have completed this step, you no longer have to worry about timing the individual exercises.

Exercise	Time	Max	1/2 Max	Date: ___	Date: ___	Date: ___	Date: ___	Date: ___	Date: ___
						Work Description			
Arm circles	30 sec								
Jumping jacks	1 min								
Push-ups	1 min								
Squats	1 min								
Curl-ups	1 min								
Side leg raises	1 min								
Heel raises	30 sec								
Upper-back flies	30 sec								
Lunges	1 min								
Back bridges	1 min								
Spine extensions	1 min								
Side bridges	1 min								
Run in place	3 min								

After your work description is set up, perform each circuit as follows:

• Warm up before you begin the circuit by doing some walking, jogging, or easy calisthenics. When you are ready to begin, note your starting time.

• Perform the exercises in order, each for the number of repetitions in the "1/2Max" column. Time no longer matters for each exercise; just work steadily.

• Monitor your intensity by checking your heart rate or monitoring your rating of perceived exertion (RPE). Do not rest between exercises unless your heart rate or RPE goes above your target zone.

• Complete three trips around the circuit. In the progress chart below, write the date and total time the three circuits took.

• Cool down.

Progress Chart

Date											
Time											

As you progress: When you can perform three circuits in 20 minutes, increase the number of repetitions (the work description) of each exercise by one-quarter of the present work description. For example, if your current work description for push-ups is 20 repetitions, your new work description will be 25. Record the date and the new work description values in the program plan table.

Developing Muscular Strength and Endurance and Flexibility

If you perform a full range of calisthenic exercises (as described in this program), you can develop muscular strength and endurance in all the major muscle groups of your body. Your gains, however, will not be as significant as those from weight training using free weights or machines (unless you add arm or leg weights to increase resistance). To develop flexibility, stretch during your cool-down, when your muscles are warm.

LAB 7.1 A Personal Fitness Program Plan and Contract

A. I, _____ , am contracting with myself to follow a physical fitness program to
   (name)

work toward the following goals:

Specific or short-term goals (include current status for each):

1. _____

2. _____

3. _____

4. _____

General or long-term goals:

1. _____

2. _____

3. _____

4. _____

B. My program plan is as follows:

Activities	Components (Check ✓)					Frequency (Check ✓)							Intensity*	Time (duration)
	CRE	MS	ME	F	BC	M	Tu	W	Th	F	Sa	Su		

*Conduct activities for achieving CRE goals in your target range for heart rate or RPE.

C. My program will begin on _____ . My program includes the following schedule of mini-goals. For each step in my
   (date)

program, I will give myself the reward listed.

_____   _____   _____
         (mini-goal 1)   (date)   (reward)

_____   _____   _____
         (mini-goal 2)   (date)   (reward)

_____   _____   _____
         (mini-goal 3)   (date)   (reward)

_____   _____   _____
         (mini-goal 4)   (date)   (reward)

_____   _____   _____
         (mini-goal 5)   (date)   (reward)

D. My program will include the addition of physical activity to my daily routine (such as climbing stairs or walking to class):

1. _____

2. _____

3. _____

4. _____

5. _____

E. I will use the following tools to monitor my program and my progress toward my goals:

_____
(list any charts, graphs, or journals you plan to use)

_____

_____

I sign this contract as an indication of my personal commitment to reach my goal.

_____   _____
(your signature)   (date)

I have recruited a helper who will witness my contract and _____

_____
(list any way your helper will participate in your program)

_____

_____   _____
(witness's signature)   (date)

Name _____ Section _____ Date _____

LAB 7.2 Getting to Know Your Fitness Facility

To help create a successful training program, take time to learn more about the fitness facility you plan to use.

Basic Information

Name and location of facility: _____

Hours of operation: _____

Times available for general use: _____

Times most convenient for your schedule: _____

Can you obtain an initial session or consultation with a trainer to help you create a program? _____ yes _____ no

If so, what does the initial planning session involve? _____

_____

Are any of the staff certified? Do any have special training? If yes, list/describe: _____

_____

What types of equipment are available for the development of cardiorespiratory endurance? Briefly list/describe: _____

_____

_____

_____

Are any group activities or classes available? If so, briefly describe: _____

_____

_____

What types of weight training equipment are available for use? _____

_____

Yes	No	
_____	_____	Is there a fee for using the facility? If so, how much? $ _____
_____	_____	Is a student ID required for access to the facility?
_____	_____	Do you need to sign up in advance to use the facility or any of the equipment?
_____	_____	Is there typically a line or wait to use the equipment during the times you use the facility?
_____	_____	Is there a separate area with mats for stretching and/or cool-down?
_____	_____	Do you need to bring your own towel?
_____	_____	Are lockers available? If so, do you need to bring your own lock? _____ yes _____ no
_____	_____	Are showers available? If so, do you need to bring your own soap and shampoo? _____ yes _____ no
_____	_____	Is drinking water available? (If not, be sure to bring your own bottle of water.)

What other amenities, such as vending machines or saunas, are available at the facility? Briefly list/describe: _____

_____

_____

Information About Equipment

Fill in the specific equipment and exercise(s) that you can use to develop cardiorespiratory endurance and each of the major muscle groups. For cardiorespiratory endurance, list the type(s) of equipment and a sample starting workout: frequency, intensity, time, and other pertinent information (such as a setting for resistance or speed). For muscular strength and endurance, list the equipment and exercises, and indicate the order in which you'll complete them during a workout session (see p. 103 for suggestions on order of weight training exercises).

Cardiorespiratory Endurance Equipment

Equipment	Sample Starting Workout

Muscular Strength and Endurance Equipment

Order	Muscle Groups	Equipment	Exercise(s)
	Neck		
	Chest		
	Shoulders		
	Upper back		
	Front of arms		
	Back of arms		
	Buttocks		
	Abdomen		
	Lower back		
	Front of thighs		
	Back of thighs		
	Calves		
	Other:		
	Other:		

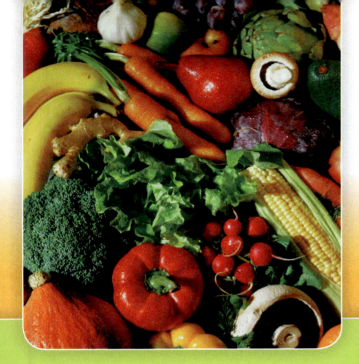

LOOKING AHEAD>>>>>

AFTER READING THIS CHAPTER, YOU SHOULD BE ABLE TO:

- List the essential nutrients and describe the functions they perform in the body
- Describe the guidelines that have been developed to help people choose a healthy diet, avoid nutritional deficiencies, and protect themselves from diet-related chronic diseases
- Discuss nutritional guidelines for vegetarians and for special population groups
- Explain how to use food labels and other consumer tools to make informed choices about foods
- Put together a personal nutrition plan based on affordable foods that you enjoy and that will promote wellness, today and in the future

NUTRITION

8

TEST YOUR KNOWLEDGE

1. **It is recommended that all adults consume 2–3 half-cup servings of fruits and vegetables every day.**

   True or false?

2. **Candy is the leading source of added sugars in the American diet.**

   True or false?

3. **Which of the following is not a whole grain?**

   a. brown rice
   b. wheat flour
   c. popcorn

ANSWERS

1. **FALSE.** For someone consuming 2000 calories, 2½ cups of vegetables and 2 cups of fruit are recommended—a total of 9 half-cup servings. Most Americans fail to meet this goal; half of all the vegetables we do eat are potatoes—and half of those are french fried.

2. **FALSE.** Regular (nondiet) sodas are the leading source of added sugars and calories, with an average of 55 gallons consumed per person per year. Each 12-ounce soda supplies about 10 teaspoons of sugar, or nearly 10% of the calories in a 2000-calorie diet.

3. **b.** Unless labeled "whole wheat," wheat flour is processed to remove the bran and germ and is not a whole grain.

WEB

FIT AND WELL ONLINE LEARNING CENTER www.mhhe.com/fahey

Visit the *Fit and Well* Online Learning Center for resources that will help you get the most out of your course!
- Study and review aids include practice quizzes, glossary flashcards, chapter summaries, learning objectives, PowerPoint presentations, Common Questions Answered, student handouts, crossword puzzles, Internet activities, and links to wellness Web sites.
- Behavior change tools include a daily fitness and nutrition journal, a behavior change workbook, sample behavior change plans, and blank behavior change logs to print and use.

In your lifetime, you will spend about 6 years eating—about 70,000 meals and 60 tons of food. What you eat affects your energy level, well-being, and overall health (see the box "Eating Habits and Total Wellness"). Of particular concern is the connection between lifetime nutritional habits and risk of the major chronic diseases, including heart disease, cancer, stroke, and diabetes. Choosing foods that provide adequate amounts of the nutrients you need while limiting the substances linked to disease should be an important part of your daily life. The food choices you make will significantly influence your health—both now and in the future.

Choosing a healthy diet that supports maximum fitness and protects against disease is a two-part process. First, you have to know which nutrients are necessary and in what amounts. Second, you have to translate those requirements into a diet consisting of foods you like to eat that are both available and affordable. Once you have an idea of what constitutes a healthy diet for you, you may need to make adjustments in your current diet to bring it into line with your goals.

This chapter explains the basic principles of **nutrition.** It introduces the six classes of essential nutrients, and examines their role in the functioning of the body. It also provides different sets of guidelines that you can use to design a healthy diet plan. Finally, it offers practical tools and advice to help you apply the guidelines to your life. Diet is an area of your life in which you have almost total control. Using your knowledge and understanding of nutrition to create a healthy diet plan is a significant step toward wellness.

NUTRITIONAL REQUIREMENTS: COMPONENTS OF A HEALTHY DIET

When you think about your diet, you probably do so in terms of the foods you like to eat—a turkey sandwich and a glass of milk or black beans and rice. What's important for your health, though, are the nutrients contained in those foods. Your body requires proteins, fats, carbohydrates, vitamins, minerals, and water—about 45 **essential nutrients.** The word *essential* in this context means that you must get these substances from food because your body either is unable to manufacture them at all or cannot do so fast enough to meet your physiological needs. The six classes of nutrients, along with their functions and major sources, are listed in Table 8.1.

Nutrients are released into the body by the process of **digestion,** which breaks food down into compounds that the gastrointestinal tract can absorb and the body can use (Figure 8.1, p. 224). A diet containing adequate amounts of all essential nutrients is vital because various nutrients provide energy, build and maintain body tissues, and regulate body functions. Some essential nutrients are needed by the body in relatively large amounts. These **macronutrients** include protein, fat, and carbohydrate. **Micronutrients,** such as vitamins and minerals, are required in much smaller amounts.

The energy in foods is expressed as **kilocalories.** One kilocalorie represents the amount of heat it takes to raise the temperature of 1 liter of water 1°C. A person needs about 2000 kilocalories a day to meet his or her energy needs. People usually refer to kilocalories as *calories,* which is a much smaller energy unit: 1 kilocalorie contains 1000 calories. This chapter uses the familiar word *calorie* to stand for the larger energy unit; you'll also find *calorie* used on food labels.

Of the six classes of essential nutrients, three supply energy:

- Fat = 9 calories per gram
- Protein = 4 calories per gram
- Carbohydrate = 4 calories per gram

Alcohol, though not an essential nutrient, also supplies energy, providing 7 calories per gram. (One gram equals a little less than 0.04 ounce.) The high caloric content of fat is one reason experts often advise against high fat consumption; most of us do not need the extra calories to meet energy needs. Regardless of their source, calories consumed in excess of energy needs can be converted to fat and stored in the body.

TERMS

nutrition   The science of food and how the body uses it in health and disease.

essential nutrients   Substances the body must get from food because it cannot manufacture them at all or fast enough to meet its needs. These nutrients include proteins, fats, carbohydrates, vitamins, minerals, and water.

digestion   The process of breaking down foods in the gastrointestinal tract into compounds the body can absorb.

macronutrients   Essential nutrients required by the body in relatively large amounts.

micronutrients   Essential nutrients required by the body in minute amounts.

kilocalorie   A measure of energy content in food; 1 kilocalorie represents the amount of heat needed to raise the temperature of 1 liter of water 1°C; commonly referred to as *calorie.*

Eating Habits and Total Wellness

Healthy eating does more than nourish your body—it enhances your ability to enjoy life to the fullest by improving overall wellness, both physical and mental. One study examined a group of adults who followed a healthy eating plan for 4 years. At the end of this period, the study subjects were more confident with their food choices and more satisfied with their lives in general than their peers who did not make any dietary changes. The reverse is also true—when people overeat, they often have feelings of guilt, anger, discouragement, and even self-loathing. Out-of-control eating can erode self-confidence and lead to depression.

Can individual foods affect the way we feel? Limited scientific evidence points to some correlation between certain foods and one's mood. Many people, especially women, seem to crave chocolate when they feel slightly depressed. Studies show that chocolate, in small quantities, may indeed give you a lift. Sugary foods tend to temporarily raise serotonin levels in the brain, which can improve mood (serotonin is a neurotransmitter associated with a calm, relaxed state). The fat found in chocolate acts to increase endorphins, brain chemicals that reduce pain and increase feelings of well-being. Chocolate also contains a variety of other less studied chemicals that may have a positive impact on mood.

A commonly held belief about the connection between food and the mind is that eating sugary foods makes people (especially children) hyperactive. Parents often comment on the wild behavior observed at parties and festive events where lots of sweets are consumed. However, several carefully controlled studies showed no correlation between behavior and the consumption of sugary foods. Researchers speculate that high-sugar foods tend to be eaten at birthday parties and other exciting occasions when children tend to

be highly stimulated regardless of what they eat.

Some recent research shows that eating certain carbohydrate-rich foods, such as a plain baked potato or a bagel with jelly, can have a temporary calming effect. This effect is most pronounced when rapidly digestible carbohydrates are consumed alone, with no fats or proteins in the meal. The practical implications of this research are uncertain.

If you are looking for a mental boost, some scientists think that eating a meal consisting primarily of protein-rich foods may be helpful. Some researchers think that eating protein-rich foods could increase the synthesis of certain neurotransmitters, which can speed reaction time and increase alertness. Whether this really works, especially in well-nourished individuals who have not been lacking these nutrients to begin with, remains to be seen. In the meantime, it wouldn't hurt, and might even help, to include some protein in the meal you eat prior to your next big exam.

What we know about how food affects mood remains limited. But evidence points to the commonsense conclusion that enjoying reasonable portions of a variety of healthy and tasty foods is a great way to optimize your physical and mental health.

Table 8.1	The Six Classes of Essential Nutrients	
Nutrient	**Function**	**Major Sources**
Proteins (4 calories/gram)	Form important parts of muscles, bone, blood, enzymes, some hormones, and cell membranes; repair tissue; regulate water and acid-base balance; help in growth; supply energy	Meat, fish, poultry, eggs, milk products, legumes, nuts
Carbohydrates (4 calories/gram)	Supply energy to cells in brain, nervous system, and blood; supply energy to muscles during exercise	Grains (breads and cereals), fruits, vegetables, milk
Fats (9 calories/gram)	Supply energy; insulate, support, and cushion organs; provide medium for absorption of fat-soluble vitamins	Animal foods, grains, nuts, seeds, fish, vegetables
Vitamins	Promote (initiate or speed up) specific chemical reactions within cells	Abundant in fruits, vegetables, and grains; also found in meat and dairy products
Minerals	Help regulate body functions; aid in growth and maintenance of body tissues; act as catalysts for release of energy	Found in most food groups
Water	Makes up 50–70% of body weight; provides medium for chemical reactions; transports chemicals; regulates temperature; removes waste products	Fruits, vegetables, liquids

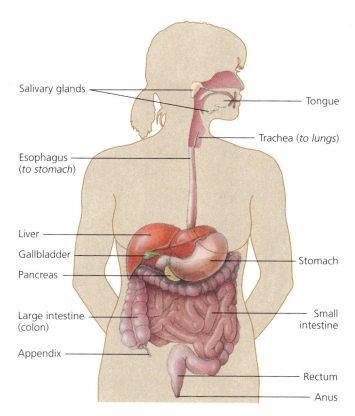

Salivary glands

Tongue

Trachea (*to lungs*)

Esophagus
(*to stomach*)

Liver

Gallbladder

Pancreas

Stomach

Large intestine
(colon)

Small
intestine

Appendix

Rectum

Anus

FIGURE 8.1 **The digestive system.** Food is partially broken down by being chewed and mixed with saliva in the mouth. After traveling to the stomach via the esophagus, food is broken down further by stomach acids. As food moves through the digestive tract, it is mixed by muscular contractions and broken down by chemicals. Most absorption of nutrients occurs in the small intestine, aided by secretions from the pancreas, gallbladder, and intestinal lining. The large intestine reabsorbs excess water; the remaining solid wastes are collected in the rectum and excreted through the anus.

Simply meeting energy needs is not enough, however; our bodies need adequate amounts of all the essential nutrients to grow and function properly. Practically all foods contain mixtures of nutrients, although foods are commonly classified according to their predominant nutrients. For example, spaghetti is considered a carbohydrate food although it contains small amounts of other nutrients. Let's take a closer look at the functions and sources of the six classes of nutrients.

Proteins—The Basis of Body Structure

Proteins form important parts of the body's main structural components: muscles and bones. Proteins also form important parts of blood, enzymes, cell membranes, and some hormones. As mentioned earlier, protein can also provide energy at 4 calories per gram of protein weight.

Amino Acids The building blocks of proteins are called **amino acids.** Twenty common amino acids are found in food; 9 of these are essential: histidine, isoleucine, leucine, lysine, methionine, phenylalanine, threonine, tryptophan,

and valine. The other 11 amino acids can be produced by the body as long as the necessary components are supplied by foods.

Complete and Incomplete Proteins Individual protein sources are considered "complete" if they supply all the essential amino acids in adequate amounts and "incomplete" if they do not. Meat, fish, poultry, eggs, milk, cheese, and soy provide complete proteins. Incomplete proteins, which come from plant sources such as **legumes** and nuts, are good sources of most essential amino acids but are usually low in one or two.

Combining two vegetable proteins, such as wheat and peanuts in a peanut butter sandwich, allows each vegetable protein to make up for the amino acids missing in the other protein. The combination yields a complete protein. It was once believed that vegetarians had to "complement" their proteins at each meal in order to receive the benefit of a complete protein. It is now known, however, that proteins consumed throughout the course of the day can complement each other to form a pool of amino acids from which the body can draw to produce the necessary proteins. Vegetarians should include a variety of vegetable protein sources in their diets to make sure they get all the essential amino acids in adequate amounts. (Healthy vegetarian diets are discussed later in the chapter.)

Recommended Protein Intake Adequate daily intake of protein for adults is 0.8 gram per kilogram (0.36 gram per pound) of body weight, corresponding to 50 grams of protein per day for someone who weighs 140 pounds and 65 grams of protein for someone who weighs 180 pounds. This amount of protein is easily obtained from popular foods: 3 ounces of lean meat, poultry, or fish or ½ cup of tofu contains about 20–25 grams of protein; 1 cup of legumes such as pinto and kidney beans, 15–20 grams; 1 cup of milk or yogurt or 1½ ounces of cheese, 8–12 grams; and cereals, grains, nuts, and vegetables, about 2–4 grams of protein per serving.

Most Americans meet or exceed the protein intake needed for adequate nutrition. Protein consumed beyond what the body needs can be synthesized into fat for energy storage or burned for energy requirements. Consuming somewhat above our needs is not harmful, but it does contribute fat to the diet because protein-rich foods are often fat-rich as well. A very high protein intake can strain the kidneys and lead to dehydration.

A fairly broad range of protein intake is associated with good health. In 2002, the Food and Nutrition Board released recommendations for the balance of energy sources in a healthful diet. These recommendations, called Acceptable Macronutrient Distribution Ranges (AMDRs), are based on ensuring adequate intake of essential nutrients while also reducing the risk of chronic diseases like heart disease and cancer. The AMDR for protein for adults is 10–35% of total daily calories. The average American diet includes about 15–16% of total daily calories as protein. (See Chapter 9 for more information about high-protein diets advocated for weight loss.)

Fats—Essential in Small Amounts

Fats, also known as *lipids,* are the most concentrated source of energy, at 9 calories per gram. The fats stored in your body represent usable energy, help insulate your body, and support and cushion your organs. Fats in the diet help your body absorb fat-soluble vitamins and add flavor and texture to foods. Fats are the major fuel for the body during periods of rest and light activity. Two fats—linoleic acid and alpha-linolenic acid—are essential to the diet; they are key regulators of such body functions as the maintenance of blood pressure and the progress of a healthy pregnancy.

Types and Sources of Fats   Most of the fats in food are in the form of triglycerides, which are composed of a glycerol molecule (an alcohol) plus three fatty acids. A fatty acid is made up of a chain of carbon atoms with oxygen attached at the end and hydrogen atoms attached along the length of the chain. Fatty acids differ in the length of their carbon atom chains and in their degree of saturation (the number of hydrogens attached to the chain). If every available bond from each carbon atom in a fatty acid chain is attached to a hydrogen atom, the fatty acid is said to be **saturated** (Figure 8.2). If not all the available bonds are taken up by hydrogens, the carbon atoms in the chain will form double bonds with each other. Such fatty acids are called *unsaturated fats.* If there is only one double bond, the fatty acid is called **monoun-saturated.** If there are two or more double bonds, the fatty acid is called **polyunsaturated.** The essential fatty acids—linoleic and alpha-linolenic acids—are both poly-unsaturated. The different types of fatty acids have different characteristics and different effects on your health.

Food fats are often composed of both saturated and unsaturated fatty acids; the dominant type of fatty acid determines the fat's characteristics. Food fats containing large amounts of saturated fatty acids are usually solid at room temperature; they are generally found naturally in animal products. The leading sources of saturated fat in the American diet are red meats (hamburger, steak, roasts), whole milk, cheese, and hot dogs and lunch meats. Food fats containing large amounts of monoun-saturated and polyunsaturated fatty acids are usually from plant sources and are liquid at room temperature. Olive, canola, safflower, and peanut oils contain mostly mono-unsaturated fatty acids. Corn, soybean, and cottonseed oils contain mostly polyunsaturated fatty acids.

There are some notable exceptions to these general-izations. When unsaturated vegetable oils undergo the process of **hydrogenation,** a mixture of saturated and unsaturated fatty acids is produced. Hydrogenation turns many of the double bonds in unsaturated fatty acids into single bonds, increasing the degree of saturation and producing a more solid fat from a liquid oil. Hydrogena-tion also changes some unsaturated fatty acids into **trans fatty acids (trans fats),** unsaturated fatty acids with an atypical shape that affects their behavior in the body. Food manufacturers use hydrogenation to increase the stability of an oil so it can be reused for deep frying; to improve the texture of certain foods (to make pastries and pie crusts flakier, for example); and to extend the shelf life of foods made with oil. Hydrogenation is also used to transform liquid vegetable oils into margarine or shortening.

FIGURE 8.2   Chemical structures of saturated and unsaturated fatty acids. This example of a triglyceride consists of a molecule of glycerol with three fatty acids attached. Fatty acids can differ in the length of their carbon chains and their degree of saturation.

protein   An essential nutrient; a compound made of amino acids that contains carbon, hydrogen, oxygen, and nitrogen.

amino acids   The building blocks of proteins.

legumes   Vegetables such as peas and beans that are high in fiber and are also important sources of protein.

saturated fat   A fat with no carbon-carbon double bonds; usually solid at room temperature.

monounsaturated fat   A fat with one carbon-carbon double bond; liquid at room temperature.

polyunsaturated fat   A fat containing two or more carbon-carbon double bonds; liquid at room temperature.

hydrogenation   A process by which hydrogens are added to unsaturated fats, increasing the degree of saturation and turning liquid oils into solid fats. Hydrogenation produces a mixture of saturated fatty acids and standard and trans forms of unsaturated fatty acids.

trans fatty acid (trans fat)   A type of unsaturated fatty acid produced during the process of hydrogenation; trans fats have an atypical shape that affects their chemical activity.

Many baked and fried foods are prepared with hydrogenated vegetable oils, so they can be relatively high in saturated and trans fatty acids. Leading sources of trans fats in the American diet are deep-fried fast foods such as french fries and fried chicken (typically fried in vegetable shortening rather than oil); baked and snack foods such as pot pies, cakes, cookies, pastries, doughnuts, and chips; and stick margarine. In general, the more solid a hydrogenated oil is, the more saturated and trans fats it contains; for example, stick margarines typically contain more saturated and trans fats than do tub or squeeze margarines. Small amounts of trans fatty acids are also found naturally in meat and milk.

Hydrogenated vegetable oils are not the only plant fats that contain saturated fats. Palm and coconut oils, although derived from plants, are also highly saturated. Yet fish oils, derived from an animal source, are rich in polyunsaturated fats.

Fats and Health   Different types of fats have very different effects on health. Many studies have examined the effects of dietary fat intake on blood **cholesterol** levels and the risk of heart disease. Saturated and trans fatty acids raise blood levels of **low-density lipoprotein (LDL),** or "bad" cholesterol, thereby increasing a person's risk of heart disease. Unsaturated fatty acids, on the other hand, lower LDL. Monounsaturated fatty acids, such as those found in olive and canola oils, may also increase levels of **high-density lipoproteins (HDL),** or "good" cholesterol, providing even greater benefits for heart health. Saturated fats have been found to impair the ability of HDLs to prevent inflammation of the blood vessels, one of the key factors in vascular disease; they have also been found to reduce the ability of the blood vessels to react normally to stress. In large amounts, trans fatty acids may lower HDL. Thus, to reduce the risk of heart disease, it is important to choose unsaturated fats instead of saturated and trans fats. (See Chapter 11 for more on cholesterol.)

Most Americans consume more saturated fat than trans fat (12% versus 2–4% of total daily calories). However, health experts are particularly concerned about trans fats because of their double negative effect on heart health—they both raise LDL and lower HDL—and because there is less public awareness of trans fats. Trans fat content wasn't required on nutrition labels until January 2006. Consumers can also check for the presence of trans fats by examining the ingredient list of a food for "partially hydrogenated oil" or "vegetable shortening."

For heart health, it's important to limit your consumption of both saturated and trans fats. The best way to reduce saturated fat in your diet is to lower your intake of meat and full-fat dairy products (whole milk, cream, butter, cheese, ice cream). To lower trans fats, decrease your intake of deep-fried foods and baked goods made with hydrogenated vegetable oils; use liquid oils for cooking; and favor tub or squeeze margarines over stick margarines. Remember, the softer or more liquid a fat is, the less saturated and trans fat it is likely to contain.

Although saturated and trans fats pose health hazards, other fats are beneficial. Monounsaturated fatty acids, as found in avocados, most nuts, and olive, canola, peanut, and safflower oils, improve cholesterol levels and may help protect against some cancers. **Omega-3 fatty acids,** a form of polyunsaturated fat found primarily in fish, may be even more healthful. An omega-3 fatty acid has its endmost double bond three carbons from the end of the fatty acid chain. (The polyunsaturated fatty acid shown in Figure 8.2 is an omega-3 form.) Omega-3s and the compounds the body makes from them have a number of heart-healthy effects: They reduce the tendency of blood to clot, inhibit inflammation and abnormal heart rhythms, and reduce blood pressure and risk of heart attack and stroke in some people. Because of these benefits, nutritionists recommend that Americans increase the proportion of omega-3s in their diet by eating fish two or more times a week. Salmon, tuna, trout, mackerel, herring, sardines, and anchovies are all good sources of omega-3s; lesser amounts are found in plant foods, including dark green leafy vegetables; walnuts; flaxseeds; and canola, walnut, and flaxseed oils.

Another form of polyunsaturated fat, omega-6 fatty acid, has its endmost double bond at the sixth carbon atom. Most of the polyunsaturated fats currently consumed by Americans are omega-6s, primarily from corn oil and soybean oil. Foods rich in omega-6s are important because they contain the essential nutrient linoleic acid. However, some nutritionists recommend that people reduce the proportion of omega-6s they consume in favor of omega-3s. To make this adjustment, use canola oil rather than corn oil in cooking, and check for corn, soybean, or cottonseed oil in products such as mayonnaise, margarine, and salad dressing.

In addition to its effects on heart disease risk, dietary fat can affect health in other ways. Diets high in fatty red meat are associated with an increased risk of certain forms of cancer, especially colon cancer. A high-fat diet can also make weight management more difficult. Because fat is a concentrated source of calories (9 calories per gram versus

TERMS

cholesterol   A waxy substance found in the blood and cells and needed for cell membranes, vitamin D, and hormone synthesis.

low-density lipoprotein (LDL)   Blood fat that transports cholesterol to organs and tissues; excess amounts result in the accumulation of fatty deposits on artery walls.

high-density lipoprotein (HDL)   Blood fat that helps transport cholesterol out of the arteries, thereby protecting against heart disease.

omega-3 fatty acids   Polyunsaturated fatty acids commonly found in fish oils that are beneficial to cardiovascular health; the endmost double bond occurs three carbons from the end of the fatty acid chain.

Type of Fatty Acid	Found In[a]	Possible Effects on Health
SATURATED (Keep Intake Low)	Animal fats (especially fatty meats and poultry fat and skin) Butter, cheese, and other high-fat dairy products Palm and coconut oils	Raises total cholesterol and LDL cholesterol levels Increases risk of heart disease May increase risk of colon and prostate cancers
TRANS (Keep Intake Low)	French fries and other deep-fried fast foods Stick margarines, shortening Packaged cookies and crackers Processed snacks and sweets	Raises total cholesterol and LDL cholesterol levels Lowers HDL cholesterol levels May increase risk of heart disease and breast cancer
MONOUNSATURATED (Choose Moderate Amounts)	Olive, canola, and safflower oils Avocados, olives Peanut butter (without added fat) Many nuts, including almonds, cashews, pecans, and pistachios	Lowers total cholesterol and LDL cholesterol levels May reduce blood pressure and lower triglyceride levels (a risk factor for CVD) May reduce risk of heart disease, stroke, and some cancers
POLYUNSATURATED (two groups)[b] Omega-3 fatty acids	Fatty fish, including salmon, white albacore tuna, mackerel, anchovies, and sardines Lesser amounts in walnut, flaxseed, canola, and soybean oils; tofu; walnuts; flaxseeds; and dark green leafy vegetables	Reduces blood clotting and inflammation and inhibits abnormal heart rhythms Lowers triglyceride levels (a risk factor for CVD) May lower blood pressure in some people May reduce risk of fatal heart attack, stroke, and some cancers
Omega-6 fatty acids	Corn, soybean, and cottonseed oils (often used in margarine, mayonnaise, and salad dressing)	Lowers total cholesterol and LDL cholesterol levels May lower HDL cholesterol levels May reduce risk of heart disease May slightly increase risk of cancer if omega-6 intake is high and omega-3 intake is low

[a] Food fats contain a combination of types of fatty acids in various proportions; for example, canola oil is composed mainly of monounsaturated fatty acids (62%) but also contains polyunsaturated (32%) and saturated (6%) fatty acids. Food fats are categorized here according to their predominant fatty acid.

[b] The essential fatty acids are polyunsaturated: Linoleic acid is an omega-6 fatty acid and alpha-linolenic acid is an omega-3 fatty acid.

FIGURE 8.3   Types of fatty acids and their possible effects on health. The health effects of dietary fats are still being investigated. In general, nutritionists recommend that we consume a diet moderate in fat overall and that we substitute unsaturated fats for saturated and trans fats. Monounsaturated fats and omega-3 polyunsaturated fats may be particularly good choices for promoting health. Eating lots of fat of any type can provide excess calories because all types of fats are rich sources of energy (9 calories per gram).

4 calories per gram for protein and carbohydrate), a high-fat diet is often a high-calorie diet that can lead to weight gain. In addition, there is some evidence that calories from fat are more easily converted to body fat than calories from protein or carbohydrate.

Although more research is needed on the precise effects of different types and amounts of fat on overall health, a great deal of evidence points to the fact that most people benefit from lowering their overall fat intake to recommended levels and choosing unsaturated fats instead of saturated and trans fats. The types of fatty acids and their effects on health are summarized in Figure 8.3.

Recommended Fat Intake   To meet the body's need for essential fats, adult men need about 17 grams per day of linoleic acid and 1.6 grams per day of alpha-linolenic acid; women need 12 grams of linoleic acid and 1.1 grams of alpha-linolenic acid. It takes only 3–4 teaspoons (15–20 grams) of vegetable oil per day incorporated into your diet to supply the essential fats. Most Americans consume sufficient amounts of the essential fats; limiting unhealthy fats is a much greater health concern.

As with protein, a range of levels of fat intake is associated with good health; the AMDR for total fat is 20–35% of total calories. Although more difficult for consumers to monitor, AMDRs have also been set for omega-6 fatty acids (5–10%) and omega-3 fatty acids (0.6–1.2%) as part of total fat intake. Because any amount of saturated and trans fat increases the risk of heart disease, the Food and Nutrition Board recommends that saturated and trans fat intake be kept as low as possible; most fat in a healthy diet should be unsaturated. American adults currently consume about 33% of total calories as fat, including 11–12% of calories as saturated fat and 2–4% as trans fat.

For advice on setting individual intake goals, see the box "Setting Intake Goals for Protein, Fat, and Carbohydrate." To determine how close you are to meeting these intake goals for fat, keep a running total over the course

Setting Intake Goals for Protein, Fat, and Carbohydrate

Goals have been established by the Food and Nutrition Board to help ensure adequate intake of the essential amino acids, fatty acids, and carbohydrate. The daily goals for adequate intake for adults are as follows:

	Men	Women
Protein	56 grams	46 grams
Fat: Linoleic acid	17 grams	12 grams
Alpha-linolenic acid	1.6 grams	1.1 grams
Carbohydrate	130 grams	130 grams

Protein intake goals can be calculated more specifically by multiplying your body weight in kilograms by 0.8 or your body weight in pounds by 0.36. (Refer to the Nutrition Resources section at the end of the chapter for information for specific age groups and life stages.)

To meet your daily energy needs, you need to consume more than the minimally adequate amounts of the energy-providing nutrients listed above, which alone supply only about 800–900 calories. The Food and Nutrition Board provides additional guidance in the form of Acceptable Macronutrient Distribution Ranges (AMDRs). These ranges can help you balance your intake of energy-providing nutrients in ways that ensure adequate intake and reduce the risk of chronic disease.

The AMDRs for protein, total fat, and carbohydrate are as follows:

Protein	10–35% of total daily calories
Total fat	20–35% of total daily calories
Carbohydrate	45–65% of total daily calories

To set individual goals, begin by estimating your total daily energy (calorie) needs; if your weight is stable, your current energy intake is the number of calories you need to maintain your weight at your current activity level. Next, select percentage goals for protein, fat, and carbohydrate. You can allocate your total daily calories among the three classes of macronutrients to suit your preferences; just make sure that the three percentages you select total 100% and that you meet the minimum intake goals listed. Two samples reflecting different total energy intake and nutrient intake goals are shown in the table below.

To translate your percentage goals into daily intake goals expressed in calories and grams, multiply the appropriate percentages by total calorie intake, and then divide the results by the corresponding calories per gram. For example, a fat limit of 35% applied to a 2200-calorie diet would be calculated as follows: $0.35 \times 2200 = 770$ calories of total fat; $770 \div 9$ calories per gram = 86 grams of total fat. (Remember that fat has 9 calories per gram and that protein and carbohydrate have 4 calories per gram.)

Two Sample Macronutrient Distributions

Nutrient	AMDR	Sample 1 Individual Goals	Sample 1 Amounts for a 1600-Calorie Diet	Sample 2 Individual Goals	Sample 2 Amounts for a 2800-Calorie Diet
Protein	10–35%	15%	240 calories = 60 grams	20%	560 calories = 140 grams
Fat	20–35%	30%	480 calories = 53 grams	20%	560 calories = 62 grams
Carbohydrate	45–65%	55%	880 calories = 220 grams	60%	1680 calories = 420 grams

Source: Food and Nutrition Board, Institute of Medicine, National Academies, 2002. *Dietary Reference Intakes: Energy, Carbohydrates, Fiber, Fat, Fatty Acids, Cholesterol, Protein, and Amino Acids*, Washington, D.C., National Academies Press. Reprinted with permission from *Dietary Reference Intakes for Energy, Carbohydrate, Fiber, Fat, Fatty Acids, Cholesterol, Protein, and Amino Acids (Macronutrients)*. Copyright © 2003 by the National Academy of Sciences. Courtesy of the National Academies Press, Washington, D.C.

of the day. For prepared foods, food labels list the number of grams of fat, protein, and carbohydrate; the breakdown for many foods and popular fast-food items can be found in Appendixes B and C. Nutrition information is also available in many grocery stores, in published nutrition guides, and online (see For Further Exploration at the end of the chapter). By checking these resources, you can keep track of the total grams of fat, protein, and carbohydrate you eat and assess how close your current diet is to the recommended intake goals.

In reducing fat intake to recommended levels, the emphasis should be on lowering saturated and trans fats (see Figure 8.3). You can still eat high-fat foods, but it makes sense to limit the size of your portions and to balance your intake with low-fat foods. For example, peanut butter is high in fat, with 8 grams (72 calories) of fat in each 90-calorie tablespoon. Two tablespoons of peanut butter eaten on whole-wheat bread and served with a banana, carrot sticks, and a glass of nonfat milk makes a nutritious lunch—high in protein and carbohydrate, relatively low in total and saturated fat (500 calories, 18 grams of total fat, 4 grams of saturated fat). Four tablespoons of peanut butter on high-fat crackers with potato chips, cookies, and whole milk is a less healthy combination (1000 calories, 62 grams of total fat, 15 grams of saturated fat). So although it's important to evaluate individual food items for their fat content, it is more important to look at them in the context of your overall diet.

Carbohydrates—An Ideal Source of Energy

Carbohydrates are needed in the diet primarily to supply energy to body cells. Some cells, such as those in the brain and other parts of the nervous system and in the blood, use only carbohydrates for fuel. During high-intensity exercise, muscles also get most of their energy from carbohydrates.

Simple and Complex Carbohydrates Carbohydrates are classified into two groups: simple and complex. Simple carbohydrates contain only one or two sugar units in each molecule; they include sucrose (table sugar), fructose (fruit sugar, honey), maltose (malt sugar), and lactose (milk sugar). Providing much of the sweetness in foods, they are found naturally in fruits and milk and are added to soft drinks, fruit drinks, candy, and sweet desserts. There is no evidence that any one type of simple sugar is more nutritious than any other.

Complex carbohydrates consist of chains of many sugar molecules; they include starches and most types of dietary fiber. Starches are found in a variety of plants, especially grains (wheat, rye, rice, oats, barley, millet), legumes (dried beans, peas, lentils), and tubers (potatoes, yams). Most other vegetables contain a mix of starches and simple carbohydrates. Fiber is found in fruits, vegetables, and grains.

During digestion in the mouth and small intestine, your body breaks down starches and double sugars into single sugar molecules, such as **glucose,** for absorption. Once the glucose is in the bloodstream, the pancreas releases insulin, which allows cells to take up glucose and use it for energy. The liver and muscles also take up glucose and store it in the form of a starch called **glycogen.** The muscles use glucose from glycogen as fuel during endurance events or long workouts. Carbohydrates consumed in excess of the body's energy needs can be changed into fat and stored. Whenever calorie intake exceeds calorie expenditure, fat storage can lead to weight gain. This is true whether the excess calories come from carbohydrates, proteins, fat, or alcohol.

Refined Carbohydrates Versus Whole Grains Complex carbohydrates can be further divided between refined, or processed, carbohydrates and unrefined carbohydrates, or whole grains. Before they are processed, all grains are **whole grains,** consisting of an inner layer of germ, a middle layer called the endosperm, and an outer layer of bran (Figure 8.4). During processing, the germ and bran are often removed, leaving just the starchy endosperm. The refinement of whole grains transforms whole-wheat flour into white flour, brown rice into white rice, and so on.

Refined carbohydrates usually retain all the calories of their unrefined counterparts, but they tend to be much lower in fiber, vitamins, minerals, and other beneficial compounds. Many refined grain products are enriched or

- **Bran** "Outer shell" protects seed Contains fiber, B vitamins, trace minerals
- **Endosperm** Provides energy Contains carbohydrates, protein
- **Germ** Provides nourishment for the seed Contains antioxidants, vitamin E, B vitamins

FIGURE 8.4 The parts of a whole grain kernel.

fortified with vitamins and minerals, but often the nutrients lost in processing are not replaced. Unrefined carbohydrates tend to take longer to chew and digest than refined ones; they also enter the bloodstream more slowly. This slower digestive pace tends to make people feel full sooner and for a longer period, lessening the chance that they will overeat. Also, a slower rise in blood glucose levels following consumption of complex carbohydrates may help in the prevention and management of diabetes. Whole grains are also high in dietary fiber. Consumption of whole grains has been linked to reduced risk for heart disease, diabetes, high blood pressure, stroke, and certain forms of cancer. For all these reasons, whole grains are recommended over those that have been refined. This does not mean that you should never eat refined carbohydrates such as white bread or white rice; it simply means that whole-wheat bread, brown rice, and other whole grains are healthier choices. See the box "Choosing More Whole-Grain Foods" for tips on increasing your intake of whole grains.

Glycemic Index Insulin and glucose levels rise and fall following a meal or snack containing any type of carbohydrate. Some foods cause a quick and dramatic rise in glucose and insulin levels; others have a slower, more moderate effect. A food that has a rapid effect on blood glucose levels is said to have a high **glycemic index.**

carbohydrate An essential nutrient; sugars, starches, and dietary fiber are all carbohydrates.

glucose A simple sugar that is the body's basic fuel.

glycogen An animal starch stored in the liver and muscles.

whole grain The entire edible portion of a grain such as wheat, rice, or oats, including the germ, endosperm, and bran.

glycemic index A measure of how the ingestion of a particular food affects blood glucose levels.

Choosing More Whole-Grain Foods

What Are Whole Grains?

The first step in increasing your intake of whole grains is to correctly identify them. The following are whole grains:

whole wheat	whole-grain corn
whole rye	popcorn
whole oats	brown rice
oatmeal	whole-grain barley

Other choices include bulgur (cracked wheat), millet, kasha (roasted buckwheat kernels), quinoa, teff, wheat and rye berries, amaranth, graham flour, whole-grain kamut, whole-grain spelt, and whole-grain triticale.

Wheat flour, unbleached flour, enriched flour, and degerminated corn meal are not whole grains. Wheat germ and wheat bran are also not whole grains, but they are the constituents of wheat typically left out when wheat is processed and so are healthier choices than regular wheat flour, which typically contains just the endosperm.

Reading Food Packages to Find Whole Grains

To find packaged foods rich in whole grains, read the list of ingredients and check for special health claims related to whole grains. *The first item on the list of ingredients should be one of the whole grains listed above.* In addition, the FDA allows manufacturers to include special health claims for foods that contain 51% or more whole-grain ingredients. Such products may contain a statement such as the following on their packaging: "Rich in whole grain," "Made with 100% whole grain," or "Diets rich in whole-grain foods may help reduce the risk of heart disease and certain cancers." However, many whole-grain products will not carry such claims.

Incorporating Whole Grains into Your Daily Diet

- **Bread.** Look for sandwich breads, bagels, English muffins, buns, and pita breads with a whole grain listed as the first ingredient.

- **Breakfast cereals.** Look for whole-grain cereals, which include oatmeal, muesli, shredded wheat, and some types of raisin bran, bran flakes, wheat flakes, toasted oats, and granola.

- **Rice.** Choose brown rice or rice blends that include brown rice.

- **Pasta.** Look for whole-wheat, whole-grain kamut, or whole-grain spelt pasta.

- **Tortillas.** Choose whole-wheat or whole-corn tortillas.

- **Crackers and snacks.** Look for varieties of crackers made from whole grains, including some flatbreads or crispbreads, woven wheat crackers, and rye crackers. Other whole-grain snack possibilities include popcorn, popcorn cakes, brown rice cakes, whole-corn tortilla chips, and whole-wheat fig cookies. Be sure to check food labels for fat content, as many popular snacks are also high in fat.

- **Mixed-grain dishes.** Combine whole grains with other foods to create healthy mixed dishes such as tabouli; soups made with hulled barley or wheat berries; and pilafs, casseroles, and salads made with brown rice, whole-wheat couscous, kasha, millet, wheat bulgur, and quinoa.

If your grocery store doesn't carry these items, try your local health food store.

Research findings have been mixed, but some studies have found that a meal containing high-glycemic-index foods may increase appetite; over the long term, diets rich in high-glycemic-index foods are linked to increased risk of diabetes and heart disease in some people. High-glycemic-index foods do not, as some popular diets claim, directly cause weight gain beyond the calories they contain.

Attempting to base food choices on glycemic index is a difficult task, however. Although unrefined complex carbohydrates and high-fiber foods tend to have a low glycemic index, patterns are less clear for other types of foods and do not follow a simple distinction such as that of simple versus complex carbohydrates. For example, some fruits with fairly high levels of simple carbohydrates have only a moderate effect on blood glucose levels, whereas white rice, potatoes, and white bread, which are rich in complex carbohydrates, have a high glycemic index. Watermelon has a glycemic index more than twice that of strawberries, and the glycemic index of a banana changes dramatically as it ripens. The acid and fat content of a food also affect glycemic index—the more acidic and higher in fat a food is, the lower its effect on glucose levels. Other factors that affect the body's response to carbohydrates include the way foods are combined and prepared and the fitness status of the individual.

This complexity is one reason major health organizations have not issued specific guidelines for glycemic index. For people with particular health concerns, glycemic index may be an important consideration; however, it should not be the sole criterion for food choices. For example, ice cream has a much lower glycemic index than brown rice or carrots—but that doesn't make it a healthier choice overall. Glycemic index and its effects on appetite and heart health are discussed further in Chapters 9 and 11. For now, remember that most unrefined grains, fruits, vegetables, and legumes are rich in nutrients and have a low-to-moderate glycemic index. Choose a variety of vegetables daily, and avoid heavy consumption of white potatoes. Limit foods that are high in added sugars but provide few other nutrients. Some studies have singled out regular soda, with its large dose of rapidly absorbable sugar, as specifically linked to increased diabetes risk.

Recommended Carbohydrate Intake On average, Americans consume 200–300 grams of carbohydrate per day, well above the 130 grams needed to meet the body's requirement for essential carbohydrate. A range of intakes is associated with good health, and experts recommend that adults consume 45–65% of total daily calories as carbohydrate, about 225–325 grams of carbohydrate for someone consuming 2000 calories per day. The focus should be on consuming a variety of foods rich in complex carbohydrates, especially whole grains.

Health experts offer separate guidelines for intake of added sugars as part of total carbohydrate consumption. The Food and Nutrition Board set an AMDR for added sugars of 25% or less of total daily calories, but many health experts recommend a substantially lower intake. Guidelines released by the World Health Organization in 2003 suggested a limit of 10% of total daily calories from added sugars. Limits set by the USDA in 2005 are even lower, with a maximum of about 8 teaspoons (32 grams) suggested for someone consuming 2000 calories per day. Foods high in added sugar are generally high in calories and low in nutrients and fiber, thus providing "empty" calories. To reduce your intake of added sugars, limit soft drinks, candy, sweet desserts, and sweetened fruit drinks. The simple carbohydrates in your diet should come from food sources in which they are found naturally—including fruits, which are excellent sources of vitamins and minerals—and from low-fat or fat-free milk and other dairy products, which are high in protein and calcium.

Athletes in training can especially benefit from high-carbohydrate diets (60–70% of total daily calories), which enhance the amount of carbohydrates stored in their muscles (as glycogen) and therefore provide more carbohydrate fuel for use during endurance events or long workouts. In addition, high-glycemic-index carbohydrates consumed during prolonged athletic events can help fuel muscles and extend the availability of the glycogen stored in muscles. Caution is in order, however, because overconsumption of carbohydrates can lead to feelings of fatigue and underconsumption of other nutrients.

Fiber—A Closer Look

Fiber is the term given to nondigestible carbohydrates provided mainly by plants. Instead of being digested, like starch, fiber passes through the intestinal tract and provides bulk for feces in the large intestine, which in turn facilitates elimination. In the large intestine, some types of fiber are broken down by bacteria into acids and gases, which explains why consuming too much fiber can lead to intestinal gas. Because humans cannot digest fiber, it is not a source of carbohydrate in the diet; however, the consumption of fiber is necessary for good health.

Types of Dietary Fiber The Food and Nutrition Board has defined two types of fiber: dietary fiber and functional fiber. **Dietary fiber** refers to nondigestible

carbohydrates and lignin that are present naturally in plants such as grains, legumes, and vegetables. **Functional fiber** refers to nondigestible carbohydrates that have been either isolated from natural sources or synthesized in a lab and then added to a food product or supplement. **Total fiber** is the sum of dietary and functional fiber.

Fibers have different properties that lead to different physiological effects in the body. **Soluble (viscous) fiber** slows the body's absorption of glucose and binds cholesterol-containing compounds in the intestine, lowering blood cholesterol levels and reducing the risk of cardiovascular disease. **Insoluble fiber** binds water, making the feces bulkier and softer so they pass more quickly and easily through the intestines.

Both kinds of fiber contribute to disease prevention. A diet high in soluble fiber can help people manage diabetes and high blood cholesterol levels. A diet high in insoluble fiber can help prevent a variety of health problems, including constipation, hemorrhoids, and **diverticulitis.** Some studies have linked diets high in fiber-rich fruits, vegetables, and grains with a lower risk of some kinds of cancer; however, it is unclear whether fiber or other food components are responsible for this reduction in risk.

Sources of Dietary Fiber All plant foods contain some dietary fiber, but fruits, legumes, oats (especially oat bran), and barley are particularly rich in it. Wheat (especially wheat bran), cereals, grains, and vegetables are all good sources of insoluble fiber. Psyllium, which is often added to cereals or used in fiber supplements and laxatives, improves intestinal health and also helps control glucose and cholesterol levels. The processing of packaged foods can remove fiber, so it's important to depend on fresh fruits and vegetables and foods made from whole grains as sources of dietary fiber.

Recommended Intake of Dietary Fiber To reduce the risk of chronic disease and maintain intestinal health, the Food and Nutrition Board recommends a daily fiber intake of 38 grams for adult men and 25 grams for adult

---

dietary fiber   Nondigestible carbohydrates and lignin that are intact in plants.

functional fiber   Nondigestible carbohydrates either isolated from natural sources or synthesized; these may be added to foods and dietary supplements.

total fiber   The total amount of dietary fiber and functional fiber in the diet.

soluble (viscous) fiber   Fiber that dissolves in water or is broken down by bacteria in the large intestine.

insoluble fiber   Fiber that does not dissolve in water and is not broken down by bacteria in the large intestine.

diverticulitis   A digestive disorder in which abnormal pouches form in the walls of the intestine and become inflamed.

women. Americans currently consume about half this amount. Fiber should come from foods, not supplements, which should be used only under medical supervision.

To increase the amount of fiber in your diet, try the following:

- Choose breads, crackers, and cereals that list whole grain first in the ingredient list: Whole-wheat flour, whole-grain oats, and whole-grain rice are whole grains; wheat flour is not. Choose a breakfast cereal with 5 or more grams of fiber per serving.
- Eat whole, unpeeled fruits rather than drinking fruit juice. Top cereals, yogurt, and desserts with berries, apple slices, or other fruit.
- Include legumes in soups and salads. Combine raw vegetables with pasta, rice, or beans in salads.
- Substitute bean dip for cheese-based or sour cream–based dips or spreads. Use raw vegetables rather than chips for dipping.

Vitamins—Organic Micronutrients

Vitamins are organic (carbon-containing) substances required in very small amounts to regulate various processes within living cells (Table 8.2). Humans need 13 vitamins. Four are fat-soluble (A, D, E, and K), and nine are water-soluble (C and the eight B-complex vitamins: thiamin, riboflavin, niacin, vitamin B-6, folate, vitamin B-12, biotin, and pantothenic acid). Solubility affects how a vitamin is absorbed, transported, and stored in the body. The water-soluble vitamins are absorbed directly into the bloodstream, where they travel freely; excess water-soluble vitamins are removed by the kidneys and excreted in urine. Fat-soluble vitamins require a more complex absorptive process; they are usually carried in the blood by special proteins and are stored in the liver and in fat tissues rather than excreted.

Functions of Vitamins Many vitamins help chemical reactions take place. They provide no energy to the body directly but help unleash the energy stored in carbohydrates, proteins, and fats. Vitamins are critical in the production of red blood cells and the maintenance of the nervous, skeletal, and immune systems. Some vitamins act as **antioxidants,** which help preserve healthy cells in the body. Key vitamin antioxidants include vitamin E,

vitamins Organic substances needed in small amounts to help promote and regulate chemical reactions and processes in the body.

antioxidant A substance that protects against the breakdown of body constituents by free radicals; actions include binding oxygen, donating electrons to free radicals, and repairing damage to molecules.

vitamin C, and the vitamin A precursor beta-carotene. (Antioxidants are described later in the chapter.)

Sources of Vitamins The human body does not manufacture most of the vitamins it requires and must obtain them from foods. Vitamins are abundant in fruits, vegetables, and grains. In addition, many processed foods, such as flour and breakfast cereals, contain added vitamins. A few vitamins are made in certain parts of the body: The skin makes vitamin D when it is exposed to sunlight, and intestinal bacteria make vitamin K. Nonetheless, you still need to get vitamin D and vitamin K from foods.

Vitamin Deficiencies and Excesses If your diet lacks sufficient amounts of a particular vitamin, characteristic symptoms of deficiency develop (see Table 8.2). For example, vitamin A deficiency can cause blindness, and vitamin B-6 deficiency can cause seizures. Vitamin deficiency diseases are most often seen in developing countries; they are relatively rare in the United States because vitamins are readily available from our food supply. However, intakes below recommended levels can have adverse effects on health even if they are not low enough to cause a deficiency disease. For example, low intake of folate increases a woman's chance of giving birth to a baby with a neural tube defect (a congenital malformation of the central nervous system). Low intake of folate and vitamins B-6 and B-12 has been linked to increased heart disease risk. Many Americans consume less-than-recommended amounts of vitamins A, C, D, and E.

Extra vitamins in the diet can be harmful, especially when taken as supplements. High doses of vitamin A are toxic and increase the risk of birth defects, for example. Vitamin B-6 can cause irreversible nerve damage when taken in large doses. Megadoses of fat-soluble vitamins are particularly dangerous because the excess will be stored in the body rather than excreted, increasing the risk of toxicity. Even when supplements are not taken in excess, relying on them for an adequate intake of vitamins can be problematic: There are many substances in foods other than vitamins and minerals, and some of these compounds may have important health effects. Later in the chapter, we discuss specific recommendations for vitamin intake and when a supplement is advisable. For now, keep in mind that it's best to obtain most of your vitamins from foods rather than supplements.

The vitamins and minerals in vegetables can be easily lost or destroyed during storage or cooking. To retain their value, eat or process vegetables immediately after buying them. If you can't do this, then store them in a cool place, covered to retain moisture—either in the refrigerator (for a few days) or in the freezer (for a longer term). To reduce nutrient losses during food preparation, minimize the amount of water used and the total cooking time. Develop a taste for a crunchier texture in cooked vegetables. Baking, steaming, broiling, grilling, and microwaving are all good methods of preparing vegetables.

Table 8.2   Facts About Vitamins

Vitamin	Important Dietary Sources	Major Functions	Signs of Prolonged Deficiency	Toxic Effects of Megadoses
Fat-Soluble				
Vitamin A	Liver, milk, butter, cheese, fortified margarine; carrots, spinach, and other orange and deep green vegetables and fruits	Maintenance of vision, skin, linings of the nose, mouth, digestive and urinary tracts, immune function	Night blindness; dry, scaling skin; increased susceptibility to infection; loss of appetite; anemia; kidney stones	Liver damage, miscarriage and birth defects, headache, vomiting and diarrhea, vertigo, double vision, bone abnormalities
Vitamin D	Fortified milk and margarine, fish oils, butter, egg yolks (sunlight on skin also produces vitamin D)	Development and maintenance of bones and teeth; promotion of calcium absorption	Rickets (bone deformities) in children; bone softening, loss, fractures in adults	Kidney damage, calcium deposits in soft tissues, depression, death
Vitamin E	Vegetable oils, whole grains, nuts and seeds, green leafy vegetables, asparagus, peaches	Protection and maintenance of cellular membranes	Red blood cell breakage and anemia, weakness, neurological problems, muscle cramps	Relatively nontoxic, but may cause excess bleeding or formation of blood clots
Vitamin K	Green leafy vegetables; smaller amounts widespread in other foods	Production of proteins essential for blood clotting and bone metabolism	Hemorrhaging	None reported
Water-Soluble				
Biotin	Cereals, yeast, egg yolks, soy flour, liver; widespread in foods	Synthesis of fat, glycogen, and amino acids	Rash, nausea, vomiting, weight loss, depression, fatigue, hair loss	None reported
Folate	Green leafy vegetables, yeast, oranges, whole grains, legumes, liver	Amino acid metabolism, synthesis of RNA and DNA, new cell synthesis	Anemia, weakness, fatigue, irritability, shortness of breath, swollen tongue	Masking of vitamin B-12 deficiency
Niacin	Eggs, poultry, fish, milk, whole grains, nuts, enriched breads and cereals, meats, legumes	Conversion of carbohydrates, fats, and proteins into usable forms of energy	Pellagra (symptoms include diarrhea, dermatitis, inflammation of mucous membranes, dementia)	Flushing of skin, nausea, vomiting, diarrhea, liver dysfunction, glucose intolerance
Pantothenic acid	Animal foods, whole grains, broccoli, potatoes; widespread in foods	Metabolism of fats, carbohydrates, and proteins	Fatigue, numbness and tingling of hands and feet, gastrointestinal disturbances	None reported
Riboflavin	Dairy products, enriched breads and cereals, lean meats, poultry, fish, green vegetables	Energy metabolism; maintenance of skin, mucous membranes, nervous system structures	Cracks at corners of mouth, sore throat, skin rash, hypersensitivity to light, purple tongue	None reported
Thiamin	Whole-grain and enriched breads and cereals, organ meats, lean pork, nuts, legumes	Conversion of carbohydrates into usable forms of energy, maintenance of appetite and nervous system function	Beriberi (symptoms include muscle wasting, mental confusion, anorexia, enlarged heart, nerve changes)	None reported
Vitamin B-6	Eggs, poultry, fish, whole grains, nuts, soybeans, liver, kidney, pork	Metabolism of amino acids and glycogen	Anemia, convulsions, cracks at corners of mouth, dermatitis, nausea, confusion	Neurological abnormalities and damage
Vitamin B-12	Meat, fish, poultry, fortified cereals	Synthesis of blood cells; other metabolic reactions	Anemia, fatigue, nervous system damage, sore tongue	None reported
Vitamin C	Peppers, cruciferous vegetables, spinach, citrus fruits, strawberries, tomatoes, potatoes, other fruits and vegetables	Maintenance and repair of connective tissue, bones, teeth, cartilage; promotion of healing; aid in iron absorption	Scurvy, anemia, reduced resistance to infection, loosened teeth, joint pain, poor wound healing, hair loss, poor iron absorption	Urinary stones in some people, acid stomach from ingesting supplements in pill form, nausea, diarrhea, headache, fatigue

SOURCES: Food and Nutrition Board, Institute of Medicine. 2006. *Dietary Reference Intakes: The Essential Guide to Nutrient Requirements.* Washington, D.C.: National Academies Press. The complete Dietary Reference Intake reports are available from the National Academies Press (http://www.nap.edu). Shils, M. E., et al., eds. 2005. *Modern Nutrition in Health and Disease,* 10th ed. Baltimore: Lippincott Williams and Wilkins.

Minerals—Inorganic Micronutrients

Minerals are inorganic (non-carbon-containing) elements you need in small amounts to help regulate body functions, aid in the growth and maintenance of body tissues, and help release energy (Table 8.3). There are about 17 essential minerals. The major minerals, those that the body needs in amounts exceeding 100 milligrams, include calcium, phosphorus, magnesium, sodium, potassium, and chloride. The essential trace minerals, those that you need in minute amounts, include copper, fluoride, iodine, iron, selenium, and zinc.

Characteristic symptoms develop if an essential mineral is consumed in a quantity too small or too large for good health. The minerals most commonly lacking in the American diet are iron, calcium, magnesium, and

Table 8.3	Facts About Selected Minerals			
Mineral	**Important Dietary Sources**	**Major Functions**	**Signs of Prolonged Deficiency**	**Toxic Effects of Megadoses**
Calcium	Milk and milk products, tofu, fortified orange juice and bread, green leafy vegetables, bones in fish	Formation of bones and teeth; control of nerve impulses, muscle contraction, blood clotting	Stunted growth in children, bone mineral loss in adults; urinary stones	Kidney stones, calcium deposits in soft tissues, inhibition of mineral absorption, constipation
Fluoride	Fluoridated water, tea, marine fish eaten with bones	Maintenance of tooth and bone structure	Higher frequency of tooth decay	Increased bone density, mottling of teeth, impaired kidney function
Iodine	Iodized salt, seafood, processed foods	Essential part of thyroid hormones, regulation of body metabolism	Goiter (enlarged thyroid), cretinism (birth defect)	Depression of thyroid activity, hyperthyroidism in susceptible people
Iron	Meat and poultry, fortified grain products, dark green vegetables, dried fruit	Component of hemoglobin, myoglobin, and enzymes	Iron-deficiency anemia, weakness, impaired immune function, gastrointestinal distress	Nausea, diarrhea, liver and kidney damage, joint pains, sterility, disruption of cardiac function, death
Magnesium	Widespread in foods and water (except soft water); especially found in grains, legumes, nuts, seeds, green vegetables, milk	Transmission of nerve impulses, energy transfer, activation of many enzymes	Neurological disturbances, cardiovascular problems, kidney disorders, nausea, growth failure in children	Nausea, vomiting, diarrhea, central nervous system depression, coma; death in people with impaired kidney function
Phosphorus	Present in nearly all foods, especially milk, cereal, peas, eggs, meat	Bone growth and maintenance, energy transfer in cells	Impaired growth, weakness, kidney disorders, cardiorespiratory and nervous system dysfunction	Drop in blood calcium levels, calcium deposits in soft tissues, bone loss
Potassium	Fruits and vegetables, especially leafy greens, cantaloupe, bananas, mushrooms, potatoes	Basic functioning of cells, water balance, acid-base balance	Elevated blood pressure, bone mineral loss, kidney stones, increased salt sensitivity, cardiac arrhythmia, muscle weakness	Cardiac arrhythmia and arrest, gastrointestinal discomfort
Selenium	Seafood, meat, eggs, whole grains	Defense against oxidative stress; regulation of thyroid hormone action	Muscle pain and weakness, heart disorders	Hair and nail brittleness and loss, nausea and vomiting, weakness, irritability
Sodium	Salt, soy sauce, fast food, processed foods, especially lunch meats, canned soups and vegetables, salty snacks, processed cheese	Body water balance, acid-base balance, nerve function	Muscle weakness, loss of appetite, nausea, vomiting; deficiency rarely seen	Increased blood pressure (even at fairly low levels of intake), renal stones, edema
Zinc	Whole grains, meat, eggs, liver, seafood (especially oysters)	Synthesis of proteins, RNA, and DNA; wound healing; immune response; ability to taste	Growth failure, loss of appetite, impaired taste acuity, skin rash, impaired immune function, poor wound healing	Vomiting, impaired immune function, decline in blood HDL levels, impaired copper absorption

SOURCES: Food and Nutrition Board, Institute of Medicine. 2006. *Dietary Reference Intakes: The Essential Guide to Nutrient Requirements*. Washington, D.C.: National Academies Press. The complete Dietary Reference Intake reports are available from the National Academies Press (http://www.nap.edu). Shils, M. E., et al., eds. 2005. *Modern Nutrition in Health and Disease*, 10th ed. Baltimore: Lippincott Williams and Wilkins.

Eating for Healthy Bones

Osteoporosis is a condition in which the bones become dangerously thin and fragile over time. An estimated 10 million Americans over age 50 have osteoporosis, and another 34 million are at risk. Women account for about 80% of osteoporosis cases. Most bone mass is built by age 18. After bone density peaks between ages 25 and 35, bone mass is slowly lost over time. To prevent osteoporosis, the best strategy is to build as much bone as possible during your youth and then do everything you can to maintain it as you age. Up to 50% of bone loss is determined by controllable lifestyle factors. Key nutrients include the following:

- **Calcium.** Consuming an adequate amount of calcium is important throughout life to build and maintain bone mass. Milk, yogurt, and calcium-fortified orange juice, bread, and cereals are all good sources.

- **Vitamin D.** Vitamin D is necessary for bones to absorb calcium; a daily intake of 5 micrograms is recommended for adults age 19–50. Vitamin D can be obtained from foods and is manufactured by the skin when exposed to sunlight. Candidates for vitamin D supplements include people who don't eat many foods in vitamin D; those who don't expose their face, arms, and hands to the sun (without sunscreen) for 5–15 minutes a few times each week; and people who live north of an imaginary line roughly between Boston and the Oregon–California border (the sun is weaker in northern latitudes).

- **Vitamin K.** Vitamin K promotes the synthesis of proteins that help keep bones strong. Broccoli and leafy green vegetables are rich in vitamin K.

- **Other nutrients.** Other nutrients that may play an important role in bone health include vitamin C, magnesium, potassium, manganese, zinc, copper, and boron.

On the flip side, there are several dietary substances that may have a *negative* effect on bone health, especially if consumed in excess: alcohol, sodium, caffeine, and retinol (a form of vitamin A). Drinking lots of soda, which often replaces milk in the diet and which is high in phosphorus (a mineral that may interfere with calcium absorption), has been shown to increase the risk of bone fracture in teenage girls.

The effect of protein intake on bone mass depends on other nutrients: Protein helps build bone as long as calcium and vitamin D intake are adequate; but if intake of calcium and vitamin D is low, high protein intake can lead to bone loss.

As described in earlier chapters, weight-bearing aerobic exercise helps maintain bone mass throughout life, and strength training improves bone density, muscle mass, strength, and balance. Drinking alcohol only in moderation, refraining from smoking, and managing depression and stress are also important for maintaining strong bones. For people who do develop osteoporosis, a variety of medications are available to treat the condition.

---

potassium. Focus on good food choices for these nutrients (see Table 8.3). Lean meats are rich in iron; low-fat or fat-free dairy products are excellent choices for calcium. Plant foods such as whole grains and leafy vegetables are good sources of magnesium. Potassium-rich foods include spinach and other leafy greens, cantaloupe, bananas, mushrooms, and white and sweet potatoes. Iron-deficiency **anemia** is a problem in some age groups, and researchers fear poor calcium intakes in childhood are sowing the seeds for future **osteoporosis,** especially in women. See the box "Eating for Healthy Bones" to learn more.

Water—Vital but Often Ignored

Water is the major component in both foods and the human body: You are composed of about 50–60% water. Your need for other nutrients, in terms of weight, is much less than your need for water. You can live up to 50 days without food but only a few days without water.

Water is distributed all over the body, among lean and other tissues and in blood and other body fluids. Water is used in the digestion and absorption of food and is the medium in which most of the chemical reactions take place within the body. Some water-based fluids, such as blood, transport substances around the body; other fluids serve as lubricants or cushions. Water also helps regulate body temperature.

Water is contained in almost all foods, particularly in liquids, fruits, and vegetables. The foods and fluids you consume provide 80–90% of your daily water intake; the remainder is generated through metabolism. You lose water each day in urine, feces, and sweat and through evaporation from your lungs.

As described in Chapter 3, severe dehydration causes weakness and can lead to death. However, most people maintain a healthy water balance by consuming beverages at meals and drinking fluids in response to thirst. In 2004, the Food and Nutrition Board set levels of adequate water intake to maintain hydration; all fluids, including those containing caffeine, can count toward your total daily fluid intake. Water and other beverages typically make up about 80% of your fluid intake; the remainder comes from foods, especially fruits and vegetables. Men need to consume about 3.7 total liters of water, with 3.0 liters (about 13 cups) coming from beverages; women need

minerals Inorganic compounds needed in small amounts for the regulation, growth, and maintenance of body tissues and functions.

anemia A deficiency in the oxygen-carrying material in the red blood cells.

osteoporosis A condition in which the bones become thin and brittle and break easily.

2.7 total liters, with 2.2 liters (about 9 cups) coming from beverages. (See Table 1 in the Nutrition Resources section at the end of the chapter for recommendations for specific age groups.) If you exercise vigorously or live in a hot climate, you need to consume additional fluids to maintain a balance between water consumed and water lost. (See p. 250 for more on the fluid needs of athletes and active people.)

Other Substances in Food

There are many substances in food that are not essential nutrients but that may influence health.

Antioxidants   When the body uses oxygen or breaks down certain fats or proteins as a normal part of metabolism, it gives rise to substances called **free radicals.** Environmental factors such as cigarette smoke, exhaust fumes, radiation, excessive sunlight, certain drugs, and stress can increase free radical production. A free radical is a chemically unstable molecule that reacts with fats, proteins, and DNA, damaging cell membranes and mutating genes. Free radicals have been implicated in aging, cancer, cardiovascular disease, and other degenerative diseases like arthritis.

Antioxidants found in foods can help protect the body by blocking the formation and action of free radicals and repairing the damage they cause. Some antioxidants, such as vitamin C, vitamin E, and selenium, are also essential nutrients; others, such as carotenoids, found in yellow, orange, and dark green leafy vegetables, are not. Researchers recently identified the top antioxidant-containing foods and beverages as blackberries, walnuts, strawberries, artichokes, cranberries, brewed coffee, raspberries, pecans, blueberries, cloves, grape juice, unsweetened baking chocolate, sour cherries, and red wine. Also high in antioxidants are Brussels sprouts, kale, cauliflower, and pomegranates.

Phytochemicals   Antioxidants fall into the broader category of **phytochemicals,** substances found in plant foods that may help prevent chronic disease. Researchers have just begun to identify and study all the different compounds found in foods, and many preliminary findings are promising. For example, certain substances found in soy foods may help lower cholesterol levels. Sulforaphane, a compound isolated from broccoli and other **cruciferous vegetables,** may render some carcinogenic compounds harmless. Allyl sulfides, a group of chemicals found in garlic and onions, appear to boost the activity of cancer-fighting immune cells. Further research on phytochemicals may extend the role of nutrition to the prevention and treatment of many chronic diseases.

To increase your intake of phytochemicals, eat a variety of fruits and vegetables rather than relying on supplements. Like many vitamins and minerals, isolated phytochemicals may be harmful if taken in high doses. In addition, it is likely that their health benefits are the result of chemical substances working in combination. The role of phytochemicals in disease prevention is discussed further in Chapters 11 and 12.

NUTRITIONAL GUIDELINES: PLANNING YOUR DIET

Various tools have been created by scientific and government groups to help people design healthy diets. The **Dietary Reference Intakes (DRIs)** are standards for nutrient intake designed to prevent nutritional deficiencies and reduce the risk of chronic disease. **Dietary Guidelines for Americans** have been established to promote health and reduce the risk for major chronic diseases through diet and physical activity. Further guidance symbolized by **MyPyramid** provides daily food intake patterns that meet the DRIs and are consistent with the Dietary Guidelines for Americans.

Dietary Reference Intakes (DRIs)

The Food and Nutrition Board establishes dietary standards, or recommended intake levels, for Americans of all ages. The current set of standards, called Dietary Reference Intakes (DRIs), is relatively new, having been introduced in 1997. The DRIs are frequently reviewed and are updated as new nutrition-related information becomes available. The DRIs present different categories of nutrients in easy-to-read table format. An earlier set of standards, called the Recommended Dietary Allowances (RDAs), focused on preventing nutritional deficiency diseases such as anemia. The DRIs have a broader focus because recent research has looked not just at the prevention of nutrient deficiencies but also at the role of nutrients in promoting optimal health and preventing chronic diseases such as cancer, osteoporosis, and heart disease.

The DRIs include standards for both recommended intakes and maximum safe intakes. The recommended intake of each nutrient is expressed as either a Recommended Dietary Allowance (RDA) or as Adequate Intake (AI). An AI is set when there is not enough information available to set an RDA value; regardless of the type of standard used, however, the DRI represents the best available estimate of intake for optimal health. The Tolerable Upper Intake Level (UL) sets the maximum daily intake by a healthy person that is unlikely to cause health problems. For example, the RDA for calcium for an 18-year-old female is 1300 milligrams per day; the UL is 2500 milligrams per day.

Because of a lack of data, ULs have not been set for all nutrients. This does not mean that people can tolerate long-term intakes of these vitamins and minerals above recommended levels. Like all chemical agents, nutrients can produce adverse effects if intakes are excessive. There is no established benefit from consuming nutrients at levels above the RDA or AI. The DRIs can be found in the Nutrition Resources section at the end of the chapter. For more information, visit the Web site of the Food and Nutrition Board (see For Further Exploration at the end of the chapter).

Should You Take Supplements?

The aim of the DRIs is to guide you in meeting your nutritional needs primarily with food, rather than with vitamin and mineral supplements. This goal is important because recommendations have not yet been set for some essential nutrients. Many supplements contain only nutrients with established recommendations, so using them to meet nutrient needs can leave you deficient in other nutrients. Supplements also lack potentially beneficial phytochemicals that are found only in whole foods. Most Americans can get most of the vitamins and minerals they need by consuming a varied, nutritionally balanced diet.

The question of whether to take supplements is a serious one. Some vitamins and minerals are dangerous when ingested in excess, as described in Tables 8.2 and 8.3. Large doses of particular nutrients can also cause health problems by affecting the absorption of other vitamins and minerals. For all these reasons, you should think carefully about whether to take high-dose supplements; consider consulting a physician or registered dietitian.

In setting the DRIs, the Food and Nutrition Board recommended supplements of particular nutrients for the following groups:

• Women who are capable of becoming pregnant should take 400 micrograms (mg) per day of folic acid (the synthetic form of the vitamin folate) from fortified foods and/or supplements in addition to folate from a varied diet. Research indicates that this level of folate intake will reduce the risk of neural tube defects. (This defect occurs early in pregnancy, before most women know they are pregnant; therefore, the recommendation for folate applies to all women of reproductive age rather than only to pregnant women.) Since 1998, enriched breads, flours, corn meals, rice, noodles, and other grain products have been fortified with small amounts of folic acid. Folate is found naturally in green leafy vegetables, legumes, oranges and orange juice, and strawberries.

• People over age 50 should consume foods fortified with vitamin B-12, B-12 supplements, or a combination of the two in order to meet the majority of the DRI of 2.4 milligrams of B-12 daily. Up to 30% of people over 50 may have problems absorbing protein-bound B-12 in foods. Vitamin B-12 in supplements and fortified foods is more readily absorbed and can help prevent a deficiency.

Because of the oxidative stress caused by smoking, the Food and Nutrition Board also recommends that smokers consume 35 milligrams *more* vitamin C per day than the DRI intake level set for their age and sex (for adults, recommended daily vitamin C intakes for nonsmokers are 90 mg for men and 75 mg for women). However, supplements are not usually needed because this extra vitamin C can easily be obtained from foods. For example, 1 cup of orange juice has about 100 milligrams of vitamin C.

Supplements may also be recommended in other cases. Women with heavy menstrual flows may need extra iron to compensate for the monthly loss. Older people, people with dark skin, and people exposed to little sunlight may need extra vitamin D from vitamin D–fortified foods and/or supplements. Some vegetarians may need supplemental calcium, iron, zinc, and vitamin B-12, depending on their food choices. Newborns need a single dose of vitamin K, which must be administered under the direction of a physician. People who consume few calories, who have certain diseases, or who take certain medications may need specific vitamin and mineral supplements; such supplement decisions must be made by a physician because some vitamins and minerals counteract the actions of certain medications.

free radical An electron-seeking compound that can react with fats, proteins, and DNA, damaging cell membranes and mutating genes in its search for electrons; produced through chemical reactions in the body and by exposure to environmental factors such as sunlight and tobacco smoke.

phytochemical A naturally occurring substance found in plant foods that may help prevent and treat chronic diseases such as heart disease and cancer; *phyto* means "plant."

cruciferous vegetables Vegetables of the cabbage family, including cabbage, broccoli, brussels sprouts, kale, and cauliflower; the flower petals of these plants form the shape of a cross, hence the name.

Dietary Reference Intakes (DRIs) An umbrella term for four types of nutrient standards: Adequate Intake (AI), Estimated Average Requirement (EAR), and Recommended Dietary Allowance (RDA) set levels of intake considered adequate to prevent nutrient deficiencies and reduce the risk of chronic disease; Tolerable Upper Intake Level (UL) sets the maximum daily intake that is unlikely to cause health problems.

Dietary Guidelines for Americans General principles of good nutrition intended to help prevent certain diet-related diseases; published by the U.S. Department of Health and Human Services and the USDA.

MyPyramid A food-group plan that provides practical advice to ensure a balanced intake of the essential nutrients.

For many Americans, general dietary changes needed to meet dietary guidelines include consuming more fruits, whole grains, and dark green vegetables. Most fats in the diet should be unsaturated, like those found in fish and nuts.

In deciding whether to take a vitamin and mineral supplement, consider whether you already regularly consume a fortified breakfast cereal. Many breakfast cereals contain almost as many nutrients as a vitamin pill. If you decide to take a supplement, choose a balanced formulation that contains 50–100% of the Daily Value for vitamins and minerals. Avoid supplements containing large doses of particular nutrients. (See p. 250 for more on choosing and using supplements.)

Daily Values Because the DRIs are too cumbersome to use as a basis for food labels, the U.S. Food and Drug Administration developed another set of dietary standards, the **Daily Values.** The Daily Values are based on several different sets of guidelines and include standards for fat, cholesterol, carbohydrate, dietary fiber, and selected vitamins and minerals. The Daily Values represent appropriate intake levels for a 2000-calorie diet. The percent Daily Value shown on a food label shows how well that food contributes to your recommended daily intake. Food labels are described in detail later in the chapter.

Dietary Guidelines for Americans

To provide general guidance for choosing a healthy diet, the U.S. Department of Agriculture (USDA) and the U.S. Department of Health and Human Services (DHHS) have jointly issued Dietary Guidelines for Americans, most recently in 2005. These guidelines are intended for healthy children age 2 and older and adults of all ages. Key recommendations include the following:

- Consume a variety of nutrient-dense foods within and among the basic food groups, while staying within energy needs.
- Control calorie intake to manage body weight.

- Be physically active every day.
- Increase daily intake of foods from certain groups: fruits and vegetables, whole grains, and fat-free or low-fat milk and milk products.
- Choose fats wisely for good health, limiting intake of saturated and trans fats.
- Choose carbohydrates wisely for good health, limiting intake of added sugars.
- Choose and prepare foods with little salt, and consume potassium-rich foods.
- If you drink alcoholic beverages, do so in moderation.
- Keep foods safe to eat.

Following these guidelines promotes health and reduces risk for chronic diseases, including heart disease, cancer, diabetes, stroke, osteoporosis, and obesity. Each of the recommendations in the 2005 Dietary Guidelines for Americans is supported by an extensive review of scientific and medical evidence. What follows is a brief summary of the guidelines.

Adequate Nutrients Within Calorie Needs Many people consume more calories than they need while failing to meet recommended intakes for all nutrients. Meeting the DRIs provides a foundation not only for current health but also for reducing chronic disease risk. Many adults don't get enough calcium, potassium, fiber, magnesium, and vitamins A, C, and E; many children don't get enough calcium, potassium, fiber, magnesium, and vitamin E. Most people need to choose meals and snacks that are high in nutrients but low to moderate in calories.

Two eating plans that translate nutrient recommendations into food choices are the USDA's MyPyramid and the DASH eating plan. MyPyramid is described in detail in the next section (pp. 242–246); the DASH plan appears in the Nutrition Resources section at the end of the chapter. You can obtain all the nutrients and other substances you need by choosing the recommended number of daily servings from basic food groups and following the advice about selecting nutrient-dense foods within the groups. Following these plans would mean that many Americans would have to make some general dietary changes:

- Eat more dark green vegetables, orange vegetables, legumes, fruits, whole grains, and low-fat and fat-free milk and milk products.
- Eat less refined grains, saturated fat, trans fat, cholesterol, added sugars, and calories.

Your nutrients should come primarily from foods that contain not only the essential vitamins and minerals but also hundreds of naturally occurring substances that may benefit health, such as antioxidants. Situations in which a supplement might be recommended were described earlier in the chapter.

For maximum nutrition, it is important to consume foods from all the food groups daily and to consume a variety of nutrient-dense foods within the groups. Nutrient-dense foods are those that provide substantial amounts of vitamins and minerals and relatively few calories. Americans currently consume many foods and beverages that are low in nutrient density, making it difficult or impossible to meet nutrient needs without overconsuming calories. Selecting nutrient-dense foods—low-fat forms of foods in each group and those free of added sugars—allows you to meet your nutrient needs without overconsuming calories and unhealthy food components such as saturated and trans fats.

People's food choices can be affected by individual and cultural preferences, moral beliefs, the cost and availability of food, and food intolerances and allergies, but healthy eating is possible no matter how foods are prepared or combined. If you avoid most or all foods from any of the major food groups, be sure to get enough nutrients from the other groups. MyPyramid can be applied to vegetarian diets.

Weight Management Overweight and obesity are a major public health problem in the United States. Calorie intake and physical activity work together to influence body weight. Most Americans need to reduce calorie intake, increase their level of physical activity, and make wiser food choices. Many adults gain weight slowly over time, but even small changes in behavior can help avoid weight gain.

Evaluate your body weight in terms of body mass index (BMI), a measure of relative body weight that also takes height into account (see Chapter 6 for instructions on how to determine your BMI). If your current weight is healthy, aim to avoid weight gain. Do so by increasing physical activity and making small cuts in calorie intake. Choose nutrient-dense foods and sensible portion sizes. Avoiding weight gain is easier than losing weight. For example, for most adults, a reduction of 50–100 calories per day may prevent gradual weight gain, whereas a reduction of 500 calories or more per day may be needed initially for weight loss.

Monitoring weight regularly helps people know if they need to adjust their food intake or physical activity to maintain a healthy weight. Those who need to lose weight should aim for slow, steady weight loss by decreasing calorie intake, maintaining adequate nutrient intake, and increasing physical activity. In terms of macronutrient intake, use the AMDR ranges described earlier in the chapter for dietary planning; within these healthy ranges, total calorie intake is what counts for weight management rather than specific percentages of particular macronutrients.

Physical Activity As described earlier, regular physical activity improves fitness, helps manage weight, promotes psychological well-being, and reduces risk of heart disease, high blood pressure, cancer, and diabetes. Become active if you are inactive, and maintain or increase physical activity if you are already active. The amount of daily physical activity recommended for you depends on your current health status and goals.

- To reduce the risk of chronic disease, aim to accumulate at least 30 minutes (adults) or 60 minutes (children) of moderate physical activity—the equivalent of brisk walking at a pace of 3–4 miles per hour—beyond your usual activity at work, home, and school. Greater health benefits can be obtained by engaging in more vigorous activity or activity of longer duration.

- To help manage body weight and prevent gradual, unhealthy weight gain, engage in 60 minutes of moderate-to-high-intensity activity on most days of the week.

- To sustain weight loss in adulthood, engage daily in at least 60–90 minutes of moderate physical activity.

You can do the activity all at once or spread it out over several 10-minute or longer bouts during the day; choose activities you enjoy and can do regularly. You can boost fitness by engaging in exercises specifically designed for the health-related fitness components: cardiorespiratory endurance exercises, stretching exercises for flexibility, and resistance training for muscular strength and endurance.

Food Groups to Encourage Many Americans do not consume the recommended amounts of fruits, vegetables, whole grains, and low-fat or fat-free milk products—all of which have health benefits.

FRUITS AND VEGETABLES Fruits and vegetables are important sources of dietary fiber, vitamins, and minerals. For a 2000-calorie diet, about 4½ cups or the equivalent (9 servings) of fruits and vegetables each day is recommended. Eat a variety of fruits—fresh, frozen, canned, or dried—rather than fruit juice for most of your fruit choices. For vegetables, choose a variety of colors and kinds. Eat more of the following types of vegetables:

- Dark green vegetables, such as broccoli, kale, and other dark leafy greens

- Orange vegetables, such as carrots, sweet potatoes, pumpkin, and winter squash

- Legumes, such as pinto beans, kidney beans, black beans, garbanzo beans, split peas, and lentils

Other fruits and vegetables that are important sources of nutrients of concern include tomatoes and tomato products, red sweet peppers, cabbage and other cruciferous vegetables, bananas, citrus fruits, berries, and melons. See the discussion of MyPyramid for more advice on choosing fruits and vegetables.

Daily Values A simplified version of the RDAs used on food labels; also included are values for nutrients with no established RDA.

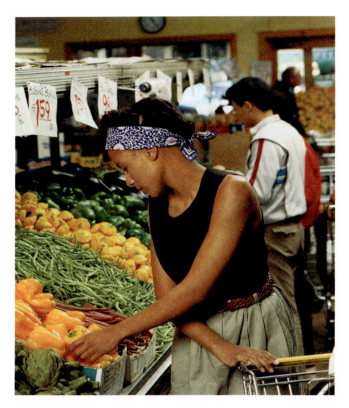

Brightly colored fruits and vegetables provide a broad range of vitamins and minerals and are excellent daily choices.

WHOLE GRAINS Whole grains provide more fiber and nutrients than refined grains, and intake of whole grains reduces the risk of chronic disease and helps with weight maintenance. For a 2000-calorie diet, 6 ounce-equivalents (6 servings) of grains each day are recommended; at least half of these servings should be whole grains. (One ounce is about 1 slice of bread, 1 cup of breakfast cereal flakes, or ½ cup of cooked pasta or rice.) The remaining grain servings should be from enriched or whole-grain products.

LOW-FAT AND FAT-FREE MILK AND MILK PRODUCTS Milk and other dairy products are important sources of calcium and other nutrients. Regular consumption of milk and milk products can reduce the risk of low bone mass throughout life. Choosing low-fat and fat-free dairy products helps to control calorie intake and reduce intake of saturated fat and cholesterol. For adults, the equivalent of 3 cups daily of fat-free or low-fat milk or milk products is recommended; 1½ ounces of cheese is the equivalent of 1 cup of milk. Yogurt and lactose-free milk are options for people who are lactose intolerant, as is use of the enzyme lactase prior to the consumption of milk products. For individuals who avoid all milk products, nondairy calcium sources include fortified cereals and beverages, tofu prepared with calcium sulfate, leafy green vegetables, soybeans, and certain types of fish.

Fats Fats and oils provide the essential fatty acids needed for a healthy diet, but, as described earlier in the chapter, the type and amount of fats consumed can make a difference for health. A diet low in saturated fat, trans fat, and cholesterol helps keep blood cholesterol low and reduces the risk for heart disease; a diet containing omega-3 fats from fish also reduces the risk for heart disease. Goals for fat intake for most adults are as follows:

Total fat: 20–35% of total daily calories

Saturated fat: Less than 10% of total daily calories

Trans fat: As little as possible

Cholesterol: Less than 300 mg per day

Most fats in the diet should come from sources of unsaturated fats, such as fish, nuts, and vegetable oils. When selecting and preparing meat, poultry, dry beans, and milk or milk products, make choices that are lean, low-fat, or fat-free. To reduce trans fat intake, limit intake of foods made with hydrogenated vegetable oils. Refer to the box "Reducing the Saturated and Trans Fats in Your Diet" for additional specific suggestions.

Cholesterol is found only in animal foods. If you need to reduce your cholesterol intake, limit your intake of foods that are particularly high in cholesterol, including egg yolks, dairy fats, certain shellfish, and liver and other organ meats; watch your serving sizes of animal foods. Food labels list the fat and cholesterol content of foods.

Two servings per week of fish rich in heart-healthy omega-3 fatty acids are also recommended for people at high risk for heart disease. However, for certain groups, intake limits are set for varieties of fish that may contain mercury (see p. 255 for more information). Fish rich in omega-3 fatty acids include salmon, mackerel, and trout.

Carbohydrates Carbohydrates are an important energy source in a healthy diet. Foods rich in carbohydrates may also be rich in dietary fiber. Fruits, vegetables, whole grains, and fat-free or low-fat milk can provide the recommended amount of carbohydrate. Choose fiber-rich foods often—for example, whole fruits, whole grains, and legumes.

People who consume foods and beverages high in added sugars tend to consume more calories but smaller amounts of vitamins and minerals than those who limit their intake of added sugars. A food is high in sugar if one of the following appears first or second in the list of ingredients or if several are listed: sugar (any type, including beet, brown, invert, raw, and cane), corn syrup or sweetener, fruit juice concentrate, honey, malt syrup, molasses, syrup, cane juice or dextrose, fructose, glucose, lactose, maltose, or sucrose.

To reduce added sugar consumption, cut back on soft drinks, candies, sweet desserts, fruit drinks, and other foods high in added sugars. Watch out for specialty coffee drinks, chai tea, smoothies, and sports drinks, which can contain hundreds of extra calories from sugar. Drink water rather than sweetened drinks, and don't let sodas and other sweets crowd out more nutritious foods, such as low-fat milk. Regular soda is the leading source of both

Reducing the Saturated and Trans Fats in Your Diet

Your overall goal is to limit total fat intake to no more than 35% of total calories. Favor unsaturated fats over saturated and trans fats.

- Be moderate in your consumption of foods high in fat, including fast foods, commercially prepared baked goods and desserts, deep-fried food, meat, poultry, nuts and seeds, and regular dairy products.

- When you eat high-fat foods, limit your portion sizes, and balance your intake with other foods that are low in fat.

- Choose lean cuts of meat, and trim any visible fat from meat before and after cooking. Remove skin from poultry before or after cooking.

- Drink fat-free or low-fat milk instead of whole milk, and use lower-fat milk in puddings, soups, and baked products. Substitute plain low-fat yogurt, blender-whipped low-fat cottage cheese, or buttermilk for sour cream.

- Use vegetable oil instead of butter or margarine. Use tub or squeeze margarine instead of stick margarine. Look for margarines that are free of trans fats. Minimize intake of coconut or palm oil.

- Season vegetables, seafood, and meats with herbs and spices rather than with creamy sauces, butter, or margarine.

- Use olive oil and lemon juice on salad, or use a yogurt-based salad dressing instead of mayonnaise or sour cream dressings.

- Steam, boil, bake, or microwave vegetables, or stir-fry them in a small amount of vegetable oil.

- Roast, bake, or broil meat, poultry, or fish so that fat drains away as the food cooks.

- Use a nonstick pan for cooking so that added fat will be unnecessary; use a vegetable spray for frying. Kitchen stores sell non-aerosol spray bottles to use with regular cooking oils.

- Chill broths from meat or poultry until the fat becomes solid. Spoon off the fat before using the broth.

- Substitute egg whites for whole eggs when baking; limit the number of egg yolks when scrambling eggs.

- Choose fruits as desserts most often.

- Eat a low-fat vegetarian main dish at least once a week.

added sugars and calories in the American diet; it provides little in the way of nutrients except sugar (Figure 8.5). The 10 teaspoons of sugar in a 12-ounce soda can exceed the recommended daily limit for added sugars for someone consuming 2000 calories per day; for more on added sugar limits, see the discussion of MyPyramid.

Nutrient	Recommended Daily Intake*	Orange Juice		Low-Fat (1%) Milk		Regular Cola		Bottled Iced Tea	
Calories	2000 calories	168 calories		150 calories		152 calories		150 calories	
Carbohydrate	300 g		40.5 g		18 g		38 g		37.5 g
Added sugars	32 g						38 g		34.5 g
Fat	65 g				3.9 g				
Protein	55 g				12 g				
Calcium	1000 mg		33 mg		450 mg		11 mg		
Potassium	4700 mg	15%	710 mg	12%	570 mg		4 mg		
Vitamin A	700 μg	4%	30 μg	31%	216 μg				
Vitamin C	75 mg		145.5 mg		3.6 mg				
Vitamin D	5 μg				3.7 μg				
Folate	400 μg		160 μg		20 μg				

*Recommended intakes and limits appropriate for a 20-year-old woman consuming 2000 calories per day.

FIGURE 8.5 Nutrient density of 12-ounce portions of selected beverages. The four beverages shown have approximately the same number of calories in a 12-ounce serving. However, regular cola and iced tea provide few nutrients besides added sugars; both contain more than the total daily recommended limit of added sugars (about 8 teaspoons). Orange juice is rich in potassium, vitamin C, and folate; low-fat milk is an excellent source of protein, calcium, potassium, vitamin A, and vitamin D. (Color bars represent percentage of recommended daily intake or limit for each nutrient.)

Keep your teeth and gums healthy by limiting consumption of sweet or starchy foods between meals and by brushing and flossing regularly; drinking fluoridated water also reduces the risk of dental caries (decay).

Sodium and Potassium   Many people can reduce their chance of developing high blood pressure or lower already elevated blood pressure by consuming less salt; reducing blood pressure lowers the risk for stroke, heart disease, and kidney disease. Salt is made up of the minerals sodium and chloride, and although both of these minerals are essential for normal body function, we need only small amounts (1500 mg per day for adults). Most Americans consume much more salt than they need. The goal is to reduce sodium intake to less than 2300 milligrams per day, the equivalent of about 1 teaspoon of salt. Certain groups, including people with hypertension, African Americans, and older adults, benefit from an even lower sodium intake of no more than 1500 milligrams per day.

Salt is found mainly in processed and prepared foods; smaller amounts may also be added during cooking or at the table. To lower your intake of salt, choose fresh or plain frozen meat, poultry, seafood, and vegetables most often; these are lower in salt than processed forms are. Check and compare the sodium content in processed foods, including frozen dinners, cheeses, soups, salad dressings, sauces, and canned mixed dishes. Add less salt during cooking and at the table, and limit your use of high-sodium condiments like soy sauce, ketchup, mustard, pickles, and olives. Use lemon juice, herbs, and spices instead of salt to enhance the flavor of foods.

Along with lowering salt intake, increasing potassium intake helps lower blood pressure. Fruits, vegetables, and most milk products are available in forms that contain no salt, and many of these are sources of potassium. Potassium-rich foods include leafy green vegetables, sweet and white potatoes, winter squash, soybeans, tomato sauce, bananas, peaches, apricots, cantaloupes, and orange juice.

Alcoholic Beverages   Alcoholic beverages supply calories but few nutrients. Drinking in moderation—that is, no more than one drink per day for women and no more than two drinks per day for men—is associated with mortality reduction among some groups, primarily males age 45 and over and women age 55 and over. Among younger people, alcohol use provides little if any health benefit, and heavy drinking is associated with motor vehicle injuries and deaths, liver disease, stroke, violence, and other health problems.

People who should not drink at all include individuals who cannot restrict their drinking to moderate levels; women who are pregnant or breastfeeding or who may become pregnant; children and adolescents; people with specific health conditions; individuals who plan to drive or operate machinery or engage in any activity that requires attention, skill, or coordination; and individuals taking prescription or over-the-counter medications that can interact with alcohol.

If you choose to drink alcoholic beverages, do so sensibly and moderately, preferably with meals. Never drink in situations in which it may put you or others at risk.

Food Safety   Safe foods are those that pose little risk from harmful bacteria, viruses, parasites, toxins, or chemical or physical contaminants. Foodborne diseases affect about 76 million Americans each year. Actions by consumers can reduce the occurrence of foodborne illness significantly. It is especially important to be careful with perishable foods such as poultry, meats, eggs, shellfish, milk products, and fresh fruits and vegetables. Refer to the section on foodborne illness (pp. 254–255) for specific food safety tips.

USDA's MyPyramid

When the first USDA daily food guide was published, in 1916, it emphasized the importance of getting enough calories from fats and sugars to support daily activity. Today, the guidelines stress the importance of limiting fats and sugars to control calorie intake. Many Americans are familiar with the USDA Food Guide Pyramid, the food guidance system that was first released in 1992. Since the initial release of the Pyramid, scientists have updated both nutrient recommendations (the DRIs) and the Dietary Guidelines for Americans. So, as the 2005 Dietary Guidelines were prepared, the USDA reassessed its overall food guidance system and released MyPyramid in April 2005 (Figure 8.6).

A variety of experts have proposed other food-group plans. Some of these address perceived shortcomings in the USDA plans, and some adapt the basic 1992 Pyramid to special populations. Two alternative food plans appear in the Nutrition Resources section at the end of the chapter: the DASH eating plan and the Harvard Healthy Eating Pyramid. The USDA Center for Nutrition Policy and Promotion (www.usda.gov/cnpp) has more on alternative food plans for special populations such as young children, older adults, and people choosing particular ethnic diets. MyPyramid is available in Spanish, and there is a special adaptation of MyPyramid for children age 6–11, called MyPyramid for Kids.

Another food plan that has received attention in recent years is the Mediterranean diet, which emphasizes vegetables, fruits, and whole grains; daily servings of beans, legumes, and nuts; moderate consumption of fish, poultry, and dairy products; and the use of olive oil over other types of fat, especially saturated fat. The Mediterranean diet has been associated with lower rates of heart disease and cancer, and a 2006 study found a link between the diet and a greatly reduced risk of Alzheimer's disease.

Key Messages of MyPyramid   The new MyPyramid symbol (see Figure 8.6) has been developed to remind

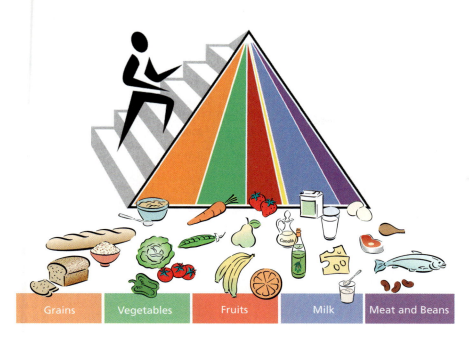

FIGURE 8.6 USDA's MyPyramid. The USDA food guidance system, called MyPyramid, can be personalized based on an individual's sex, age, and activity level; visit MyPyramid. gov to obtain a food plan appropriate for you. MyPyramid contains five main food groups plus oils (yellow band). Key consumer messages include the following:

- Grains: Make half your grains whole.
- Vegetables: Vary your veggies.
- Fruits: Focus on fruits.
- Oils: Know your fats.
- Milk: Get your calcium-rich foods.
- Meat and Beans: Go lean with protein.

SOURCE: U.S. Department of Agriculture. 2005. *MyPyramid* (http://mypyramid.gov; retrieved May 27, 2007).

consumers to make healthy food choices and to be active every day. Key messages include the following:

- *Personalization* is represented by the person on the steps and the MyPyramid.gov site, which includes individualized recommendations, interactive assessments of food intake and physical activity, and tips for success.
- *Daily physical activity,* represented by the person climbing the steps, is important for maintaining a healthy weight and reducing the risk of chronic disease.
- *Moderation* of food intake is represented by the narrowing of each food group from bottom to top.
- *Proportionality* is represented by the different widths of the food group bands. The widths provide a general guide for how much food a person should choose from each group.
- *Variety* is represented by the six color bands representing the five food groups of MyPyramid and oils. Foods from all groups are needed daily for good health.
- *Gradual improvement* is a good strategy; people can benefit from taking small steps to improve their diet and activity habits each day.

The MyPyramid chart in Figure 8.7 shows the food intake patterns recommended for different levels of calorie intake; Table 8.4 provides guidance for determining an appropriate calorie intake for weight maintenance. Use the table to identify an energy intake that is about right for you; then refer to the appropriate column in Figure 8.7. You can also get a personalized version of MyPyramid recommendations by visiting MyPyramid.gov. Each food group is described briefly in the following sections. Many Americans have trouble identifying serving sizes, so recommended daily intakes from each group are now given in terms of cups and ounces; see the box "Judging Portion Sizes" for additional advice.

Grains Foods from this group are usually low in fat and rich in complex carbohydrates, dietary fiber (if grains are unrefined), and many vitamins and minerals, including thiamin, riboflavin, iron, niacin, folic acid (if enriched or fortified), and zinc. Someone eating 2000 calories a day should include 6 ounce-equivalents each day, with half of those servings from whole grains such as whole-grain bread, whole-wheat pasta, high-fiber cereal, and brown rice. The following count as 1 ounce-equivalent:

- 1 slice of bread
- 1 small (2½-inch diameter) muffin
- 1 cup ready-to-eat cereal flakes
- ½ cup cooked cereal, rice, grains, or pasta
- 1 6-inch tortilla

Choose foods that are typically made with little fat or sugar (bread, rice, pasta) over those that are high in fat and sugar (croissants, chips, cookies, doughnuts).

Vegetables Vegetables contain carbohydrates, dietary fiber, vitamin A, vitamin C, folate, potassium, and other nutrients. They are also naturally low in fat. In a 2000-calorie diet, 2½ cups (5 servings) of vegetables should be included daily. Each of the following counts as ½ cup or equivalent (1 serving) of vegetables:

- ½ cup raw or cooked vegetables
- 1 cup raw leafy salad greens
- ½ cup vegetable juice

Because vegetables vary in the nutrients they provide, it is important to consume a variety of types of vegetables to

Daily Amount of Food from Each Group

Food group amounts shown in cups (c) or ounce-equivalents (oz-eq), with number of daily servings (srv) shown in parentheses; vegetable subgroup amounts are per week

Calorie level	1600	1800	2000	2200	2400	2600	2800	3000
Grains	5 oz-eq	6 oz-eq	6 oz-eq	7 oz-eq	8 oz-eq	9 oz-eq	10 oz-eq	10 oz-eq
Whole grains	3 oz-eq	3 oz-eq	3 oz-eq	3.5 oz-eq	4 oz-eq	4.5 oz-eq	5 oz-eq	5 oz-eq
Other grains	2 oz-eq	3 oz-eq	3 oz-eq	3.5 oz-eq	4 oz-eq	4.5 oz-eq	5 oz-eq	5 oz-eq
Vegetables	2 c (4 srv)	2.5 c (5 srv)	2.5 c (5 srv)	3c (6 srv)	3 c (6 srv)	3.5 c (7 srv)	3.5 c (7 srv)	4 c (8 srv)
Dark green	2 c/wk	3 c/wk	3 c/wk	3 c/wk	3 c/wk	3 c/wk	3 c/wk	3 c/wk
Orange	1.5 c/wk	2 c/wk	2 c/wk	2 c/wk	2 c/wk	2.5 c/wk	2.5 c/wk	2.5 c/wk
Legumes	2.5 c/wk	3 c/wk	3 c/wk	3 c/wk	3 c/wk	3.5 c/wk	3.5 c/wk	3.5 c/wk
Starchy	2.5 c/wk	3 c/wk	3 c/wk	6 c/wk	6 c/wk	7 c/wk	7 c/wk	9 c/wk
Other	5.5 c/wk	6.5 c/wk	6.5 c/wk	7 c/wk	7 c/wk	8.5 c/wk	8.5 c/wk	10 c/wk
Fruits	1.5 c (3 srv)	1.5 c (3 srv)	2 c (4 srv)	2 c (4 srv)	2 c (4 srv)	2 c (4 srv)	2.5 c (5 srv)	2.5 c (5 srv)
Milk	3 c	3 c	3 c	3 c	3 c	3 c	3 c	3 c
Lean meat and beans	5 oz-eq	5 oz-eq	5.5 oz-eq	6 oz-eq	6.5 oz-eq	6.5 oz-eq	7 oz-eq	7 oz-eq
Oils	5 tsp	5 tsp	6 tsp	6 tsp	7 tsp	8 tsp	8 tsp	10 tsp

The discretionary calorie allowances shown below are the calories remaining at each level after nutrient-dense foods in each food group are selected. Those trying to lose weight may choose not to use discretionary calories. For those wanting to maintain weight, discretionary calories may be used to increase the amount of food from each food group; to consume foods that are not in the lowest fat form or that contain added sugars; to add oil, fat, or sugars to foods; or to consume alcohol. The amounts below show how discretionary calories may be divided between solid fats and added sugars.

Discretionary calories	132	195	267	290	362	410	426	512
Solid fats	11 g	15 g	18 g	19 g	22 g	24 g	24 g	29 g
Added sugars	12 g (3 tsp)	20 g (5 tsp)	32 g (8 tsp)	38 g (9 tsp)	48 g (12 tsp)	56 g (14 tsp)	60 g (15 tsp)	72 g (18 tsp)

FIGURE 8.7 MyPyramid food intake patterns. To determine an appropriate amount of food from each group, find the column with your approximate daily energy intake. That column lists the daily recommended intake from each food group. Visit MyPyramid.gov for a personalized intake plan and for intakes for other calorie levels.

SOURCE: U.S. Department of Health and Human Services and U.S. Department of Agriculture. 2005. *Dietary Guidelines for Americans, 2005, Appendix A. Eating Patterns* (http://www.health.gov/dietaryguidelines/dga2005/document/html/appendixA.htm; retrieved May 27, 2007).

obtain maximum nutrition. Many Americans consume only a few types of vegetables, with white potatoes (baked or served as french fries) being the most popular. To help boost variety, MyPyramid recommends servings from five different subgroups within the vegetables group; choose vegetables from several subgroups each day. (For clarity, Figure 8.7 shows servings from the subgroups in terms of weekly consumption.)

- Dark green vegetables like spinach, chard, collards, bok choy, broccoli, kale, romaine lettuce, and turnip and mustard greens
- Orange and deep yellow vegetables like carrots, winter squash, sweet potatoes, and pumpkin
- Legumes like pinto beans, kidney beans, black beans, lentils, chickpeas, soybeans, split peas, and

Judging Portion Sizes

TAKE CHARGE

Studies have shown that most people underestimate the size of their food portions, in many cases by as much as 50%. If you need to retrain your eye, try using measuring cups and spoons and an inexpensive kitchen scale when you eat at home. With a little practice, you'll learn what the difference between 3 and 8 ounces of chicken or meat is, and what a half-cup of rice really looks like. For quick estimates, use the following equivalents:

- 1 teaspoon of margarine = the tip of your thumb
- 1 ounce of cheese = your thumb, four dice stacked together, or an ice cube
- 3 ounces of chicken or meat = a deck of cards or an audio-cassette tape.

- 1 cup of pasta = a small fist or a tennis ball
- ½ cup of rice or cooked vegetables = an ice cream scoop or one-third of a can of soda
- 2 tablespoons of peanut butter = a Ping-Pong ball or large marshmallow
- 1 medium potato = a computer mouse
- 1–2-ounce muffin or roll = a plum or large egg
- 2-ounce bagel = a hockey puck or yo-yo
- 1 medium fruit (apple or orange) = a baseball
- ¼ cup nuts = a golf ball
- Small cookie or cracker = a poker chip

tofu; legumes can be counted as servings of vegetables *or* as alternatives to meat
- Starchy vegetables like corn, green peas, and white potatoes

- Other vegetables: tomatoes, bell peppers (red, orange, yellow, or green), green beans, and cruciferous vegetables like cauliflower are good choices

Fruits Fruits are rich in carbohydrates, dietary fiber, and many vitamins, especially vitamin C. For someone eating a 2000-calorie diet, 2 cups (4 servings) of fruits are recommended daily. The following each count as ½ cup or equivalent (1 serving) of fruit:

- ½ cup fresh, canned, or frozen fruit
- ½ cup fruit juice (100% juice)
- 1 small whole fruit
- ¼ cup dried fruit

Good choices from this group are citrus fruits and juices, melons, pears, apples, bananas, and berries. Choose whole fruits often—they are higher in fiber and often lower in calories than fruit juices. Fruit *juices* typically contain more nutrients and less added sugar than fruit *drinks*. Choose canned fruits packed in 100% fruit juice or water rather than in syrup.

Milk This group includes all milk and milk products, such as yogurt, cheeses (except cream cheese), and dairy desserts, as well as lactose-free and lactose-reduced products. Foods from this group are high in protein, carbohydrate, calcium, riboflavin, and vitamin D (if fortified). Those consuming 2000 calories per day should include 3 cups of milk or the equivalent daily. Each of the following counts as the equivalent of 1 cup:

- 1 cup milk or yogurt
- ½ cup ricotta cheese
- 1½ ounces natural cheese
- 2 ounces processed cheese

Cottage cheese is lower in calcium than most other cheeses; ½ cup is equivalent to ¼ cup milk. Ice cream is also lower in calcium and higher in sugar and fat than many other dairy products; one scoop counts as ⅓ cup milk. To limit

Table 8.4	MyPyramid Daily Calorie Intake Levels		
Age (years)	Sedentary*	Moderately Active**	Active†
Child			
2–3	1000	1000–1400	1000–1400
Female			
4–8	1200–1400	1400–1600	1400–1800
9–13	1400–1600	1600–2000	1800–2200
14–18	1800	2000	2400
19–30	1800–2000	2000–2200	2400
31–50	1800	2000	2200
51+	1600	1800	2000–2200
Male			
4–8	1200–1400	1400–1600	1600–2000
9–13	1600–2000	1800–2200	2000–2600
14–18	2000–2400	2400–2800	2800–3200
19–30	2400–2600	2600–2800	3000
31–50	2200–2400	2400–2600	2800–3000
51+	2000–2200	2200–2400	2400–2800

*A lifestyle that includes only the light physical activity associated with typical day-to-day life.
**A lifestyle that includes physical activity equivalent to walking about 1.5–3 miles per day at 3–4 miles per hour (30–60 minutes a day of moderate physical activity), in addition to the light physical activity associated with typical day-to-day life.
†A lifestyle that includes physical activity equivalent to walking more than 3 miles per day at 3–4 miles per hour (60 or more minutes a day of moderate physical activity), in addition to the light physical activity associated with typical day-to-day life.

SOURCE: U.S. Department of Agriculture, 2005. *MyPyramid Food Intake Pattern Calorie Levels* (http://www.mypyramid.gov/downloads/mypyramid_calorie_levels.pdf; retrieved May 27, 2007).

calories and saturated fat in your diet, it is best to choose servings of low-fat and fat-free items from this group.

Meat and Beans   This group includes meat, poultry, fish, dry beans and peas, eggs, nuts, and seeds. These foods provide protein, niacin, iron, vitamin B-6, zinc, and thiamin; the animal foods in the group also provide vitamin B-12. For someone consuming a 2000-calorie diet, 5½ ounce-equivalents is recommended. Each of the following counts as equivalent to 1 ounce:

- 1 ounce cooked lean meat, poultry, or fish
- ¼ cup cooked dry beans (legumes) or tofu
- 1 egg
- 1 tablespoon peanut butter
- ½ ounce nuts or seeds

One egg at breakfast, ½ cup of pinto beans at lunch, and a 3-ounce (cooked weight) hamburger at dinner would add up to the equivalent of 6 ounces of lean meat for the day. To limit your intake of fat and saturated fat, choose lean cuts of meat and skinless poultry, and watch your serving sizes carefully. Choose at least one serving of plant proteins, such as black beans, lentils, or tofu, every day.

Oils   The oils group represents the oils that are added to foods during processing or cooking or at the table; oils and soft margarines include vegetable oils and soft vegetable oil table spreads that have no trans fats. These are major sources of vitamin E and unsaturated fatty acids, including the essential fatty acids. For a 2000-calorie diet, 6 teaspoons of oils per day are recommended. One teaspoon is the equivalent of the following:

- 1 teaspoon vegetable oil or soft margarine
- 1 tablespoon salad dressing or light mayonnaise

Foods that are mostly oils include nuts, olives, avocados, and some fish. The following portions include about 1 teaspoon of oil: 8 large olives, ⅙ medium avocado, ½ tablespoon peanut butter, and ⅓ ounce roasted nuts. Food labels can help you identify the type and amount of fat in various foods.

Discretionary Calories, Solid Fats, and Added Sugars

The suggested intakes from the basic food groups in My-Pyramid assume that nutrient-dense foods are selected from each group; nutrient-dense foods are those that are fat-free or low-fat and that contain no added sugars. If this pattern is followed, then a small amount of additional calories can be consumed—the *discretionary calorie allowance*. Figure 8.7 shows the discretionary calorie allowance at each calorie level in MyPyramid.

People who are trying to lose weight may choose not to use discretionary calories. For those wanting to maintain weight, discretionary calories may be used to increase the amount of food from a food group; to consume foods that are not in the lowest fat form or that contain added sugars;

to add oil, fat, or sugars to foods; or to consume alcohol. The amounts shown in Figure 8.7 show how discretionary calories may be divided between solid fats and added sugars. The values for additional fat target no more than 30% of total calories from fat and less than 10% of calories from saturated fat. Examples of discretionary solid fat calories include higher-fat meats such as sausages or chicken with skin, whole milk instead of fat-free milk, and foods topped with butter. For example, 1 cup of whole milk has 60 calories more than 1 cup of fat-free milk; these 60 calories would be counted as discretionary calories.

As described earlier in the chapter, added sugars are the sugars added to foods and beverages in processing or preparation, not the naturally occurring sugars in fruits or milk. The suggested amounts of added sugars may be helpful limits for including some sweetened foods or beverages in the daily diet without exceeding energy needs or underconsuming other nutrients. For example, in a 2000-calorie diet, MyPyramid lists 32 grams (8 teaspoons) for discretionary intake of added sugars. In the American diet, added sugars are often found in sweetened beverages (regular soda, sweetened teas, fruit drinks), dairy products (ice cream, some yogurts), and grain products (bakery goods). For example, a 20-ounce regular soda has 260 calories from added sugars that would be counted as discretionary calories. The current American diet includes higher-than-recommended levels of sugar intake.

Remember, the amounts listed in Figure 8.7 for solid fats and added sugars assume that you select nutrient-dense foods from the major food groups; don't just add fats and sugars to your diet. The average American diet is overich in foods that contain relatively large amounts of added sugars and fats and that are low in essential nutrients (Table 8.5). To control weight and obtain adequate amounts of essential nutrients, it is important to choose nutrient-dense foods for most of your daily servings.

Table 8.5	Top Ten Sources of Calories in the American Diet

Food	Percent of Total Calories
Regular soft drinks	7.1
Cake, sweet rolls, doughnuts, pastries	3.6
Hamburgers, cheeseburgers, meatloaf	3.1
Pizza	3.1
Potato chips, corn chips, popcorn	2.9
Rice	2.7
Rolls, buns, English muffins, bagels	2.7
Cheese or cheese spread	2.6
Beer	2.6
French fries, fried potatoes	2.2

SOURCE: Block, G. 2004. Foods contributing to energy intake in the US: Data from NHANES III and NHANES 1999–2000. *Journal of Food Composition and Analysis* 17(2004): 439–447.

The Vegetarian Alternative

Some people choose a diet with one essential difference from the diets we've already described: Foods of animal origin (meat, poultry, fish, eggs, milk) are eliminated or restricted. Many do so for health reasons; vegetarian diets tend to be lower in saturated fat, cholesterol, and animal protein and higher in complex carbohydrates, dietary fiber, folate, vitamins C and E, carotenoids, and phytochemicals. Some people adopt a vegetarian diet out of concern for the environment, for financial considerations, or for reasons related to ethics or religion.

Types of Vegetarian Diets   There are various vegetarian styles; the wider the variety of the diet eaten, the easier it is to meet nutritional needs. **Vegans** eat only plant foods. **Lacto-vegetarians** eat plant foods and dairy products. **Lacto-ovo-vegetarians** eat plant foods, dairy products, and eggs. According to some polls, about 5 million American adults never eat meat, poultry, or fish and fall into one of these three groups. Others can be categorized as **partial vegetarians, semivegetarians,** or **pescovegetarians;** these individuals eat plant foods, dairy products, eggs, and usually a small selection of poultry, fish, and other seafood. Many other people choose vegetarian meals frequently but are not strictly vegetarian. Including some animal protein (such as dairy products) in a mostly vegetarian diet makes planning easier, but it is not necessary.

A Food Plan for Vegetarians   MyPyramid can be adapted for use by vegetarians with only a few key modifications. For the meat and beans group, vegetarians can focus on the nonmeat choices of dry beans (legumes), nuts, seeds, eggs, and soy foods like tofu (soybean curd) and tempeh (a cultured soy product). Vegans and other vegetarians who do not consume any dairy products must find other rich sources of calcium (see the following list). Fruits, vegetables, and whole grains are healthy choices for people following all types of vegetarian diets.

A healthy vegetarian diet emphasizes a wide variety of plant foods. Although plant proteins are generally incomplete, choosing a variety of plant foods will supply all of the essential amino acids. Choosing minimally processed and unrefined foods will maximize nutrient value and provide ample dietary fiber. Daily consumption of a variety of plant foods in amounts that meet total energy needs can provide all needed nutrients except vitamin B-12 and possibly vitamin D. Strategies for obtaining these and other nutrients of concern include the following:

- *Vitamin B-12* is found naturally only in animal foods; if dairy products and eggs are limited or avoided, B-12 can be obtained from fortified foods such as ready-to-eat cereals, soy beverages, meat substitutes, and special yeast products, or from supplements.

- *Vitamin D* can be obtained by spending 5–15 minutes a day in the sun, by consuming vitamin D–fortified products like ready-to-eat cereals and soy or rice milk, or by taking a supplement.

- *Calcium* is found in legumes, tofu processed with calcium, dark-green leafy vegetables, nuts, tortillas made from lime-processed corn, fortified orange juice, soy milk, bread, and other foods.

- *Iron* is found in whole grains, fortified bread and breakfast cereals, dried fruits, leafy green vegetables, nuts and seeds, legumes, and soy foods. The iron in plant foods is more difficult for the body to absorb than the iron from animal sources; consuming a good source of vitamin C with most meals is helpful because vitamin C improves iron absorption.

- *Zinc* is found in whole grains, nuts, legumes, and soy foods.

It takes a little planning and common sense to put together a good vegetarian diet. If you are a vegetarian or are considering becoming one, devote some extra time and thought to your diet. It's especially important to eat as wide a variety of foods as possible to ensure that all your nutritional needs are satisfied. Consulting with a registered dietitian will make your planning easier. Vegetarian diets for children, teens, and pregnant and lactating women warrant professional guidance.

Dietary Challenges for Special Population Groups

MyPyramid and the Dietary Guidelines for Americans provide a basis that everyone can use to create a healthy

vegan   A vegetarian who eats no animal products at all.

lacto-vegetarian   A vegetarian who includes milk and cheese products in the diet.

lacto-ovo-vegetarian   A vegetarian who eats no meat, poultry, or fish, but does eat eggs and milk products.

partial vegetarian, semivegetarian, or **pescovegetarian**   A vegetarian who includes eggs, dairy products, and small amounts of poultry and seafood in the diet.

diet. However, some population groups face special dietary challenges.

Women Women tend to be smaller and to weigh less than men, meaning they have lower energy needs and so need fewer calories. Because of this, women may have more difficulty getting adequate amounts of all the essential nutrients and need to focus on nutrient-dense foods. Two nutrients of special concern are calcium and iron, minerals for which many women fail to meet the RDAs. Low calcium intake may be linked to the development of osteoporosis in later life. The *Healthy People 2010* report sets a goal of increasing from 40% to 75% the proportion of women age 20–49 who meet the dietary recommendation for calcium. Nonfat and low-fat dairy products and fortified cereal, bread, and orange juice are good choices.

Iron is also a concern: Menstruating women have higher iron requirements than other groups, and a lack of iron in the diet can lead to iron-deficiency anemia. Lean red meat, leafy green vegetables, and fortified breakfast cereals are good sources of iron. As discussed earlier, all women capable of becoming pregnant should consume adequate folate or folic acid from fortified foods and/or supplements.

Men Men are seldom thought of as having nutritional deficiencies because they generally have high-calorie diets. However, many men have a diet that does not follow recommended food intake patterns and that includes more red meat and fewer fruits, vegetables, and grains than recommended. This dietary pattern is linked to heart disease and some types of cancer. A high intake of calories can lead to weight gain in the long term if a man's activity level decreases as he ages. Men should use MyPyramid as a basis for their overall diet and focus on increasing their consumption of fruits, vegetables, and grains to obtain vitamins, minerals, dietary fiber, and phytochemicals.

The "Fruits and Veggies Matter" program was created by the Centers for Disease Control and Prevention (CDC) and partner agencies to promote increased intake of fruits and vegetables. For strategies and guidelines for consuming more fruits and vegetables, visit http://www.fruitsandveggiesmatter.gov.

College Students Foods that are convenient for college students are not always the healthiest choices. However, it is possible to make healthy eating both convenient and affordable (see the tips in the box "Eating Strategies for College Students"). Two settings of concern often found on college campuses are buffet-style dining halls and fast-food restaurants. Both may offer foods that are low in nutrient density—and in very large portions. While no foods are entirely "bad," consuming moderate portions of a wide variety of foods is critical for a healthy diet.

Older Adults As people age, they tend to become less active, so they require fewer calories to maintain their weight. At the same time, the absorption of nutrients tends to be lower in older adults because of age-related changes in the digestive tract. Thus, they must consume nutrient-dense foods to meet their nutritional requirements. As discussed earlier, foods fortified with vitamin B-12 and/or B-12 supplements are recommended for people over age 50. Because constipation is a common problem, consuming foods high in dietary fiber and obtaining adequate fluids are important goals.

Athletes Key dietary concerns for athletes are meeting increased energy and fluid requirements for training and making healthy food choices throughout the day.

ENERGY INTAKE Individuals engaged in vigorous training programs expend more energy (calories) than sedentary and moderately active individuals and may have energy needs ranging from 2000 to more than 6000 calories per day. For athletes, the American Dietetic Association recommends a diet with 60–65% of calories coming from carbohydrates, 10–15% from protein, and no more than 30% from fat. Athletes for whom maintaining low body weight and body fat is important—such as gymnasts, skaters, and wrestlers—should consume adequate calories and nutrients and avoid falling into unhealthy patterns of eating. The combination of low levels of body fat, high physical activity, disordered eating habits—and, in women, amenorrhea—is associated with stress fractures and other injuries and with osteoporosis. (The female athlete triad was discussed in Chapter 6; see Chapter 9 for more on eating disorders.)

CARBOHYDRATE Endurance athletes involved in competitive events lasting longer than 90 minutes may benefit from increasing carbohydrate intake to 65–70% of total calories; this increase should come in the form of complex, rather than simple, carbohydrates. High carbohydrate intake builds and maintains muscle glycogen stores, resulting in greater endurance and delayed fatigue during competitive events. Some endurance athletes engage in "carbohydrate loading"—a practice that involves increasing carbohydrate intake in the days before a competition. Before exercise, the ACSM recommends that an active adult or athlete consume a meal or snack that is relatively high in carbohydrates, moderate in protein, and low in fat. Soon after exercise, particularly following a strenuous competition or training session, a mixed meal containing carbohydrates, protein, and fat should be consumed to replace muscle glycogen and provide amino acids for building and repairing muscle tissue. Consuming some simple carbohydrates immediately after exercise can help replenish glycogen stores in the liver and muscles.

PROTEIN For endurance athletes, the ACSM recommends a protein intake of 1.2–1.4 grams of protein per kilogram (0.55–0.64 gram per pound) of body weight per day, up from the standard DRI of 0.8 gram per kilogram (0.36 gram per pound); for athletes engaged in heavy strength

Eating Strategies for College Students

General Guidelines

- Eat slowly and enjoy your food. Set aside a separate time to eat. Don't eat while you study.

- Eat a colorful, varied diet. The more colorful your diet is, the more varied and rich in fruits and vegetables it will be. Don't limit your vegetable choices to french fries, which are typically high in saturated and trans fats.

- Consider nutrient density in your food choices, and avoid large servings of foods that provide calories but few essential nutrients. Spend your daily calorie budget wisely.

- Check out the labels and ingredient lists of foods you commonly eat so that you are aware of their general nutrient profile.

- Eat breakfast. You'll have more energy in the morning and be less likely to grab an unhealthy snack later on. Whole-grain cereals or whole-grain toast are excellent breakfast choices.

- Choose healthy snacks—fruits, vegetables, grains, and cereals—as often as you can.

- Drink water more often than soft drinks or other sweetened beverages. Rent a mini-refrigerator for your dorm room, and stock up on healthy beverages.

- Pay attention to portion sizes. Read food labels carefully, and take special note of serving sizes and the total number of servings in the package. You may find that your favorite bottled drinks and packaged snack foods provide multiple servings and that you are consuming more calories, fat, and added sugars than you realize.

Eating in the Dining Hall

- Choose a meal plan that includes breakfast—and don't skip it.

- Accept that dining hall food is not going to be as good as home cooking. Find dishes that you like that are nutritious.

- If menus are posted or distributed, decide what you want to eat before getting in line and stick to your choices. Consider what you plan to do and eat for the rest of the day before making your choices.

- Ask for large servings of vegetables and small servings of meat and other high-fat main dishes. Build your meals around grains and vegetables.

- Choose whole grains.

- Choose leaner poultry, fish, or bean dishes rather than high-fat meats and fried entrees.

- Ask that gravies and sauces be served on the side; limit your intake.

- Choose broth-based or vegetable soups rather than cream soups.

- At the salad bar, load up on leafy greens, beans, and fresh vegetables. Avoid mayonnaise-coated salads (macaroni salad, potato salad), bacon, croutons, and high-fat dressings. Put dressing on the side; dip your fork into it rather than pouring it over the salad.

- Drink nonfat milk, water, mineral water, or 100% fruit juice rather than heavily sweetened fruit drinks, whole milk, soft drinks, or beer.

- Choose fruit for dessert rather than pastries, cookies, or cakes.

Eating in Fast-Food Restaurants

- Most fast-food chains can provide a brochure with a nutritional breakdown of the foods on the menu. Ask for it and identify the healthiest options. (See also the information in Appendix C.)

- Order small single burgers with no cheese instead of double burgers with many toppings.

- Ask for items to be prepared without mayonnaise, tartar sauce, sour cream, or other high-fat sauces. Ketchup, mustard, and fat-free mayonnaise or sour cream are available at many fast-food restaurants.

- Choose whole-grain buns or bread for burgers, hot dogs, and sandwiches.

- Choose chicken items made from chicken breast, not processed chicken.

- Order vegetable pizzas without extra cheese.

- If you order french fries or onion rings, get the smallest size and/or share them with a friend. Better yet, get a salad or a fruit cup instead.

Fast-food meals are a health concern. A large cheeseburger, large order of fries, and large (32 oz) nondiet soda may provide about 1600 calories, 75 grams of fat, and 30 teaspoons of added sugars. If you have a fast-food meal, balance it with healthy, nutrient-rich foods during the rest of the day.

Eating on the Run

Are you chronically short of time? Pack these items for a quick snack or meal: fresh or dried fruit, fruit juices, raw fresh vegetables, plain bagels, bread sticks, whole-wheat fig bars, low-fat cheese sticks or cubes, low-fat crackers or granola bars, nonfat or low-fat yogurt, snack-size cereal boxes, pretzels, rice or corn cakes, plain popcorn, soup (if you have access to a microwave), or water.

---

training, protein needs may be as high as 1.6–1.7 grams per kilogram (0.73–0.77 gram per pound) of body weight. This level of protein intake is easily obtainable from foods, however. A 160-pound athlete consuming 3500 calories per day needs to obtain only 12% of total calories as pro-

tein to achieve the upper end of the range for endurance athletes. The average American diet includes about 16% of total calories as protein, and a balanced high-carbohydrate, moderate-protein, moderate-fat diet can provide the nutrients athletes need.

There is no evidence that consuming supplements containing vitamins, minerals, protein, or specific amino acids will build muscle or improve sports performance. Strength and muscle are built with exercise, not extra protein, and carbohydrates provide the fuel needed for muscle-building exercise. Strenuous physical activity does increase the need for protein and some vitamins and minerals; however, the increased energy intake of athletes more than compensates for this increased need.

FLUIDS Moderately active people should consume adequate fluids as described earlier in the chapter. People who exercise heavily and/or live in a hot climate need to consume additional fluids to maximize performance and prevent heat illness. For a strenuous endurance event, prepare yourself the day before by drinking plenty of fluids. On the day of the event, the ACSM recommends that you consume 14–22 ounces (400–600 ml) of fluid about 2 hours before exercise, and then 6–12 ounces (150–350 ml) of fluid every 15–20 minutes during exercise—or as much of this amount as you can tolerate. Afterward, drink enough to replace lost fluids—16–24 ounces for every pound of weight lost. (Weight loss during a workout or athletic event comes primarily from fluid loss through sweat; as described in Chapter 3, checking your weight can help you monitor your fluid balance.)

Water is a good choice for fluid replacement for workouts and events lasting less than 60–90 minutes, especially if you are trying to avoid the additional calories in many other beverages. However, for workouts or events lasting longer, a sports drink can be a good choice. These contain water, electrolytes, and carbohydrates. The advantage of sports drinks is that they can provide you with some extra energy (in the form of rapidly digestible carbohydrates that help maintain blood glucose levels) and replace electrolytes like sodium that are lost in sweat.

People with Special Health Concerns Many Americans have special health concerns that affect their dietary needs. For example, women who are pregnant or breastfeeding require extra calories, vitamins, and minerals. People with diabetes benefit from a well-balanced diet that is low in simple sugars, high in complex carbohydrates, and relatively rich in monounsaturated fats. People with

high blood pressure need to limit their sodium consumption and control their weight. If you have a health problem or concern that may require a special diet, discuss your situation with a physician or registered dietitian.

NUTRITIONAL PLANNING: MAKING INFORMED CHOICES ABOUT FOOD

Knowing about nutrition is a good start to making sound choices about food. It also helps if you can interpret food labels, understand food additives, and avoid foodborne illnesses.

Reading Food Labels

Food labels can help you apply the principles of MyPyramid and the Dietary Guidelines for Americans. Since 1994, all processed foods regulated by either the FDA or the USDA have included standardized nutrition information on their labels. Every food label shows serving sizes and the amount of fat, saturated fat, trans fat, cholesterol, protein, dietary fiber, and sodium in each serving. To make intelligent choices about food, learn to read and understand food labels (see the box "Using Food Labels"). The FDA's Web site features an interactive tutorial on reading food labels; to use this online tool, visit http://www.cfsan.fda.gov/~ear/hwm/labelman.html.

Because most meat, poultry, fish, fruits, and vegetables are not processed, they were not covered by the 1994 law. You can get information on the nutrient content of these items from basic nutrition books, registered dietitians, nutrient analysis computer software, the Web, and the companies that produce or distribute these foods. Also, supermarkets often have posters or pamphlets listing the nutrient contents of these foods. In Lab 8.3, you compare foods using the information on their labels.

Reading Dietary Supplement Labels

Dietary supplements include vitamins, minerals, amino acids, herbs, enzymes, and other compounds. Although dietary supplements are often thought of as safe and natural, they contain powerful bioactive chemicals that have the potential for harm. About one-quarter of all pharmaceutical drugs are derived from botanical sources, and even essential vitamins and minerals can have toxic effects if consumed in excess.

In the United States, supplements are not legally considered drugs and are not regulated the way drugs are. Before they are approved by the FDA and put on the market, drugs undergo clinical studies to determine safety, effectiveness, side effects and risks, possible interactions with other substances, and appropriate dosages. The FDA does not authorize or test dietary supplements, and supplements are not required to demonstrate either safety or

? QUESTIONS FOR CRITICAL THINKING AND REFLECTION

What factors influence your food choices—convenience, cost, availability, habit? Do you ever consider nutritional content or nutritional recommendations like the Dietary Guidelines for Americans or MyPyramid? If not, how big a change would it be for you to think of nutritional content first when choosing food? Is it something you could do easily?

CRITICAL CONSUMER

Using Food Labels

Food labels are designed to help consumers make food choices based on the nutrients that are most important to good health. In addition to listing nutrient content by weight, the label puts the information in the context of a daily diet of 2000 calories that includes no more than 65 grams of fat (approximately 30% of total calories). For example, if a serving of a particular product has 13 grams of fat, the label will show that the serving represents 20% of the daily fat allowance. If your daily diet contains fewer or more than 2000 calories, you need to adjust these calculations accordingly.

Food labels contain uniform serving sizes. This means that if you look at different brands of salad dressing, for example, you can compare calories and fat content based on the serving amount. (Food label serving sizes may be larger or smaller than MyPyramid serving size equivalents, however.) Regulations also require that foods meet strict definitions if their packaging includes the terms *light, low-fat,* or *high-fiber* (see below). Health claims such as "good source of dietary fiber" or "low in saturated fat" on packages are signals that those products can wisely be included in your diet. Overall, the food label is an important tool to help you choose a diet that conforms to MyPyramid and the Dietary Guidelines.

Selected Nutrient Claims and What They Mean

- **Healthy.** A food that is low in fat, is low in saturated fat, has no more than 360–480 mg of sodium and 60 mg of cholesterol, *and* provides 10% or more of the Daily Value for vitamin A, vitamin C, protein, calcium, iron, or dietary fiber.

- **Light or lite.** 33% fewer calories or 50% less fat than a similar product.

- **Reduced or fewer.** At least 25% less of a nutrient than a similar product; can be applied to fat ("reduced fat"), saturated fat, cholesterol, sodium, and calories.

- **Extra or added.** 10% or more of the Daily Value per serving when compared to what a similar product has.

- **Good source.** 10–19% of the Daily Value for a particular nutrient per serving.

- **High, rich in, or excellent source of.** 20% or more of the Daily Value for a particular nutrient per serving.

- **Low calorie.** 40 calories or less per serving.

- **High fiber.** 5 g or more of fiber per serving.

- **Good source of fiber.** 2.5–4.9 g of fiber per serving.

- **Fat-free.** Less than 0.5 g of fat per serving.

- **Low-fat.** 3 g of fat or less per serving.

- **Saturated fat-free.** Less than 0.5 g of saturated fat and 0.5 g of trans fatty acids per serving.

- **Low saturated fat.** 1 g or less of saturated fat per serving and no more than 15% of total calories.

- **Cholesterol-free.** Less than 2 mg of cholesterol and 2 g or less of saturated fat per serving.

- **Low cholesterol.** 20 mg or less of cholesterol and 2 g or less of saturated fat per serving.

- **Low sodium.** 140 mg or less of sodium per serving.

- **Very low sodium.** 35 mg or less of sodium per serving.

- **Lean.** Cooked seafood, meat, or poultry with less than 10 g of fat, 4.5 g or less of saturated fat, and less than 95 mg of cholesterol per serving.

- **Extra lean.** Cooked seafood, meat, or poultry with less than 5 g of fat, 2 g of saturated fat, and 95 mg of cholesterol per serving.

Note: As of June 2005, the FDA had not yet defined nutrient claims relating to carbohydrates, so foods labeled low- or reduced-carbohydrate do not conform to any approved standard.

1. Serving size: Determine how many servings there are in the food package and compare it to how much you actually eat. You may need to adjust the rest of the nutrient values based on your typical serving size.

2. Calories and calories from fat: Note whether a serving is high in calories and fat. The sample food shown here is low in fat, with only 30 of its 235 calories from fat.

3. Daily Values: Based on a 2000-calorie diet, Daily Value percentages tell you whether the nutrients in a serving of food contribute a lot or a little to your total daily diet.
  5% or less is low
  20% or more is high

4. Limit these nutrients: Look for foods low in fat, saturated fat, trans fat, cholesterol, and sodium.

5. Get enough of these nutrients: Look for foods high in dietary fiber, vitamin A, vitamin C, calcium, and iron.

Nutrition Facts
Serving Size 1 cup (265g)
Servings per Container 2

Amount per Serving

Calories 235   Calories from Fat 30

% Daily Value*

Total Fat 3g	**5%**
Saturated Fat 1g	**5%**
Trans Fat 0.5g	
Cholesterol 30mg	**10%**
Sodium 775mg	**32%**
Total Carbohydrate 34g	**11%**
Dietary Fiber 9g	**36%**
Sugars 5g	
Protein 18g	

Vitamin A 25%	•	Vitamin C 0%	
Calcium 12%	•	Iron 20%	

*Percent Daily Values are based on a 2,000 calorie diet. Your daily values may be higher or lower depending on your calorie needs:

		Calories	2,000	2,500
Total Fat	Less than		65g	80g
Sat Fat	Less than		20g	25g
Cholesterol	Less than		300mg	300mg
Sodium	Less than		2,400mg	2,400mg
Total Carbohydrate			300g	375g
Dietary Fiber			25g	30g

Calories per gram:
Fat 9 • Carbohydrate 4 • Protein 4

TURKEY CHILI

Footnote: This section shows recommended daily intake for two levels of calorie consumption and values for dietary calculations; it's the same on all labels.

effectiveness before they are marketed. Although dosage guidelines exist for some of the compounds in dietary supplements, dosages for many are not well established.

Many ingredients in dietary supplements are classified by the FDA as "generally recognized as safe," but some have been found to be dangerous on their own or to interact with prescription or over-the-counter drugs in dangerous ways. Garlic supplements, for example, can cause bleeding if taken with anticoagulant (blood-thinning) medications. Even products that are generally considered safe can have side effects—St. John's wort, for example, increases the skin's sensitivity to sunlight and may decrease the effectiveness of oral contraceptives, drugs used to treat HIV infection, and many other medications.

There are also key differences in this way drugs and supplements are manufacture: FDA-approved medications are standardized for potency, and quality control and proof of purity are required. Dietary supplement manufacture is not as closely regulated, and there is no guarantee that a product even contains a given ingredient, let alone in the appropriate amount. The potency of herbal supplements can vary widely due to differences in growing and harvesting conditions, preparation methods, and storage. Contamination and misidentification of plant compounds are also potential problems.

In an effort to provide consumers with more reliable and consistent information about supplements, the FDA has developed labeling regulations. Labels similar to those found on foods are now required for dietary supplements; for more information, see the box "Using Dietary Supplement Labels".

Food Additives

Today, some 2800 substances are intentionally added to foods for one or more of the following reasons: (1) to maintain or improve nutritional quality, (2) to maintain freshness, (3) to help in processing or preparation, or (4) to alter taste or appearance. Additives make up less than 1% of our food. The most widely used are sugar, salt, and corn syrup; these three, plus citric acid, baking soda, vegetable colors, mustard, and pepper, account for 98% by weight of all food additives used in the United States.

Food additives pose no significant health hazard to most people because the levels used are well below any that could produce toxic effects. Two additives of potential concern for some people are sulfites, used to keep vegetables from turning brown, and monosodium glutamate (MSG), used as a flavor enhancer. Sulfites can cause severe reactions in some people, and the FDA strictly limits their use and requires clear labeling on any food containing

Careful food handling greatly reduces the risk of foodborne illness. Helpful strategies include washing hands and all fruits and vegetables, using separate cutting boards for meat and for foods that will be eaten raw, cooking meat thoroughly, and refrigerating leftovers promptly.

sulfites. MSG may cause some people to experience episodes of sweating and increased blood pressure. If you have any sensitivity to an additive, check food labels when you shop and ask questions when you eat out.

Foodborne Illness

Many people worry about additives or pesticide residues in their food. However, a greater threat to the safety of the food supply comes from microorganisms that cause foodborne illnesses. Raw or undercooked animal products, such as chicken, hamburger, and oysters, pose the greatest risk for contamination. The CDC estimates that 76 million Americans become sick each year as a result of foodborne illness, 325,000 are hospitalized, and 5000 die. In most cases, foodborne illness produces acute gastroenteritis, characterized by diarrhea, vomiting, fever, and weakness. People often mistake foodborne illness for a bout of the flu. Although the effects of foodborne illness are usually not serious, some groups, such as children and older people, are at risk for severe complications, including rheumatic diseases, kidney failure, seizures, blood poisoning, and death.

Causes of Foodborne Illnesses   Most cases of foodborne illness are caused by **pathogens**, disease-causing microorganisms that contaminate food, usually from

Using Dietary Supplement Labels

Since 1999, specific types of information have been required on the labels of dietary supplements. In addition to basic information about the product, labels include a "Supplement Facts" panel, modeled after the "Nutrition Facts" panel used on food labels (see the figure). Under the Dietary Supplement Health and Education Act (DSHEA) and food labeling laws, supplement labels can make three types of health-related claims:

• *Nutrient-content claims,* such as "high in calcium," "excellent source of vitamin C," or "high potency." The claims "high in" and "excellent source of" mean the same as they do on food labels. A "high potency" single-ingredient supplement must contain 100% of its Daily Value; a "high potency" multi-ingredient product must contain 100% or more of the Daily Value of at least two-thirds of the nutrients present for which Daily Values have been established.

• *Health claims,* if they have been authorized by the FDA or another authoritative scientific body. The association between adequate calcium intake and lower risk of osteoporosis is an example of an approved health claim. Since 2003, the FDA has also allowed so-called *qualified* health claims for situations in which there is emerging but as yet inconclusive evidence for a particular claim. Such claims must include qualifying language such as "scientific evidence suggests but does not prove."

• *Structure-function claims,* such as "antioxidants maintain cellular integrity" or "this product enhances energy levels." Because these claims are not reviewed by the FDA, they must carry a disclaimer (see the sample label).

Tips for Choosing and Using Dietary Supplements

• Check with your physician before taking a supplement. Many are not meant for children, older people, women who are pregnant or breastfeeding, people with chronic illnesses or upcoming surgery, or people taking prescription or OTC medications.

• Follow the cautions, instructions for use, and dosage given on the label.

• Look for the USP verification mark on the label, indicating that the product meets minimum safety and purity standards developed under the Dietary Supplement Verification Program by the United States Pharmacopeia (USP). The USP mark means that the product (1) contains the ingredients stated on the label, (2) has the declared amount and strength of ingredients, (3) will dissolve effectively, (4) has been screened for harmful contaminants, and (5) has been manufactured using safe, sanitary, and well-controlled procedures. The Natural Products Association has a self-regulatory testing program for its members; other, smaller associations and labs, including ConsumerLab. Com, also test and rate dietary supplements.

• Choose brands made by nationally known food and drug manufacturers or "house brands" from large retail chains. Due to their size and visibility, such sources are likely to have higher manufacturing standards.

• If you experience side effects, discontinue use of the product and contact your physician. Report any serious reactions to the FDA's MedWatch monitoring program (1-800-FDA-1088; http://www.fda.gov/medwatch).

For More Information About Dietary Supplements

ConsumerLab.Com: http://www.consumerlab.com

Food and Drug Administration: http://cfsan.fda.gov/~dms/ supplmnt.html

National Institutes of Health, Office of Dietary Supplements: http://dietary-supplements.info.nih.gov

Natural Products Association: http://www.naturalproductsassoc.org

U.S. Department of Agriculture: http://www.nal.usda.gov/fnic/etext/000015.html

U.S. Pharmacopeia: http://www.usp.org/uspverified

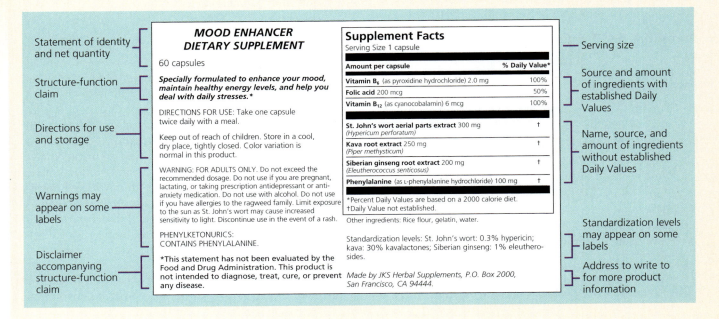

improper handling. The threats are numerous and varied; among them are the sometimes deadly *Escherichia coli (E. coli)* O157:H7 in meat and water; *Salmonella* in eggs, on vegetables, and on poultry; *Vibrio* in shellfish; *Cyclospora* and hepatitis A virus on fruit; *Cryptosporidium* in drinking water; *Campylobacter jejuni* in meat and poultry; and *Listeria monocytogenes* in lunch meats, sausages, and hot dogs.

You can't tell by taste, smell, or sight whether a food is contaminated. In 2003, *Consumer Reports* tested 484 chickens purchased in grocery stores and found that half were contaminated with *Campylobacter* and/or *Salmonella*. Although pathogens are usually destroyed during cooking, the U.S. government is taking steps to bring down levels of contamination by improving national testing and surveillance. Raw meat and poultry products are now sold with safe-handling and -cooking instructions, and all packaged, unpasteurized fresh fruit and vegetable juices carry warnings about potential contamination. It is important to note that while foodborne illness outbreaks associated with food-processing plants make headlines, most cases of illness trace back to poor food handling in the home or in restaurants.

A potential threat from food is bovine spongiform encephalopathy (BSE), or "mad cow disease," a fatal degenerative neurological disease caused by an abnormal protein that forms deposits in the brain. A variant form of this disease, known as Creutzfeldt-Jakob disease (CJD), is believed to be caused by eating beef contaminated with central nervous system tissue from BSE-infected cows. To date, there have been about 150 confirmed cases worldwide of CJD among the hundreds of thousands of people who may have consumed BSE-contaminated products. In December 2003, the first BSE-infected cow was identified in the United States. Although the USDA states that the risk to human health from BSE is extremely low, additional steps are being taken to prevent the BSE protein from entering the food supply; visit the USDA Web site for more information (www.usda.gov).

Preventing and Treating Foodborne Illness

The key to protecting yourself from foodborne illness is to handle, cook, and store foods in ways that prevent bacteria from spreading and multiplying:

- Don't buy food in containers that leak, bulge, or are severely dented. Refrigerated foods should be cold, and frozen foods should be solid.

- Refrigerate perishable items as soon as possible after purchase. Use or freeze fresh meats within 3–5 days and fresh poultry, fish, and ground meat within 1–2 days.

- Thaw frozen food in the refrigerator or in the microwave oven, not on the kitchen counter.

- Thoroughly wash your hands with warm, soapy water for 20 seconds before and after handling food, especially raw meat, fish, poultry, or eggs.

- Make sure counters, cutting boards, dishes, and other equipment are thoroughly cleaned before and after use. If possible, use separate cutting boards for meat and for foods that will be eaten raw, such as fruits and vegetables. Wash dishcloths and kitchen towels frequently.

- Thoroughly rinse and scrub fruits and vegetables with a brush, if possible, or peel off the skin.

- Cook foods thoroughly, especially beef, poultry, fish, pork, and eggs. Cooking kills most microorganisms, as long as an appropriately high temperature is reached. The USDA now recommends that consumers, especially high-risk individuals, use a food thermometer to verify that hamburgers are cooked to 160°F. When eating out, order red meat cooked "well done."

- Cook stuffing separately from poultry; or wash poultry thoroughly, stuff immediately before cooking, and transfer the stuffing to a clean bowl immediately after cooking.

- Refrigerate foods at or below 40°F and freeze at or below 0°F. Do not leave cooked or refrigerated foods, such as meats or salads, at room temperature for more than 2 hours. Use refrigerated leftovers within 3–4 days.

- Don't eat raw animal products, including raw eggs in Caesar salad, hollandaise sauce, or eggnog. Use only pasteurized milk and juice, and look for pasteurized eggs, which are now available in some states.

- Cook eggs until they're firm, and fully cook foods containing eggs. Store eggs in the coldest part of the refrigerator, not on the door, and use them within 3–5 weeks.

- Because of possible contamination with *E. coli* O157:H7 and *Salmonella,* avoid raw sprouts, or eat sprouts only after submerging them in boiling water for 10 seconds.

- According to the USDA, "When in doubt, throw it out."

Additional precautions are recommended for people at particularly high risk for foodborne illness—pregnant women, young children, older persons, and people with weakened immune systems or certain chronic illnesses. If you are a member of one of these groups, don't eat or drink any of the following products: unpasteurized juices; raw sprouts; raw (unpasteurized) milk and products made from unpasteurized milk; raw or undercooked meat, poultry, eggs, fish, and shellfish; and soft cheeses such as feta, Brie, Camembert, or blue-veined varieties. It's also important to avoid ready-to-eat foods such as hot dogs, luncheon meats, and cold cuts unless they are reheated until they are steaming hot.

If you think you may be having a bout of foodborne illness, drink plenty of clear fluids to prevent dehydration and rest to speed recovery. To prevent further contamination, wash your hands often and always before handling food until you recover. A fever higher than 102°F, blood in the stool, or dehydration deserves a physician's evaluation, especially if the symptoms persist for more than 2–3 days. In cases of suspected botulism—characterized by symptoms such as double vision, paralysis, dizziness, and vomiting—consult a physician immediately.

Irradiated Foods

Food irradiation is the treatment of foods with gamma rays, X-rays, or high-voltage electrons to kill potentially harmful pathogens, including bacteria, parasites, insects, and fungi that cause foodborne illness. It also reduces spoilage and extends shelf life. Even though irradiation has been generally endorsed by agencies such as the World Health Organization, the Centers for Disease Control and Prevention, and the American Medical Association, few irradiated foods are currently on the market due to consumer resistance and skepticism. Studies haven't conclusively identified any harmful effects of food irradiation, and newer methods of irradiation involving electricity and X-rays do not require the use of any radioactive materials. Studies indicate that when consumers are given information about the process of irradiation and the benefits of irradiated foods, most want to purchase them.

All primary irradiated foods (meat, vegetables, and so on) are labeled with the flowerlike radura symbol and a brief information label; spices and foods that are merely ingredients do not have to be labeled. It is important to remember that although irradiation kills most pathogens, it does not completely sterilize foods. Proper handling of irradiated foods is still critical for preventing foodborne illness.

Environmental Contaminants and Organic Foods

Contaminants are present in the food-growing environment, but few of them ever enter the food and water supply in amounts sufficient to cause health problems. Environmental contaminants include various minerals, antibiotics, hormones, pesticides, and industrial chemicals. Safety regulations attempt to keep our exposure to contaminants at safe levels, but monitoring is difficult, and many substances (such as pesticides) persist in the environment long after being banned from use.

Organic Foods Some people who are concerned about pesticides and other environmental contaminants choose to buy foods that are **organic.** To be certified as organic, foods must meet strict production, processing, handling, and labeling criteria. Organic crops must meet limits on pesticide residues; for meat, milk, eggs, and other animal prod-

ucts to be certified organic, animals must be given organic feed and access to the outdoors and may not be given antibiotics or growth hormones. The use of genetic engineering, ionizing radiation, and sewage sludge is prohibited. Products can be labeled "100% organic" if they contain all organic ingredients and "organic" if they contain at least 95% organic ingredients; all such products may carry the USDA organic seal. A product with at least 70% organic ingredients can be labeled "made with organic ingredients" but cannot use the USDA seal.

Foods that are organic may not be chemical-free, however. They may be contaminated with pesticides used on neighboring lands or on foods transported in the same train or truck. However, they tend to have lower levels of pesticide residues than conventionally grown crops. Some experts recommend that consumers who want to buy organic fruits and vegetables spend their money on those that carry higher pesticide residues than their conventional counterparts (the "dirty dozen"): apples, bell peppers, celery, cherries, imported grapes, nectarines, peaches, pears, potatoes, red raspberries, spinach, and strawberries. Experts also recommend buying organic beef, poultry, eggs, dairy products, and baby food. Fruits and vegetables that carry little pesticide residue whether grown conventionally or organically include asparagus, avocadoes, bananas, broccoli, cauliflower, corn, kiwi, mangoes, onions, papaya, pineapples, and peas. All foods are subject to strict pesticide limits; the debate about the health effects of small amounts of residue is ongoing.

Whether or not organic foods are better for your health, organic farming is better for the environment. It helps maintain biodiversity of crops and replenish Earth's resources; it is also less likely to degrade soil, contaminate water, or expose farm workers to toxic chemicals. As multinational food companies get into the organic food business, however, consumers who want to support environmentally friendly farming methods should look for foods that are not only organic but locally grown.

Guidelines for Fish Consumption A specific area of concern has been possible mercury contamination in fish. Overall, fish and shellfish are healthy sources of protein, omega-3 fats, and other nutrients; prudent choices can minimize the risk of any possible negative health effects. High mercury concentrations are most likely to be found in predator fish—large fish that eat smaller fish. Mercury can cause brain damage to fetuses and young children. In

food irradiation The treatment of foods with gamma rays, X-rays, or high-voltage electrons to kill potentially harmful pathogens and increase shelf life.

organic A designation applied to foods grown and produced according to strict guidelines limiting the use of pesticides, nonorganic ingredients, hormones, antibiotics, genetic engineering, irradiation, and other practices.

2004, the FDA and Environmental Protection Agency (EPA) released an advisory with specific guidelines for certain groups. To reduce exposure to the harmful effects of mercury, women who are or who may become pregnant and nursing mothers should follow these guidelines:

- Do not eat shark, swordfish, king mackerel, or tilefish.
- Eat up to 12 ounces a week of a variety of fish and shellfish that is lower in mercury, such as shrimp, canned light tuna, salmon, pollock, and catfish. Limit consumption of albacore tuna to 6 ounces per week.
- Check advisories about the safety of recreationally caught fish from local lakes, rivers, and coastal areas; if no information is available, limit consumption to 6 ounces per week.

The same FDA/EPA guidelines apply to children, although they should consume smaller servings.

Some experts have also expressed concern about the presence of toxins such as PCBs in farmed fish, especially farmed salmon. Although no federal guidelines have been set, some researchers suggest that consumers limit themselves to 8 ounces of farmed salmon per month. Fish should be labeled with its country of origin and whether it is wild or farmed; most canned salmon is wild.

A PERSONAL PLAN: APPLYING NUTRITIONAL PRINCIPLES

Based on your particular nutrition and health status, there probably is an ideal diet for you, but no single type of diet provides optimal health for everyone. Many cultural dietary patterns can meet people's nutritional requirements (see the box "Ethnic Foods"). Customize your food plan based on your age, gender, weight, activity level, medical risk factors—and, of course, personal tastes.

Assessing and Changing Your Diet

The first step in planning a healthy diet is to examine what you currently eat. Labs 8.1 and 8.2 help you analyze your current diet and compare it with optimal dietary goals. (This analysis can be completed using Appendix B, a nutritional analysis software program, or one of several Web sites.)

To put your plan into action, use the behavioral self-management techniques and tips described in Chapter 1. If you identify several changes you want to make, focus on one at a time. You might start, for example, by substituting nonfat or low-fat milk for whole milk. When you become used to that, you can try substituting whole-wheat bread for white bread. The information on eating behavior in Lab 8.1 will help you identify and change unhealthy patterns of eating.

Staying Committed to a Healthy Diet

Beyond knowledge and information, you also need support in difficult situations. Keeping to your plan is easiest when you choose and prepare your own food at home. Advance planning is the key: mapping out meals and shopping appropriately, cooking in advance when possible, and preparing enough food for leftovers. A tight budget does not necessarily make it more difficult to eat healthy meals. It makes good health sense and good budget sense to use only small amounts of meat and to have a few meatless meals each week.

In restaurants, keeping to food plan goals becomes somewhat more difficult. Portion sizes in restaurants tend to be larger than MyPyramid serving size equivalents, but by remaining focused on your goals, you can eat only part of your meal and take the rest home for a meal later in the week. Don't hesitate to ask questions when you're eating in a restaurant. Most restaurant personnel are glad to explain how menu selections are prepared and to make small adjustments, such as serving salad dressings and sauces on the side so they can be avoided or used sparingly.

Strategies like these are helpful, but small changes cannot change a fundamentally high-fat, high-calorie meal into a moderate, healthful one. Often, the best advice is to bypass a large steak with potatoes au gratin for a flavorful but low-fat entree. Many of the selections offered in ethnic restaurants are healthy choices (refer to the box on ethnic foods for suggestions).

Ethnic Foods

There is no one ethnic diet that clearly surpasses all others in providing people with healthful foods. However, every diet has its advantages and disadvantages, and within each cuisine, some foods are better choices. The dietary guidelines described in this chapter can be applied to any ethnic cuisine. For additional guidance, refer to the table below.

Choose More Often	Choose Less Often
CHINESE Dishes that are steamed, poached (jum), boiled (chu), roasted (kow), barbecued (shu), or lightly stir-fried Hoisin sauce, oyster sauce, wine sauce, plum sauce, velvet sauce, or hot mustard Fresh fish and seafood, skinless chicken, tofu Mixed vegetables, Chinese greens Steamed rice, steamed spring rolls, soft noodles	Fried wontons or egg rolls Crab rangoon Crispy (Peking) duck or chicken Sweet-and-sour dishes made with breaded and deep-fried meat, poultry, or fish Fried rice Fried or crispy noodles
FRENCH Dishes prepared au vapeur (steamed), en brochette (skewered and broiled), or grillé (grilled) Fresh fish, shrimp, scallops, or mussels or skinless chicken, without sauces Clear soups	Dishes prepared à la crème (in cream sauce), au gratin or gratinée (baked with cream and cheese), or en croûte (in pastry crust) Drawn butter, hollandaise sauce, and remoulade (mayonnaise-based sauce)
GREEK Dishes that are stewed, broiled, or grilled, including shish kabobs (souvlaki) Dolmas (grape leaves) stuffed with rice Tzatziki (yogurt, cucumbers, and garlic) Tabouli (bulgur-based salad) Pita bread, especially whole wheat	Moussaka, saganaki (fried cheese) Vegetable pies such as spanakopita and tyropita Baba ghanoush (eggplant and olive oil) Deep-fried falafel (chickpea patties) Gyros stuffed with ground meat Baklava
INDIAN Dishes prepared masala (curry), tandoori (roasted in a clay oven), or tikke (pan roasted); kabobs Raita (yogurt and cucumber salad) and other yogurt-based dishes and sauces Dal (lentils), pullao or pilau (basmati rice) Chapati (baked bread)	Ghee (clarified butter) Korma (meat in cream sauce) Samosas, pakoras (fried dishes) Molee and other coconut milk–based dishes Poori, bhatura, or paratha (fried breads)
ITALIAN Pasta primavera or pasta, polenta, risotto, or gnocchi with marinara, red or white wine, white or red clam, or light mushroom sauce Dishes that are grilled or prepared cacciatore (tomato-based sauce), marsala (broth and wine sauce), or piccata (lemon sauce) Cioppino (seafood stew) Vegetable soup, minestrone or fagioli (beans)	Antipasto (cheese, smoked meats) Dishes that are prepared alfredo, frito (fried), crema (creamed), alla panna (with cream), or carbonara Veal scaloppini Chicken, veal, or eggplant parmigiana Italian sausage, salami, and prosciutto Buttered garlic bread Cannoli
JAPANESE Dishes prepared nabemono (boiled), shabu-shabu (in boiling broth), mushimono (steamed), nimono (simmered), yaki (broiled), or yakimono (grilled) Sushi or domburi (mixed rice dish) Steamed rice or soba (buckwheat), udon (wheat), or rice noodles	Tempura (battered and fried) Agemono (deep fried) Katsu (fried pork cutlet) Sukiyaki Fried tofu
MEXICAN Soft corn or wheat tortillas Burritos, fajitas, enchiladas, soft tacos, and tamales filled with beans, vegetables, or lean meats Refried beans, nonfat or low-fat; rice and beans Ceviche (fish marinated in lime juice) Salsa, enchilada sauce, and picante sauce Gazpacho, menudo, or black bean soup Fruit or flan for dessert	Crispy, fried tortillas Dishes that are fried, such as chile relleños, chimichangas, flautas, and tostadas Nachos and cheese, chili con queso, and other dishes made with cheese or cheese sauce Guacamole, sour cream, and extra cheese Refried beans made with lard Fried ice cream
THAI Dishes that are barbecued, sautéed, broiled, boiled, steamed, braised, or marinated Sàté (skewered and grilled meats) Fish sauce, basil sauce, chili or hot sauces Bean thread noodles, Thai salad	Coconut milk soup Peanut sauce or dishes topped with nuts Mee-krob (crispy noodles) Red, green, and yellow curries, which typically contain coconut milk

SOURCES: National Heart, Lung and Blood Institute. 2006. *Guidelines on Overweight and Obesity: Electronic Textbook* (http://www.nhlbi.nih.gov/guidelines/obesity/e_txtbk/appndx/6a3b.htm; retrieved May 27, 2007). Duyff, R. L. 2006. *The American Dietetic Association's Complete Food and Nutrition Guide*, 2nd ed. Hoboken, N.J.: Wiley.

Knowledge of food and nutrition is essential to the success of your program. The information provided in this chapter should give you the tools you need to design and implement a diet that promotes long-term health and well-being. If you need additional information or have questions about nutrition, be sure the source you consult is reliable.

TIPS FOR TODAY AND THE FUTURE

Opportunities to improve your diet present themselves every day, and small changes add up.

RIGHT NOW YOU CAN

- Substitute a healthy snack for an unhealthy one.
- Drink a glass of water and put a bottle of water in your backpack for tomorrow.
- Plan to make healthy selections when you eat out, such as steamed vegetables instead of french fries or salmon instead of steak.

IN THE FUTURE, YOU CAN

- Visit the MyPyramid Web site at www.mypyramid.gov and use the online tools to create a personalized nutrition plan and begin tracking your eating habits.
- Learn to cook healthier meals. There are hundreds of free Web sites and low-cost cookbooks that provide recipes for healthy dishes.

SUMMARY

- The six classes of nutrients are carbohydrates, proteins, fats, vitamins, minerals, and water.

- The nutrients essential to humans are released into the body through digestion. Nutrients in foods provide energy, measured in kilocalories (commonly called calories); build and maintain body tissues; and regulate body functions.

- Protein, an important component of body tissue, is composed of amino acids; nine are essential to good health. Foods from animal sources provide complete proteins; plants provide incomplete proteins.

- Fats, a major source of energy, also insulate the body and cushion the organs; 3–4 teaspoons of vegetable oil per day supply the essential fats. For most people, dietary fat intake should be 20–35% of total calories, and unsaturated fats should be favored over saturated and trans fats.

- Carbohydrates provide energy to the brain, nervous system, and blood and to muscles during high-intensity exercise. Naturally occurring simple carbohydrates and unrefined complex carbohydrates should be favored over added sugars and refined carbohydrates.

- Fiber includes plant substances that are impossible for the human body to digest. It helps reduce cholesterol levels and promotes the passage of wastes through the intestines.

- The 13 essential vitamins are organic substances that promote specific chemical and cell processes and act as antioxidants. The 17 known essential minerals are inorganic substances that regulate body functions, aid in growth and tissue maintenance, and help in the release of energy from food. Deficiencies in vitamins and minerals can cause severe symptoms over time, but excess doses are also dangerous.

- Water aids in digestion and food absorption, allows chemical reactions to take place, serves as a lubricant or cushion, and helps regulate body temperature.

- Foods contain other substances, such as phytochemicals, that may not be essential nutrients but that may protect against chronic diseases.

- The Dietary Reference Intakes, Dietary Guidelines for Americans, and MyPyramid food guidance system provide standards and recommendations for getting all essential nutrients from a varied, balanced diet and for eating in ways that protect against chronic disease.

- The Dietary Guidelines for Americans advise us to consume a variety of foods while staying within calorie needs; manage body weight through calorie control and regular physical activity; eat more fruits, vegetables, whole grains, and reduced-fat dairy products; choose fats and carbohydrates wisely; eat less salt and more potassium; be moderate with alcohol intake; and handle foods safely.

- Choosing foods from each group in MyPyramid every day helps ensure the appropriate amounts of necessary nutrients.

- A vegetarian diet requires special planning but can meet all human nutritional needs.

- Different population groups, such as college students and athletes, face special dietary challenges and should plan their diets to meet their particular needs.

- Consumers can get help applying nutritional principles by reading the standardized labels that appear on all packaged foods and on dietary supplements.

- Although nutritional basics are well established, no single diet provides wellness for everyone. Individuals should focus on their particular needs and adapt general dietary principles to meet them.

For reliable nutrition advice, talk to a faculty member in the nutrition department on your campus, a registered dietitian (RD), or your physician. Many large communities have a telephone service called Dial a Dietitian. By calling this number, you can receive free nutrition information from an RD.

Experts on quackery suggest that you steer clear of anyone who puts forth any of the following false statements: Most diseases are caused primarily by faulty nutrition, large doses of vitamins are effective against many diseases, hair analysis can be used to determine a person's nutritional state, or a computer-scored nutritional deficiency test is a basis for prescribing vitamins. Any practitioner—licensed or not—who sells supplements in his or her office should be thoroughly scrutinized.

BOOKS

Duyff, R. L. 2006. *ADA Complete Food and Nutrition Guide,* 3rd ed. Hoboken, N. J.: Wiley. *An excellent review of current nutrition information.*

Insel, P., R. E. Turner, and D. Ross. 2006. *Discovering Nutrition,* 2nd ed. Sudbury, Mass.: Jones and Bartlett. *A comprehensive review of major concepts in nutrition.*

Nestle, M. 2007. *What to Eat.* New York: North Point Press. *A nutritionist examines the marketing of food and explains how to interpret food-related information while shopping.*

Selkowitz, A. 2005. *The College Student's Guide to Eating Well on Campus,* rev. ed. Bethesda, Md.: Tulip Hill Press. *Provides practical advice for students, including how to make healthy choices when eating in a dorm or restaurant and how to stock a first pantry.*

Wardlaw, G. M., and A. M. Smith. 2006. *Perspectives in Nutrition,* 7th ed. New York: McGraw-Hill. *An easy-to-understand review of major concepts in nutrition.*

Warshaw, H. 2006. *What to Eat When You're Eating Out.* Alexandria, Vir.: American Diabetes Association. *A registered dietician explains how to eat well when dining in restaurants; designed especially for those trying to manage their weight or a chronic condition such as diabetes.*

NEWSLETTERS

Environmental Nutrition (800-424-7887; http://www. environmentalnutrition.com)

Nutrition Action Health Letter (202-332-9110; http://www.cspinet. org/nah)

Tufts University Health and Nutrition Letter (800-274-7581; http:// www.healthletter.tufts.edu)

ORGANIZATIONS, HOTLINES, AND WEB SITES

American Dietetic Association. Provides a wide variety of educational materials on nutrition.
800-877-1600
http://www.eatright.org

American Heart Association: Delicious Decisions. Provides basic information about nutrition, tips for shopping and eating out, and heart-healthy recipes.
http://www.deliciousdecisions.org

FDA Center for Food Safety and Applied Nutrition. Offers information and interactive tools about topics such as food labeling, food additives, dietary supplements, and foodborne illness.
http://www.cfsan.fda.gov

Food Safety Hotlines. Provide information on the safe purchase, handling, cooking, and storage of food.
888-SAFEFOOD (FDA)
800-535-4555 (USDA)

Fruits and Veggies Matter. Hosted by a partnership of the CDC, DHHS, and National Cancer Institute; promotes the consumption of fruits and vegetables every day.
http://www.fruitsandveggiesmatter.gov

Gateways to Government Nutrition Information. Provides access to government resources relating to food safety, including consumer advice and information on specific pathogens.
http://www.nutrition.gov
http://www.foodsafety.gov

Harvard School of Public Health: Nutrition Source. Provides advice on interpreting news on nutrition; an overview of the Healthy Eating Pyramid, an alternative to the basic USDA pyramid; and suggestions for building a healthy diet.
http://www.hsph.harvard.edu/nutritionsource

International Food Information Council. Provides information on food safety and nutrition for consumers, journalists, and educators.
http://www.ific.org

MedlinePlus: Nutrition. Provides links to information from government agencies and major medical associations on a variety of nutrition topics.
http://www.nlm.nih.gov/medlineplus/nutrition.html

MyPyramid. Provides personalized dietary plans and interactive food and activity tracking tools.
http://www.mypyramid.gov

National Academies' Food and Nutrition Board. Provides information about the Dietary Reference Intakes and related guidelines.
http://www.iom.edu/CMS/3788.aspx

National Institutes of Health: Osteoporosis and Related Bone Diseases—National Resource Center. Provides information about osteoporosis prevention and treatment; includes a special section on men and osteoporosis.
http://www.osteo.org

National Osteoporosis Foundation. Provides information on the causes, prevention, detection, and treatment of osteoporosis.
http://www.nof.org

USDA Center for Nutrition Policy and Promotion. Click on the Healthy Eating Index for an assessment of Americans' diets and a comparison with the Dietary Guidelines and the Food Guide Pyramid.
http://www.cnpp.usda.gov

USDA Food and Nutrition Information Center. Provides a variety of materials relating to the Dietary Guidelines, food labels, Food Guide Pyramid, MyPyramid, and many other topics.
http://www.nal.usda.gov/fnic

Vegetarian Resource Group. Provides information and links for vegetarians and people interested in learning more about vegetarian diets.
http://www.vrg.org

Q Which should I eat—butter or margarine?

A Both butter and margarine are concentrated sources of fat, containing about 11 grams of fat and 100 calories per tablespoon. Butter is higher in saturated fat, which raises levels of artery-clogging LDL ("bad" cholesterol). Each tablespoon of butter has about 8 grams of saturated fat; margarine has about 2. Butter also contains cholesterol, which margarine does not.

Margarine, on the other hand, contains trans fat, which not only raises LDL but lowers HDL ("good" cholesterol). A tablespoon of stick margarine contains about 2 grams of trans fat. Butter contains a small amount of trans fat as well. Although butter has a combined total of saturated and trans fats that is twice that of stick margarine, the trans fat in stick margarine may be worse for you. Clearly, you should avoid both butter and stick margarine. To solve this dilemma, remember that softer is better. The softer or more liquid a margarine or spread is, the less hydrogenated it is and the less trans fat it contains. Tub and squeeze margarines contain less trans fat than stick margarines; some margarines are modified to be low-trans or trans-free and are labeled as such. Vegetable oils are an even better choice for cooking and for table use (such as olive oil for dipping bread) because most are low in saturated fat and completely free of trans fats.

Q MyPyramid recommends such large amounts of vegetables and fruit. How can I possibly eat that many servings without gaining weight?

A First, consider your typical portion sizes—you may be closer to meeting the recommendations than you think. Many people consume large servings of foods and underestimate the size of their portions. For example, a large banana may contain the equivalent of a cup of fruit, or half the recommended daily total for someone consuming 2000–2600 calories per day. Likewise, a medium baked potato (3-inch diameter) or an ear of corn (8-inch length) counts as a cup of vegetables. Use a measuring cup or a food scale for a few days to train your eye to accurately estimate food portion sizes. The MyPyramid.gov Web site includes charts of portion-size equivalents for each food group.

If an analysis of your diet indicates that you need to increase your overall intake of fruits and vegetables, look for healthy substitutions. If you are like most Americans, you are consuming more than the recommended number of calories from added sugars and solid fats; trim some of these calories to make room for additional servings of fruits and vegetables. Your beverage choices may be a good place to start. Do you routinely consume regular sodas, sweetened bottled teas or fruit drinks, or whole milk? One regular 12-ounce soda contains the equivalent of about 150 calories of added sugars; one 8-ounce glass of whole milk provides about 75 calories as discretionary fats. Substituting water, diet soda, or low-fat milk would free up calories for additional servings of fruits and vegetables. A half-cup of carrots, tomatoes, apples, or melon has only about 25 calories; you could consume 6 cups of these foods for the calories in one can of regular soda. Substituting lower-fat condiments for such full-fat items as butter, mayonnaise, and salad dressing is another good way to trim calories to make room for additional servings of nutrient-rich fruits and vegetables.

Also consider your portion sizes and/or the frequency with which you consume foods high in discretionary calories: You may not need to eliminate a favorite food—instead, just cut back. For example, cut your consumption of fast-food fries from four times a week to once a week, or reduce the size of your ice cream dessert from a cup to half a cup. Treats should be consumed appropriately—infrequently, and in small amounts.

For additional help on improving food choices to meet dietary recommendations, visit the MyPyramid.gov Web site and the family-friendly chart of "Go, Slow, and Whoa" foods at the site for the National Heart, Lung, and Blood Institute (www.nhlbi.nih.gov/health/public/heart/obesity/wecan/downloads/gswtips.pdf).

Q What exactly are genetically modified foods? Are they safe? How can I recognize them on the shelf, and how can I know when I'm eating them?

A Genetic engineering involves altering the characteristics of a plant, animal, or microorganism by adding, rearranging, or replacing genes in its DNA; the result is a genetically modified (GM) organism. New DNA may come from related species or organisms or from entirely different types of organisms.

You can find nutrient breakdowns of individual food items at the following sites:

Nutrition Analysis Tools and System (NATS)
   http://nat.crgq.com

USDA Nutrient Data Laboratory
   http://www.ars.usda.gov/ba/bhnrc/ndl

See also the resources listed in Chapters 9, 11, and 12.

SELECTED BIBLIOGRAPHY

A guide to the best and worst drinks. 2006. *Consumer Reports on Health*, July, 8–9.

Aldana, S. G., et al. 2005. Effects of an intensive diet and physical activity modification program on the health risks of adults. *Journal of the American Dietetic Association* 105(3): 371–381.

American College of Sports Medicine. 2007. American College of Sports Medicine position stand: Exercise and fluid replacement. *Medicine and Science in Sports and Exercise* 39(2): 377–390.

Many GM crops are already grown in the United States: About 75% of the current U.S. soybean crop has been genetically modified to be resistant to an herbicide used to kill weeds, and about a third of the U.S. corn crop carries genes for herbicide resistance or to produce a protein lethal to a destructive type of caterpillar. Products made with GM organisms include juice, soda, nuts, tuna, frozen pizza, spaghetti sauce, canola oil, chips, salad dressing, and soup.

The potential benefits of GM foods cited by supporters include improved yields overall and in difficult growing conditions, increased disease resistance, improved nutritional content, lower prices, and less use of pesticides. Critics of biotechnology argue that unexpected effects may occur: Gene manipulation could elevate levels of naturally occurring toxins or allergens, permanently change the gene pool and reduce biodiversity, and produce pesticide-resistant insects through the transfer of genes. In 2000, a form of GM corn approved for use only in animal feed was found to have commingled with other varieties of corn and to have been used in human foods; this mistake sparked fears of allergic reactions and led to recalls. Opposition to GM foods is particularly strong in Europe; in many developing nations that face food shortages, responses to GM crops have tended to be more positive.

In April 2000, the National Academy of Sciences released a report stating that there is no proof that GM food on the market is unsafe but that changes are needed to better coordinate regulation of GM foods and to assess potential problems.

Labeling has been another major concern. Surveys indicate that the majority of Americans want to know if their foods contain GM organisms. However, under current rules, the FDA requires special labeling only when a food's composition is changed significantly or when a known allergen is introduced. For example, soybeans that contain a gene from a peanut would have to be labeled because peanuts are a common allergen. The only foods guaranteed not to contain GM ingredients are those certified as organic.

Q How can I tell if I'm allergic to a food?

A A true food allergy is a reaction of the body's immune system to a food or food ingredient, usually a protein. This immune reaction can occur within minutes of ingesting the food, resulting in symptoms such as hives, diarrhea, difficulty breathing, or swelling of the lips or tongue. The most severe response is a systemic reaction called anaphylaxis, which involves a potentially life-threatening drop in blood pressure. Food allergies affect only about 2% of the adult population and about 4–6% of infants. Just eight foods account for more than 90% of the food allergies in the United States: cow's milk, eggs, peanuts, tree nuts (walnuts, cashews, and so on), soy, wheat, fish, and shellfish. Food manufacturers are now required to state the presence of these eight allergens in plain language in the list of ingredients on food labels.

Many people who believe they have food allergies may actually suffer from a food intolerance, a much more common source of adverse food reactions that typically involves problems with metabolism rather than with the immune system. The body may not be able to adequately digest a food or the body may react to a particular food compound. Food intolerances have been attributed to lactose (milk sugar), gluten (a protein in some grains), tartrazine (yellow food coloring), sulfite (a food additive), MSG, and the sweetener aspartame. Although symptoms of a food intolerance may be similar to those of a food allergy, they are typically more localized and not life-threatening. Many people with food intolerance can safely and comfortably consume small amounts of the food that affects them.

If you suspect you have a food allergy or intolerance, a good first step is to keep a food diary. Note everything you eat or drink, any symptoms you develop, and how long after eating the symptoms appear. Then make an appointment with your physician to go over your diary and determine if any additional tests are needed. People at risk for severe allergic reactions must diligently avoid trigger foods and carry medications to treat anaphylaxis.

For more Common Questions Answered about nutrition, visit the Online Learning Center.

American Heart Association. 2006. *Our 2006 Diet and Lifestyle Recommendations* (http://www.americanheart.org/presenter.jhtml?identifier=851; retrieved May 28, 2007).

Block, G. 2004. Foods contributing to energy intake in the US: Data from NHANES III and NHANES 1999–2000. *Journal of Food Composition and Analysis* 17(2004): 439–447.

Burke, L. M. 2007. Nutrition strategies for the marathon: Fuel for training and racing. *Sports Medicine* 37(4–5): 344–347.

Centers for Disease Control and Prevention. 2007. *Nutrition for Everyone* (http://www.cdc.gov/nccdphp/dnpa/nutrition/nutrition_for_everyone/index.htm; retrieved May 28, 2007).

Chun, O. K., et al. 2007. Estimated dietary flavonoid intake and major food sources of U.S. adults. *The Journal of Nutrition* 137(5): 1244–1252.

Clifton, P. M., J. B. Keogh, and M. Noakes. 2004. Trans fatty acids in adipose tissue and the food supply are associated with myocardial infarction. *Journal of Nutrition* 134: 874–879.

Ervin, R. B., et al. 2004. Dietary intake of selected minerals for the United States Population: 1999–2000. *Advance Data from Vital and Health Statistics,* 341.

Food and Drug Administration. 2004. *Fact Sheet: Carbohydrates* (http://www.fda.gov/oc/initiatives/obesity/factsheet.html; retrieved May 28, 2007).

Food and Nutrition Board, Institute of Medicine. 2005. *Dietary Reference Intakes for Water, Potassium, Sodium, Chloride, and Sulfate.* Washington, D.C.: National Academies Press.

Food and Nutrition Board, Institute of Medicine. 2005. *Dietary Reference Intakes for Energy, Carbohydrate, Fiber, Fat, Fatty Acids, Cholesterol, Protein, and Amino Acids.* Washington, D.C.: National Academies Press.

Hanley, D. A., and K. S. Davison. 2005. Vitamin D insufficiency in North America. *Journal of Nutrition* 135(2): 332–337.

Harvard School of Public Health, Department of Nutrition. 2007. *The Nutrition Source: Knowledge for Healthy Eating* (http://www.hsph.harvard.edu/nutritionsource/; retrieved May 28, 2007).

Hites, R. A., et al. 2004. Global assessment of organic contaminants in farmed salmon. *Science* 303(5655): 226–229.

Houston, D. K., et al. 2005. Dairy, fruit, and vegetable intakes and functional limitations and disability in a biracial cohort. *American Journal of Clinical Nutrition* 81(2): 515–522.

Kranz, S., et al. 2005. Adverse effect of high added sugar consumption on dietary intake in American preschoolers. *Journal of Pediatrics* 46(1): 105–111.

Krebs-Smith, S. M., and P. Kris-Etherton. 2007. How does MyPyramid compare to other population-based recommendations for controlling chronic disease? *Journal of the American Dietetic Association* 107(5): 830–837.

Ma, Y., et al. 2005. Association between dietary carbohydrates and body weight. *American Journal of Epidemiology* 161(4): 359–367.

Nanney, M. S., et al. 2004. Rationale for a consistent "powerhouse" approach to vegetable and fruit messages. *Journal of the American Dietetic Association* 104(3): 352–356.

National Academy of Sciences, Institute of Medicine, Food and Nutrition Board. 2006. *Dietary Reference Intakes: Recommended Intakes for Individuals* (http://www.iom.edu/Object.File/Master/7/300/Webtablemacro.pdf; retrieved May 28, 2007).

Opotowsky, A. R., et al. 2004. Serum vitamin A concentration and the risk of hip fracture among women 50 to 74 years old in the United States. *American Journal of Medicine* 117(3): 169–174.

U.S. Department of Agriculture. 2007. *Bovine Spongiform Encephalopathy* (http://www.fas.usda.gov/dlp/bse/bse.html; retrieved May 28, 2007).

U.S. Department of Agriculture. 2007. *Inside the Pyramid* (http://www.mypyramid.gov/pyramid/index.html; retrieved May 28, 2007).

U.S. Department of Health and Human Services and U.S. Department of Agriculture. 2005. *Dietary Guidelines for Americans 2005* (http://www.health.gov/dietaryguidelines/dga2005/document/; retrieved May 28, 2007).

U.S. Department of Health and Human Services and U.S. Department of Agriculture. 2005. Finding your way to a healthier you: Based on the Dietary Guidelines for Americans. *Home and Garden Bulletin* No. 232-CP.

Vartanian, L. R., et al. 2007. Effects of soft drink consumption on nutrition and health: A systematic review and meta-analysis. *American Journal of Public Health* 97(4): 667–675.

Table 1 — Dietary Reference Intakes (DRIs): Recommended Levels for Individual Intake

Life Stage	Group	Biotin (µg/day)	Choline (mg/day)[a]	Folate (µg/day)[b]	Niacin (mg/day)[c]	Pantothenic Acid (mg/day)	Riboflavin (mg/day)	Thiamin (mg/day)	Vitamin A (µg/day)[d]	Vitamin B-6 (mg/day)	Vitamin B-12 (µg/day)	Vitamin C (mg/day)[e]	Vitamin D (µg/day)[f]	Vitamin E (mg/day)[g]
Infants	0–6 months	5	125	65	2	1.7	0.3	0.2	400	0.1	0.4	40	5	4
	7–12 months	6	150	80	4	1.8	0.4	0.3	500	0.3	0.5	50	5	5
Children	1–3 years	8	200	150	6	2	0.5	0.5	300	0.5	0.9	15	5	6
	4–8 years	12	250	200	8	3	0.6	0.6	400	0.6	1.2	25	5	7
Males	9–13 years	20	375	300	12	4	0.9	0.9	600	1.0	1.8	45	5	11
	14–18 years	25	550	400	16	5	1.3	1.2	900	1.3	2.4	75	5	15
	19–30 years	30	550	400	16	5	1.3	1.2	900	1.3	2.4	90	5	15
	31–50 years	30	550	400	16	5	1.3	1.2	900	1.3	2.4	90	5	15
	51–70 years	30	550	400	16	5	1.3	1.2	900	1.7	2.4[h]	90	10	15
	>70 years	30	550	400	16	5	1.3	1.2	900	1.7	2.4[h]	90	15	15
Females	9–13 years	20	375	300	12	4	0.9	0.9	600	1.0	1.8	45	5	11
	14–18 years	25	400	400[i]	14	5	1.0	1.0	700	1.2	2.4	65	5	15
	19–30 years	30	425	400[i]	14	5	1.1	1.1	700	1.3	2.4	75	5	15
	31–50 years	30	425	400[i]	14	5	1.1	1.1	700	1.3	2.4	75	5	15
	51–70 years	30	425	400[i]	14	5	1.1	1.1	700	1.5	2.4[h]	75	10	15
	>70 years	30	425	400	14	5	1.1	1.1	700	1.5	2.4[h]	75	15	15
Pregnancy	≤18 years	30	450	600[i]	18	6	1.4	1.4	750	1.9	2.6	80	5	15
	19–30 years	30	450	600[j]	18	6	1.4	1.4	770	1.9	2.6	85	5	15
	31–50 years	30	450	600[j]	18	6	1.4	1.4	770	1.9	2.6	85	5	15
Lactation	≤18 years	35	550	500	17	7	1.6	1.4	1200	2.0	2.8	115	5	19
	19–30 years	35	550	500	17	7	1.6	1.4	1300	2.0	2.8	120	5	19
	31–50 years	35	550	500	17	7	1.6	1.4	1300	2.0	2.8	120	5	19
Tolerable Upper Intake Levels for Adults (19–70)			3500	1000[k]	35[k]				3000	100		2000	50	1000[k]

Note: The table includes values for the type of DRI standard—Adequate Intake (AI) or Recommended Dietary Allowance (RDA)—that has been established for that particular nutrient and life stage; RDAs are shown in **bold type.** The final row of the table shows the Tolerable Upper Intake Levels (ULs) for adults; refer to the full DRI report for information on other ages and life stages. A UL is the maximum level of daily nutrient intake that is likely to pose no risk of adverse effects. There is insufficient data to set ULs for all nutrients, but this does not mean that there is no potential for adverse effects; source of intake should be from food only to prevent high levels of intake of nutrients without established ULs. In healthy individuals, there is no established benefit from nutrient intakes above the RDA or AI.

[a] Although AIs have been set for choline, there are few data to assess whether a dietary supply of choline is needed at all stages of the life cycle, and it may be that the choline requirement can be met by endogenous synthesis at some of these stages.

[b] As dietary folate equivalents (DFE): 1 DFE = 1 µg food folate = 0.6 µg folate from fortified food or as a supplement consumed with food = 0.5 µg of a supplement taken on an empty stomach.

[c] As niacin equivalents (NE): 1 mg niacin = 60 mg tryptophan.

Table 1 — Dietary Reference Intakes (DRIs): Recommended Levels for Individual Intake (continued)

Life Stage	Group	Vitamin K (µg/day)	Calcium (mg/day)	Chromium (µg/day)	Copper (µg/day)	Fluoride (mg/day)	Iodine (mg/day)	Iron (mg/day)[l]	Magnesium (mg/day)	Manganese (mg/day)	Molybdenum (µg/day)	Phosphorus (mg/day)	Selenium (µg/day)	Zinc (mg/day)[m]
Infants	0–6 months	2.0	210	0.2	200	0.01	110	0.27	30	0.003	2	100	15	2
	7–12 months	2.5	270	5.5	220	0.5	130	11	75	0.6	3	275	20	3
Children	1–3 years	30	500	11	340	0.7	90	7	80	1.2	17	460	20	3
	4–8 years	55	800	15	440	1	90	10	130	1.5	22	500	30	5
Males	9–13 years	60	1300	25	700	2	120	8	240	1.9	34	1250	40	8
	14–18 years	75	1300	35	890	3	150	11	410	2.2	43	1250	55	11
	19–30 years	120	1000	35	900	4	150	8	400	2.3	45	700	55	11
	31–50 years	120	1000	35	900	4	150	8	420	2.3	45	700	55	11
	51–70 years	120	1200	30	900	4	150	8	420	2.3	45	700	55	11
	>70 years	120	1200	30	900	4	150	8	420	2.3	45	700	55	11
Females	9–13 years	60	1300	21	700	2	120	8	240	1.6	34	1250	40	8
	14–18 years	75	1300	24	890	3	150	15	360	1.6	43	1250	55	9
	19–30 years	90	1000	25	900	3	150	18	310	1.8	45	700	55	8
	31–50 years	90	1000	25	900	3	150	18	320	1.8	45	700	55	8
	51–70 years	90	1200	20	900	3	150	8	320	1.8	45	700	55	8
	>70 years	90	1200	20	900	3	150	8	320	1.8	45	700	55	8
Pregnancy	≤18 years	75	1300	29	1000	3	220	27	400	2.0	50	1250	60	13
	19–30 years	90	1000	30	1000	3	220	27	350	2.0	50	700	60	11
	31–50 years	90	1000	30	1000	3	220	27	360	2.0	50	700	60	11
Lactation	≤18 years	75	1300	44	1300	3	290	10	360	2.6	50	1250	70	14
	19–30 years	90	1000	45	1300	3	290	9	310	2.6	50	700	70	12
	31–50 years	90	1000	45	1300	3	290	9	320	2.6	50	700	70	12
Tolerable Upper Intake Levels for Adults (19–70)			2500		10,000	10	1100	45	350[k]	11	2000	4000	400	40

[d]As retinol activity equivalents (RAEs): 1 RAE = 1 µg retinol, 12 µg β-carotene, or 24 µg α-carotene or β-cryptoxanthin. Preformed vitamin A (retinol) is abundant in animal-derived foods; provitamin A carotenoids are abundant in some dark yellow, orange, red, and deep-green fruits and vegetables. For preformed vitamin A and for provitamin A carotenoids in supplements, IRE = 1 RAE; for provitamin A carotenoids in foods, divide the REs by 2 to obtain RAEs. The UL applies only to preformed vitamin A.

[e]Individuals who smoke require an additional 35 mg/day of vitamin C over that needed by nonsmokers; nonsmokers regularly exposed to tobacco smoke should ensure they meet the RDA for vitamin C.

[f]As cholecalciferol: 1 µg cholecalciferol = 40 IU vitamin D. DRI values are based on the absence of adequate exposure to sunlight.

[g]As α-tocopherol. Includes naturally occurring RRR-α-tocopherol and the 2R-stereoisomeric forms from supplements; does not include the 25-stereoisomeric forms from supplements.

[h]Because 10–30% of older people may malabsorb food-bound B-12, those over age 50 should meet their RDA mainly with supplements or foods fortified with B-12.

[i]In view of evidence linking folate intake with neural tube defects in the fetus. It is recommended that all women capable of becoming pregnant consume 400 µg from supplements or fortified foods in addition to consuming folate from a varied diet.

[j]It is assumed that women will continue consuming 400 µg from supplements or fortified food until their pregnancy is confirmed and they enter prenatal care, which ordinarily occurs after the end of the periconceptional period—the critical time for formation of the neural tube.

[k]The UL applies only to intake from supplements, fortified foods, and/or pharmacological agents and not to intake from foods.

[l]Because the absorption of iron from plant foods is low compared to that from animal foods, the RDA for strict vegetarians is approximately 1.8 times higher than the values established for omnivores (14 mg/day for adult male vegetarians; 33 mg/day for premenopausal female vegetarians). Oral contraceptives (OCs) reduce menstrual blood losses, so women taking them need less daily iron; the RDA for premenopausal women taking OCs is 10.9 mg/day. For more on iron requirements for other special situations, refer to Dietary Reference Intakes for Vitamin A, Vitamin K, Arsenic, Boron, Chromium, Copper, Iodine, Iron, Manganese, Molybdenum, Nickel, Silicon, Vanadium, and Zinc (visit http://www.nap.edu for the complete report).

[m]Zinc absorption is lower for those consuming vegetarian diets so the zinc requirement for vegetarians is approximately twofold greater than for those consuming a nonvegetarian diet.

Table 1 — Dietary Reference Intakes (DRIs): Recommended Levels for Individual Intake (continued)

Life Stage	Group	Potassium (g/day)	Sodium (g/day)	Chloride (g/day)	Carbohydrate RDA/AI (g/day)	Carbohydrate AMDR[o] (%)	Total Fiber RDA/AI (g/day)	Total Fat AMDR[o] (%)	Linoleic Acid RDA/AI (g/day)	Linoleic Acid AMDR[o] (%)	Alpha-linolenic Acid RDA/AI (g/day)	Alpha-linolenic Acid AMDR[o] (%)	Protein[n] RDA/AI (g/day)	Protein[n] AMDR[o] (%)	Water[p] (L/day)
Infants	0–6 months	0.4	0.12	0.18	60	ND[q]	ND	r	4.4	ND[q]	0.5	ND[q]	9.1	ND[q]	0.7
	7–12 months	0.7	0.37	0.57	95	ND[q]	ND	r	4.6	ND[q]	0.5	ND[q]	13.5	ND[q]	0.8
Children	1–3 years	3.0	1.0	1.5	130	45–65	19	30–40	7	5–10	0.7	0.6–1.2	13	5–20	1.3
	4–8 years	3.8	1.2	1.9	130	45–65	25	25–35	10	5–10	0.9	0.6–1.2	19	10–30	1.7
Males	9–13 years	4.5	1.5	2.3	130	45–65	31	25–35	12	5–10	1.2	0.6–1.2	34	10–30	2.4
	14–18 years	4.7	1.5	2.3	130	45–65	38	25–35	16	5–10	1.6	0.6–1.2	52	10–30	3.3
	19–30 years	4.7	1.5	2.3	130	45–65	38	20–35	17	5–10	1.6	0.6–1.2	56	10–35	3.7
	31–50 years	4.7	1.5	2.3	130	45–65	38	20–35	17	5–10	1.6	0.6–1.2	56	10–35	3.7
	51–70 years	4.7	1.3	2.0	130	45–65	30	20–35	14	5–10	1.6	0.6–1.2	56	10–35	3.7
	>70 years	4.7	1.2	1.8	130	45–65	30	20–35	14	5–10	1.6	0.6–1.2	56	10–35	3.7
Females	9–13 years	4.5	1.5	2.3	130	45–65	26	25–35	10	5–10	1.0	0.6–1.2	34	10–30	2.1
	14–18 years	4.7	1.5	2.3	130	45–65	26	25–35	11	5–10	1.1	0.6–1.2	46	10–30	2.3
	19–30 years	4.7	1.5	2.3	130	45–65	25	20–35	12	5–10	1.1	0.6–1.2	46	10–35	2.7
	31–50 years	4.7	1.5	2.3	130	45–65	25	20–35	12	5–10	1.1	0.6–1.2	46	10–35	2.7
	51–70 years	4.7	1.3	2.0	130	45–65	21	20–35	11	5–10	1.1	0.6–1.2	46	10–35	2.7
	>70 years	4.7	1.2	1.8	130	45–65	21	20–35	11	5–10	1.1	0.6–1.2	46	10–35	2.7
Pregnancy	≤18 years	4.7	1.5	2.3	175	45–65	28	20–35	13	5–10	1.4	0.6–1.2	71	10–35	3.0
	19–30 years	4.7	1.5	2.3	175	45–65	28	20–35	13	5–10	1.4	0.6–1.2	71	10–35	3.0
	31–50 years	4.7	1.5	2.3	175	45–65	28	20–35	13	5–10	1.4	0.6–1.2	71	10–35	3.0
Lactation	≤18 years	5.1	1.5	2.3	210	45–65	29	20–35	13	5–10	1.3	0.6–1.2	71	10–35	3.8
	19–30 years	5.1	1.5	2.3	210	45–65	29	20–35	13	5–10	1.3	0.6–1.2	71	10–35	3.8
	31–50 years	5.1	1.5	2.3	210	45–65	29	20–35	13	5–10	1.3	0.6–1.2	71	10–35	3.8
Tolerable Upper Intake Level for Adults (19–70)			2.3	3.6											

[n] Daily protein recommendations are based on body weight for reference body weights. To calculate for a specific body weight, use the following values: 1.5 g/kg for infants, 1.1 g/kg for 1–3 years, 0.95 g/kg for 4–13 years, 0.85 g/kg for 14–18 years, 0.8 g/kg for adults, and 1.1 g/kg for pregnant (using prepregnancy weight) and lactating women.

[o] Acceptable Macronutrient Distribution Range (AMDR), expressed as a percent of total daily calories, is the range of intake for a particular energy source that is associated with reduced risk of chronic disease while providing intakes of essential nutrients. If an individual consumes in excess of the AMDR, there is a potential for increasing the risk of chronic diseases and/or insufficient intakes of essential nutrients.

[p] Total water intake from fluids and food.

[q] Not determinable due to lack of data of adverse effects in this age group and concern with regard to lack of ability to handle excess amounts. Source of intake should be from food only to prevent high levels of intake.

[r] For infants, Adequate Intake of total fat is 31 grams/day (0–6 months) and 30 grams per day (7–12 months) from breast milk and, for infants 7–12 months, complementary food and beverages.

Source: Food and Nutrition Board, Institute of Medicine, National Academies. 2004. *Dietary Reference Intakes Tables* (http://www.iom.edu/file.asp?id = 21372; retrieved June 1, 2007). The complete Dietary Reference Intake reports are available from the National Academy Press (http://www.nap.edu).

*Reprinted with permission from *Dietary Reference Intakes Applications in Dietary Planning*. Copyright © 2004 by the National Academy of Sciences. Reprinted with permission from the National Academies Press, Washington, D.C.

Nutrition Resources

Number of servings per day (or per week, as noted)

Food groups	1600 calories	2000 calories	2600 calories	3100 calories	Serving sizes and notes
Grains	6	6–8	10–11	12–13	1 slice bread, 1 oz dry cereal, $1/2$ cup cooked rice, pasta, or cereal; choose whole grains
Vegetables	3–4	4–5	5–6	6	1 cup raw leafy vegetables, $1/2$ cup cooked vegetables, $1/2$ cup vegetable juice
Fruits	4	4–5	5–6	6	$1/2$ cup fruit juice, 1 medium fruit, $1/4$ cup dried fruit, 1/2 cup fresh, frozen, or canned fruit
Low-fat or fat-free dairy foods	2–3	2–3	3	3–4	1 cup milk; 1 cup yogurt, 1-$1/2$ oz cheese; choose fat-free or lowfat types
Meat, poultry, fish	3–6	6 or less?	6	6–9	1 oz cooked meats, poultry, or fish: select only lean; trim away visible fats; broil, roast, or boil instead of frying; remove skin from poultry
Nuts, seeds, legumes	3 servings per week	4–5 servings per week	1	1	$1/3$ cup or 1-$1/2$ oz nuts, 2 Tbsp or $1/2$ oz seeds, $1/2$ cup cooked dry beans/peas, 2 Tbsp peanut butter
Fats and oils	2	2–3	3	4	1 tsp soft margarine; 1 Tbsp low-fat mayonnaise, 2 Tbsp light salad dressing, 1 tsp vegetable oil; DASH has 27% of calories as fat (low in saturated fat)
Sweets	0	5 servings/week or less	2	2	1 Tbsp sugar, 1 Tbsp jelly or jam, $1/2$ cup sorbet, 1 cup lemonade; sweets should be low in fat

FIGURE 1   The DASH Eating Plan.   SOURCE: National Institutes of Health, National Heart, Lung, and Blood Institute. 2006. *Your Guide to Lowering Your Blood Pressure with DASH: How Do I Make the Dash?* (http://www. nhlbi.nih.gov/health/public/heart/hbp/dash/how_make_dash html; retrieved May 27, 2007).

FIGURE 2   Healthy Eating Pyramid. The Healthy Eating Pyramid is an alternative food-group plan developed by researchers at the Harvard School of Public Health; this pyramid reflects many major research studies that have looked at the relationship between diet and long-term health. The Healthy Eating Pyramid differentiates between the various dietary sources of fat, protein, and carbohydrates, and it emphasizes whole grains, vegetable oils, fruits and vegetables, nuts, and dried peas and beans.

SOURCE: Reprinted by permission of Simon & Schuster Adult Publishing Group from *Eat, Drink, and Be Healthy: The Harvard Medical School Guide to Healthy Eating* by Walter C. Willett, M.D. Copyright © 2001 by the President and Fellows of Harvard College.

Red Meat and Butter *USE SPARINGLY*

White Rice, White Bread, Potatoes, Pasta, and Sweets *USE SPARINGLY*

Dairy or Calcium Supplement

Alcohol *IN MODERATION UNLESS CONTRAINDICATED*

Fish, Poultry, and Eggs *0–2 SERVINGS*

Multiple Vitamins *FOR MOST*

Nuts and Legumes *1–3 SERVINGS*

Fruit *2–3 SERVINGS*

Vegetables *IN ABUNDANCE*

Plant Oils (olive, canola, soy, corn, sunflower, peanut, and other vegetable oils) *AT MOST MEALS*

Whole-Grain Foods *AT MOST MEALS*

Daily exercise and weight control

LAB 8.1 Your Daily Diet Versus MyPyramid

Make three photocopies of the worksheet in this lab and use them to keep track of everything you eat for 3 consecutive days. Break down each food item into its component parts, and list them separately in the column labeled "Food." Then enter the portion size you consumed in the correct food-group column. For example, a turkey sandwich might be listed as follows: whole-wheat bread, 2 oz-equiv of whole grains; turkey, 2 oz-equiv of meat/beans; tomato, $\frac{1}{3}$ cup other vegetables; romaine lettuce, $\frac{1}{4}$ cup dark green vegetables; 1 tablespoon mayonnaise dressing, 1 teaspoon oils. It can be challenging to track values for added sugars and, especially, oils and fats, but use food labels and the information in Appendix B to be as accurate as you can. MyPyramid.gov has additional guidelines for counting discretionary calories.

For vegetables, enter your portion sizes in both the "Total" column and the column corresponding to the correct subgroup; for example, the spinach in a spinach salad would be entered under "Dark Green" and carrots would be entered under "Orange." For the purpose of this 3-day activity, you will compare only your total vegetable consumption against MyPyramid guidelines; as described in the chapter, vegetable subgroup recommendations are based on weekly consumption. However, it is important to note which vegetable subgroups are represented in your diet; over a 3-day period, you should consume several servings from each of the subgroups.

This activity can also be completed online using the Pyramid Tracker program at the MyPyramid.gov Web site.

Date: _____

| Food | Grains (oz-eq) | | Vegetable (cups) | | | | | | Fruits (cups) | Milk (cups) | Meat/ Beans (oz-eq) | Oils (tsp) | Discretionary Calories | |
	Whole	Other	Total	Dark Green	Orange	Legume	Starchy	Other					Solid Fats (g)	Added Sugars (g/tsp)
Daily TOTAL														

Next, average your daily intake totals for the 3 days and enter them in the chart below. For example, if your three daily totals for the fruit group were 1 cup, 1½ cups, and 2 cups, your average daily intake would be 1½ cups. Fill in the recommended intake totals that apply to you from Figure 8.6 and Table 8.4.

MyPyramid Food Group	Recommended Daily Amounts or Limits	Your Actual Average Daily Intake
Grains (total)	oz-eq	oz-eq
Whole grains	oz-eq	oz-eq
Other grains	oz-eq	oz-eq
Vegetables (total)	cups	cups
Fruits	cups	cups
Milk	cups	cups
Meat and beans	oz-eq	oz-eq
Oils	tsp	tsp
Solid fats	g	g
Added sugars	g/tsp	g/tsp

Using Your Results

How did you score? How close is your diet to that recommended by MyPyramid? Are you surprised by the actual amount of food you're consuming from each food group or from added sugars and solid fats?

What should you do next? If the results of the assessment indicate that you could boost your level of wellness by improving your diet, set realistic goals for change. Do you need to increase or decrease your consumption of any food groups? List any areas of concern below, along with a goal for change and strategies for achieving the goal you've set. If you see that you are falling short in one food group, such as fruits or vegetables, but have many foods that are rich in discretionary calories from solid fats and added sugars, you might try decreasing those items in favor of an apple, a bunch of grapes, or some baby carrots. Think carefully about the reasons behind your food choices. For example, if you eat doughnuts for breakfast every morning because you feel rushed, make a list of ways to save time to allow for a healthier breakfast.

Problem: _____

Goal: _____

Strategies for change: _____

_____

_____

Problem: _____

Goal: _____

Strategies for change: _____

_____

_____

Problem: _____

Goal: _____

Strategies for change: _____

_____

_____

Enter the results of this lab in the Preprogram Assessment column in Appendix D. If you've set goals and identified strategies for change, begin putting your plan into action. Additional dietary tracking grids are available on the Online Learning Center. After several weeks of your program, complete this lab again and enter the results in the Postprogram Assessment column of Appendix D. How do the results compare?

LAB 8.2 Dietary Analysis

You can complete this activity using either a nutrition analysis software program or the food composition data in Appendix B and the charts printed below. Information about the nutrient content of foods is also available online; see the For Further Exploration section for recommended Web sites. (This lab asks you to analyze one day's diet. For a more complete and accurate assessment of your diet, analyze the results from several different days, including a weekday and a weekend day.)

DATE _____   DAY: M Tu W Th F Sa Su

Food	Amount	Calories	Protein (g)	Carbohydrate (g)	Dietary fiber (g)	Fat, total (g)	Saturated fat (g)	Cholesterol (mg)	Sodium (mg)	Vitamin A (RE)	Vitamin C (mg)	Calcium (mg)	Iron (mg)
Recommended totals*			10–35%	45–65%	25–38 g	20–35%	<10%	≤300 mg	≤2300 mg	RE	mg	mg	mg
Actual totals**	cal		g / %	g / %	g	g / %	g / %	mg	mg	RE	mg	mg	mg

*Fill in the appropriate DRI values for vitamin A, vitamin C, calcium, and iron from Table 1 in the Nutrition Resources section.

**Total the values in each column. To calculate the percentage of total calories from protein, carbohydrate, fat, and saturated fat, use the formula on p. 272. Protein and carbohydrate provide 4 calories per gram; fat provides 9 calories per gram. For example, if you consume a total of 270 grams of carbohydrates and 2000 calories, your percentage of total calories from carbohydrates would be (270 g × 4 cal/g) ÷ 2000 cal = 54%. Do not include data for alcoholic beverages in your calculations. Percentages may not total 100% due to rounding.

Using Your Results

How did you score? How close is your diet to that recommended by the Dietary Guidelines, Dietary Reference Intakes, and other guidelines? Are you surprised by any of the results of this assessment?

What should you do next? Enter the results of this lab in the Preprogram Assessment column in Appendix D. If your daily diet meets all the recommended intakes, congratulations—and keep up the good work. If the results of the assessment pinpoint areas of concern, then work with your food record on the previous page to determine what changes you could make to meet all the guidelines. Make changes, additions, and deletions until it conforms to all or most of the guidelines. Or, if you prefer, start from scratch to create a day's diet that meets the guidelines. Use the chart below to experiment and record your final, healthy sample diet for one day. Then put what you learned from this exercise into practice in your daily life. After several weeks of your program, complete this lab again and enter the results in the Postprogram Assessment column of Appendix D. How do the results compare?

DATE _____   DAY: M Tu W Th F Sa Su

Food	Amount	Calories	Protein (g)	Carbohydrate (g)	Dietary fiber (g)	Fat, total (g)	Saturated fat (g)	Cholesterol (mg)	Sodium (mg)	Vitamin A (RE)	Vitamin C (mg)	Calcium (mg)	Iron (mg)
Recommended totals			10–35%	45–65%	25–38 g	20–38%	<10%	≤300 mg	≤2300 mg	RE	mg	mg	mg
Actual totals		cal	g / %	g / %	g	g / %	g / %	mg	mg	RE	mg	mg	mg

LAB 8.3 Informed Food Choices

Part I   Using Food Labels

Choose three food items to evaluate. You might want to select three similar items, such as regular, low-fat, and nonfat salad dressing, or three very different items. Record the information from their food labels in the table below.

Food Items			
Serving size			
Total calories	cal	cal	cal
Total fat—grams	g	g	g
—% Daily Value	%	%	%
Saturated fat—grams	g	g	g
—% Daily Value	%	%	%
Trans fat—grams	g	g	g
Cholesterol—milligrams	mg	mg	mg
—% Daily Value	%	%	%
Sodium—milligrams	mg	mg	mg
—% Daily Value	%	%	%
Carbohydrates (total)—grams	g	g	g
—% Daily Value	%	%	%
Dietary fiber—grams	g	g	g
—% Daily Value	%	%	%
Sugars—grams	g	g	g
Protein—grams	g	g	g
Vitamin A—% Daily Value	%	%	%
Vitamin C—% Daily Value	%	%	%
Calcium—% Daily Value	%	%	%
Iron—% Daily Value	%	%	%

How do the items you chose compare? You can do a quick nutrient check by totaling the Daily Value percentages for nutrients you should limit (total fat, cholesterol, sodium) and the nutrients you should favor (dietary fiber, vitamin A, vitamin C, calcium, iron) for each food. Which food has the largest percent Daily Value sum for nutrients to limit? For nutrients to favor?

Food Items			
Calories	cal	cal	cal
% Daily Value total for nutrients to limit (total fat, cholesterol, sodium)	%	%	%
% Daily Value total for nutrients to favor (fiber, vitamin A, vitamin C, calcium, iron)	%	%	%

Part II   Evaluating Fast Food

Use the information from Appendix C, "Nutritional Content of Popular Items from Fast-Food Restaurants," to complete the chart on this page for the last fast-food meal you ate. Add up your totals for the meal. Compare the values for fat, protein, carbohydrate, cholesterol, and sodium content for each food item and for the meal as a whole with the levels suggested by the Dietary Guidelines for Americans. Calculate the percent of total calories derived from fat, saturated fat, protein, and carbohydrate using the formulas given.

If you haven't recently been to one of the restaurants included in the appendix, fill in the chart for any sample meal you might eat. If some of the food items you selected don't appear in Appendix C, ask for a nutrition information brochure when you visit the restaurant, or check out online fast-food information: Arby's (http://www.arbysrestaurant.com), Burger King (http://www.burgerking.com), Domino's Pizza (http://www.dominos.com), Jack in the Box (http://www.jackinthebox.com), KFC (http://www.kfc.com), McDonald's (http://www.mcdonalds.com), Subway (http://www.subway.com), Taco Bell (http://www.tacobell.com), Wendy's (http://www.wendys.com).

FOOD ITEMS

	Dietary Guidelines							Total**
Serving size (g)		g	g	g	g	g	g	g
Calories		cal	cal	cal	cal	cal	cal	cal
Total fat—grams		g	g	g	g	g	g	g
—% calories*	20–35%	%	%	%	%	%	%	%
Saturated fat—grams		g	g	g	g	g	g	g
—% calories*	<10%	%	%	%	%	%	%	%
Protein—grams		g	g	g	g	g	g	g
—% calories*	10–35%	%	%	%	%	%	%	%
Carbohydrate—grams		g	g	g	g	g	g	g
—% calories*	45–65%	%	%	%	%	%	%	%
Cholesterol†	100 mg	mg	mg	mg	mg	mg	mg	mg
Sodium†	800 mg	mg	mg	mg	mg	mg	mg	mg

*To calculate the percent of total calories from each food energy source (fat, carbohydrate, protein), use the following formula:

$$\frac{\text{(number of grams of energy source)} \times \text{(number of calories per gram of energy source)}}{\text{(total calories in serving of food item)}}$$

(*Note:* Fat and saturated fat provide 9 calories per gram; protein and carbohydrate provide 4 calories per gram.) For example, the percent of total calories from protein in a 150-calorie dish containing 10 grams of protein is

$$\frac{\text{(10 grams of protein)} \times \text{(4 calories per gram)}}{\text{(150 calories)}} = \frac{40}{150} = 0.27, \text{ or } 27\% \text{ of total calories from protein}$$

**For the Total column, add up the total grams of fat, carbohydrate, and protein contained in your sample meal and calculate the percentages based on the total calories in the meal. (Percentages may not total 100% due to rounding.) For cholesterol and sodium values, add up the total number of milligrams.

†Recommended daily limits of cholesterol and sodium are divided by 3 here to give an approximate recommended limit for a single meal.

Unintentional injuries are the fifth leading cause of death among Americans overall and the leading killer of young people. Injuries affect all segments of the population, but they are particularly common among minorities and people with low incomes, primarily due to social, environmental, and economic factors. The economic cost of injuries in the United States is high, with nearly $600 billion spent each year for medical care and rehabilitation of injured people.

Injuries are generally classified into four categories, based on where they occur: motor vehicle injuries, home injuries, leisure injuries, and work injuries.

MOTOR VEHICLE INJURIES

According to the CDC, more than 37,000 Americans were killed and 3 million injured in motor vehicle crashes in 2004. Motor vehicle accidents are a leading cause of paralysis due to spinal injury and the leading cause of severe brain injury.

Factors in Motor Vehicle Injuries

Driving Habits   Nearly two-thirds of motor vehicle injuries are caused by bad driving, especially speeding. As speed increases, momentum and force of impact increase and the time available for the driver to react decreases. Speed limits are posted to establish the safest *maximum* speed limit for a given area under *ideal* conditions. Aggressive driving—characterized by speeding, frequent and abrupt lane changes, tailgating, and passing on the shoulder—also increases the risk of crashes.

Anything that distracts a driver—sleepiness, bad mood, children or pets in the car, use of a cell phone—can increase the risk of a crash. Sleepiness reduces reaction time, coordination, and speed of information processing and can be as dangerous as drug and alcohol use. Even mild sleep deprivation causes a deterioration in driving ability comparable to that caused by a 0.05% blood alcohol concentration.

Cell phone users respond to hazards about 20% slower than undistracted drivers and are about twice as likely to rear-end a braking car in front of them. A 2006 study showed that drivers who use cell phones are nearly six times as likely to be involved in a crash as drivers who don't. Hands-free devices do not help significantly; the mental distraction of talking is the factor in crashes rather than holding a phone.

Safety Belts and Air Bags   A person who doesn't wear a safety belt is twice as likely to be injured in a crash as a person who does wear a safety belt. Safety belts not only prevent occupants from being thrown from the car at the time of the crash but also provide protection from the "second collision," which occurs when the occupant of the car hits something inside the car, such as the steering column or windshield. The safety belt also spreads the stopping force of a collision over the body.

Since 1998, all new cars have been equipped with dual air bags—one for the driver and one for the front passenger seat. Air bags provide supplemental protection in a collision but are most useful in head-on collisions. (Many newer vehicles feature side air bags to offer protection in a side-impact crash.) They also deflate immediately after inflating and so do not provide protection in collisions involving multiple impacts. To ensure that air bags work as intended, follow these guidelines:

- Place infants in rear-facing infant seats in the backseat.
- Transport children age 12 and under in the backseat.
- Always use safety belts or appropriate safety seats.
- Keep at least 10 inches between the air bag cover and the breastbone of the driver or passenger.

A person who cannot comply with these guidelines, can apply to the National Highway Traffic Safety Administration for permission to install an on-off switch that temporarily disables the air bag.

Alcohol and Other Drugs   Alcohol is involved in about 40% of all fatal crashes. Alcohol-impaired driving, defined by blood alcohol concentration (BAC), is illegal. The legal BAC limit is 0.08% in all states, but driving ability is impaired at much lower BACs. All psychoactive drugs have the potential to impair driving ability.

Preventing Motor Vehicle Injuries

About 75% of all motor vehicle collisions occur within 25 miles of home and at speeds lower than 40 mph. These crashes often occur because the driver believes safety measures are not necessary for short trips. Clearly, the statistics prove otherwise.

To prevent motor vehicle injuries:
- Obey the speed limit. If you have to speed to get to your destination on time, you're not allowing enough time.
- Always wear a safety belt and ask passengers to do the same. Strap infants and toddlers into government-approved car seats in the backseat. Children who have outgrown child safety seats but who are still too small for adult safety belts alone (usually age 4–8) should be secured using booster seats. All children under 12 should ride in the backseat.
- Never drive under the influence of alcohol or other drugs with a driver who is.

- Do not drive when you are sleepy or have been awake for 18 or more hours.
- Avoid using your cell phone while driving—your primary obligation is to pay attention to the road. If you do make calls, follow laws set by your city or state. Place calls when you are at a stop, and keep them short. Pull over if the conversation is stressful or emotional.
- Keep your car in good working order. Regularly inspect tires, oil and fluid levels, windshield wipers, spare tire, and so on.
- Always allow enough following distance. Follow the "3-second rule": When the vehicle ahead passes a reference point, count out 3 seconds. If you pass the reference point before you finish counting, drop back and allow more following distance.
- Always increase following distance and slow down if weather or road conditions are poor.
- Choose interstate highways rather than rural roads. Highways are much safer because of better visibility, wider lanes, fewer surprises, and other factors.
- Always signal before turning or changing lanes.
- Stop completely at stop signs. Follow all traffic laws.
- Take special care at intersections. Always look left, right, and then left again. Make sure you have plenty of time to complete your maneuver in the intersection.
- Don't pass on two-lane roads unless you're in a designated passing area and have a clear view ahead.

Motorcycles and Mopeds

About 1 out of every 10 traffic fatalities among people age 15–34 involves someone riding a motorcycle. Injuries from motorcycle collisions are generally more severe than those involving automobiles because motorcycles provide little, if any, protection. Moped riders face additional challenges. Mopeds usually have a maximum speed of 30–35 mph and have less power for maneuverability.

To prevent motorcycle and moped injuries:
- Make yourself easier to see by wearing light-colored clothing, driving with your headlights on, and correctly positioning yourself in traffic.
- Develop the necessary skills. Lack of skill, especially when evasive action is needed to avoid a collision, is a major factor in motorcycle and moped injuries. Skidding from improper braking is the most common cause of loss of control.
- Wear a close-fitting helmet, one marked with the symbol DOT (for Department of Transportation).
- Protect your eyes with goggles, a face shield, or a windshield.
- Drive defensively and never assume that other drivers see you.

Pedestrians and Bicycles

Injuries to pedestrians and bicyclists are considered motor vehicle–related because they are usually caused by motor vehicles. About 1 in 8 motor vehicle deaths each year involves a pedestrian; more than 80,000 pedestrians are injured each year.

To prevent injuries when walking or jogging:
- Walk or jog in daylight.
- Make yourself easier to see by wearing light-colored, reflective clothing.
- Face traffic when walking or jogging along a roadway, and follow traffic laws.
- Avoid busy roads or roads with poor visibility.
- Cross only at marked crosswalks and intersections.
- Don't use headphones while walking or jogging.
- Don't hitchhike; it places you in a potentially dangerous situation.

Bicycle injuries result primarily from not knowing or understanding the rules of the road, failing to follow traffic laws, and not having sufficient skill or experience to handle traffic conditions. Bicycles are considered vehicles; bicycle riders must obey all traffic laws that apply to automobile drivers, including stopping at traffic lights and stop signs.

To prevent injuries when riding a bike:
- Wear safety equipment, including a helmet, eye protection, gloves, and proper footwear. Secure the bottom of your pant legs with clips and secure your shoelaces so they don't get tangled in the chain.
- Make yourself easier to see by wearing light-colored, reflective clothing. Equip your bike with reflectors and use lights, especially at night or when riding in wooded or other dark areas.
- Ride with the flow of traffic, not against it, and follow traffic laws. Use bike paths when they are available.
- Ride defensively; never assume that drivers see you. Be especially careful when turning or crossing at corners and intersections. Watch for cars turning right.
- Stop at all traffic lights and stop signs. Know and use hand signals.
- Continue pedaling at all times when moving (don't coast) to help keep the bike stable and to maintain your balance.
- Properly maintain your bike.

Aggressive Driving

Aggressive driving, known as *road rage,* has increased more than 50% since 1990. Aggressive drivers increase the risk of crashes for themselves and others. They further increase the risk of injuries if they stop their vehicles and confront each other. Even if you are successful at controlling your own aggressive driving impulses, you may still encounter an aggressive driver.

To avoid being the victim of an aggressive driver:
- Always keep distance between your car and others. If you are behind a very slow driver and can't pass, slow down to increase distance in case that driver does something unexpected. If you are being tailgated, do not increase your speed; instead, let the other driver pass you. If you are in the left lane when being tailgated, signal and pull over to let the other driver go by, even if you are traveling at the speed limit. When you are merging, make sure you have plenty of room. If you are cut off by a merging driver, slow down to make room.

- Be courteous, even if the other driver is not. Use your horn rarely, if ever. Avoid making gestures of irritation, even shaking your head. When parking, let the other driver have the space that you both found.
- Refuse to join in a fight. Avoid eye contact with an angry driver. If someone makes a rude gesture, ignore it. If you think another car is following you and you have a cell phone, call the police. Otherwise, drive to a public place and honk your horn to get someone's attention.
- If you make a mistake while driving, apologize. Raise or wave your hand or touch or knock your head with the palm of your hand to indicate "What was I thinking?" You can also mouth the words "I'm sorry."

HOME INJURIES

Contrary to popular belief, home is one of the most dangerous places to be. The most common fatal home injuries are caused by falls, poisoning, fires, suffocation and choking, and incidents involving firearms.

Falls

Falls are second only to motor vehicle injuries in terms of causing deaths. They are a significant cause of unintentional death for people under age 25. Most deaths occurring from falls involve falling on stairs or steps or from one level to another. Falls also occur on the same level, from tripping, slipping, or stumbling. Alcohol is a contributing factor in many falls.

To prevent injuries from falls:
- Install handrails and nonslip surfaces in the shower and bathtub. Place skidproof backing on rugs and carpets.
- Keep floors clear of objects or conditions that could cause slipping or tripping, such as heavy wax coating, electrical cords, and toys.
- Put a light switch by the door of every room so that no one has to walk across a room to turn on a light. Use night-lights in bedrooms, halls, and bathrooms.
- Outside the house, clear dangerous surfaces created by ice, snow, fallen leaves, or rough ground.
- Install handrails on stairs. Keep stairs well lit and clear of objects.
- When climbing a ladder, use both hands. Never stand higher than the third step from the top. When using a stepladder, make sure the spreader brace is in the locked position. With straight ladders, set the base 1 foot out for every 4 feet of height. Don't stand on chairs to reach things.
- If there are small children in the home, place gates at the top and bottom of stairs. Never leave a baby unattended on a bed or table.

Poisoning

More than 2.4 million poisonings occur every year in the United States.

To prevent poisoning:
- Store all medicines out of the reach of children. Use medicines only as directed on the label or by a physician.
- Use cleaners, pesticides, and other dangerous substances only in areas with proper ventilation. Store them out of the reach of children.
- Never operate a vehicle in an enclosed space. Have your furnace inspected yearly. Use caution with any substance that produces potentially toxic fumes, such as kerosene. If appropriate, install carbon monoxide detectors.
- Keep poisonous plants out of the reach of children. These include azalea, oleander, rhododendron, wild mushrooms, daffodil and hyacinth bulbs, mistletoe berries, apple seeds, morning glory seeds, wisteria seeds, and the leaves and stems of potato, rhubarb, and tomato plants.

To be prepared in case of poisoning:
- Keep the number of the nearest Poison Control Center (or emergency room) in an accessible location. A call to the national poison control hotline (800-222-1222) will be routed to a local center.

Emergency first aid for poisonings:
1. Remove the poison from contact with eyes, skin, or mouth, or remove the victim from contact with poisonous fumes or gases.
2. Call the Poison Control Center immediately for instructions. Have the container with you.
3. Do not follow emergency instructions on labels. Some may be out-of-date and carry incorrect treatment information.
4. If you are instructed to go to an emergency room, take the poisonous substance or its container with you.

Guidelines for specific types of poisons:
- *Swallowed poisons.* If the person is awake and able to swallow, give water only; then call the Poison Control Center or a physician for advice.
- *Poisons on the skin.* Remove any affected clothing. Flood affected parts of the skin with warm water, wash with soap and water, and rinse. Then call for advice.
- *Poisons in the eye.* For children, flood the eye with lukewarm water poured from a pitcher held 3–4 inches above the eye for 15 minutes; alternatively, irrigate the eye under a faucet. For adults, get in the shower and flood the eye with a gentle stream of lukewarm water for 15 minutes. Then call for advice.
- *Inhaled poisons.* Immediately carry or drag the person to fresh air and, if necessary, give rescue breaths (Figure A.1). If the victim is not breathing easily, call 911 for help. Ventilate the area. Then call the Poison Control Center for advice.

Fires

Each year, about 80% of fire deaths and 65% of fire injuries occur in the home. Careless smoking is the leading cause of fire deaths.

To prevent fires:
- Dispose of all cigarettes in ashtrays. Never smoke in bed.
- Do not overload electrical outlets. Do not place extension cords under rugs or where people walk. Replace worn or frayed extension cords.

EMERGENCY CARE FOR CHOKING

- If the victim is coughing, encourage the coughing to clear the object from the airway.
- If the victim is not coughing, follow the steps in "Choking Care for Responsive Adult or Child."

Choking Care for Responsive Adult or Child

1 Stand behind an adult victim with one leg forward between the victim's legs. (With a child, kneel behind the victim.) Keep your head slightly to one side. Reach around the abdomen with both arms. Make a fist with one hand and place the thumb side of the fist against the abdomen just above the navel.

2 Grasp your fist with your other hand and thrust inward and up-ward into the victim's abdomen with quick jerks. Continue abdominal thrusts until the victim expels the object or becomes unresponsive. If the victim becomes unresponsive while you are administering abdominal thrusts, lower the victim to the floor onto his or her back, and follow the steps in "Choking Care for Unresponsive Adult or Child."

Choking Care for Unresponsive Adult or Child: CPR

1 Call 911 and begin CPR.

2 Open the airway to see if the victim is breathing. Use the "head tilt–chin lift" maneuver to open the airway: Push down on the forehead and lift the chin.

3 If the victim is not breathing, give two rescue breaths, each lasting 1 second. Pinch the victim's nose shut and blow a normal breath into the victim's mouth. If the first breath does not go in (the chest does not rise), reposition the head to open the airway and try again. Each time you give a rescue breath, look for an object in the victim's mouth and remove it if present.

4 If the obstruction remains, begin chest compressions. Place the heel of one hand in the center of the chest between the nipples and the other hand on top of the first. Position your shoulders over your hands and lock your elbows. Give 30 chest compressions at a rate of 100 per minute. The chest should go down by 1½ to 2 inches. Then give two breaths, looking in the mouth for an expelled object. Continue chest compressions until help arrives. **Remember: Push hard and push fast at a rate of 100 compressions per minute.**

EMERGENCY CARE FOR CARDIAC ARREST

For cardiac arrest, the American Heart Association's revised (2005) Emergency Cardiac Care guidelines are as follows:

1 Call 911.

2 Start CPR (100 compressions per minute, stopping every 30 to 60 seconds to give two rescue breaths).

3 If an automatic external defibrillator (AED) is available, or when one arrives, give one shock to restart the victim's heart.

4 Go back to CPR immediately after the shock.

Don't wait for an emergency to learn how to use an AED or perform CPR.
To find a course in your area, contact the American Heart Association (800 242-8721) or the American Red Cross (202 303-4498).

FIGURE A.1 Emergency care for choking and for cardiac arrest.

SOURCES: Adapted from National Safety Council, 2007. *First Aid: Taking Action.* New York: McGraw-Hill, American Heart Association, 2005. Adult basic life support. *Circulation* 112: 19–34. New CPR guidelines. Simplicity to the rescue, 2006. *Harvard Health Letter,* March. Streamlined CPR guidelines a life-taking move, 2006. *Harvard Heart Letter,* February.

- Place a wire screen in front of fireplaces and woodstoves. Remove ashes carefully and store them in airtight metal containers, not paper bags.
- Properly maintain electrical appliances, kerosene heaters, and furnaces. Clean flues and chimneys annually.
- Keep portable heaters at least 3 feet away from curtains, bedding, towels, or anything that might catch fire. Never leave heaters on when you're out of the room or sleeping.

To be prepared for a fire:
- Plan at least two escape routes out of each room. Designate a location outside the home as a meeting place. Stage a home fire drill.
- Install a smoke detection device on every level of your home. Clean the detectors and test batteries once a month, and replace the batteries at least once a year.
- Keep a fire extinguisher in your home and know how to use it.

To prevent injuries from fire:
- Get out as quickly as possible and go to the designated meeting place. Don't stop for a keepsake or a pet. Never hide in a closet or under a bed. Once outside, count heads to see if everyone is out. If you think someone is still inside the burning building, tell the firefighters. Never go back inside a burning building.
- If you're trapped in a room, feel the door. If it is hot or if smoke is coming in through the cracks, don't open it; use the alternative escape route. If you can't get out of a room, go to the window and shout or wave for help.
- Avoid inhaling smoke. Smoke inhalation is the largest cause of death and injury in fires. To avoid inhaling smoke, crawl along the floor away from the heat and smoke. Cover your mouth and nose, ideally with a wet cloth, and take short, shallow breaths.
- If your clothes catch fire, don't run. Drop to the ground, cover your face, and roll back and forth to smother the flames. Remember: Stop-drop-roll.

Suffocation and Choking

Suffocation accounts for about 4000 deaths annually in the United States. Young children account for nearly half of these deaths. Children can suffocate if they put small items in their mouths, get tangled in their crib bedding, or get trapped in airtight appliances like old refrigerators. Keep small objects out of reach of children under age 3, and don't give them raw carrots, hot dogs, popcorn, peanuts, or hard candy. Examine toys carefully for small parts that could come loose; don't give plastic bags or balloons to small children.

Adults can also become choking victims, especially if they fail to chew food properly, eat hurriedly, or try to talk and eat at the same time. Many choking victims can be saved with abdominal thrusts, also called the Heimlich maneuver (see Figure A.1). Infants who are choking can be saved with blows to the upper back, followed by chest thrusts if necessary.

Incidents Involving Firearms

Firearms pose a significant threat of unintentional injury, especially to people between ages 5 and 29.

To prevent firearm injuries:
- Never point a loaded gun at something you do not intend to shoot.
- Always unload a firearm before storing it. Store unloaded firearms under lock and key in a place separate from ammunition.
- Inspect firearms carefully before handling them.
- If you ever plan to handle a gun, take a firearms safety course first.

LEISURE INJURIES

Leisure injuries take place in public places (but do not involve motor vehicles) and include recreational, sports, and transportation injuries. Many injuries in this category involve such recreational activities as boating and swimming, playground activities, in-line skating, and sports.

Drowning and Boating Injuries

Although most drownings are reported in lakes, ponds, rivers, and oceans, more than half the drownings of young children take place in residential pools. Among adolescents and adults, alcohol plays a significant role in many boating injuries and drownings.

To prevent drowning and boating injuries:
- Develop adequate swimming skill and make sure children learn to swim.
- Make sure residential pools are fenced and that children are never allowed to swim without supervision.
- Don't swim alone or in unsupervised places.
- Use caution when swimming in unfamiliar surroundings or for an unusual length of time. To avoid being chilled, don't swim in water colder than 70°F.
- Don't swim or boat under the influence of alcohol or other drugs. Don't chew gum or eat while in the water.
- Check the depth of water before diving.
- When on a boat, use a life jacket (personal flotation device).

In-Line Skating and Scooter Injuries

Most in-line skating injuries occur because users are not familiar with the equipment and do not wear appropriate safety gear. Injuries to the wrist and head are the most common. To reduce your risk of being injured while skating, wear a helmet, elbow and knee pads, wrist guards, a long-sleeved shirt, and long pants.

Wearing a helmet and knee and elbow pads is also important for preventing scooter injuries. The rise in popularity of lightweight scooters has seen a corresponding increase in associated injuries. Scooters should not be viewed as toys, and young children should be closely supervised. Be sure that handlebars, steering column, and all nuts and bolts are securely fastened. Ride on smooth, paved surfaces away from motor vehicle traffic. Avoid streets and surfaces with water, sand, gravel, or dirt.

Sports Injuries

Since more people have begun exercising to improve their health, there has been an increase in sports-related injuries.

To prevent sports injuries:

- Develop the skills required for the activity. Recognize and guard against the hazards associated with it.
- Always warm up and cool down.
- Make sure facilities are safe.
- Follow the rules and practice good sportsmanship.
- Use proper safety equipment, including, where appropriate, helmets, eye protection, knee and elbow pads, and wrist guards. Wear correct footwear.
- When it is excessively hot and humid, avoid heat stress by following the guidelines given in the box "Exercising in Hot Weather" in Chapter 3.

WORK INJURIES

Many aspects of workplace safety are monitored by the Occupational Safety and Health Administration (OSHA), a federal agency. The highest rate of work-related injuries occurs among laborers, whose jobs usually involve extensive manual labor and lifting—two areas not addressed by OSHA safety standards. Back injuries are the most common work injury.

To protect your back when lifting:

- Don't try to lift beyond your strength. If you need it, get help.
- Get a firm footing, with your feet shoulder-width apart. Get a firm grip on the object.
- Keep your torso in a relatively upright position and crouch down, bending at the knees and hips. Avoid bending at the waist. To lift, stand up or push up with your leg muscles. Lift gradually, keeping your arms straight. Keep the object close to your body.
- Don't twist. If you have to turn with an object, change the position of your feet.
- Put the object down gently, reversing the rules for lifting.

Another type of work-related injury is damage to the musculoskeletal system from repeated strain on the hand, arm, wrist, or other part of the body. Such repetitive-strain injuries are proliferating due to increased use of computers. One type, carpal tunnel syndrome, is characterized by pain and swelling in the tendons of the wrists and sometimes numbness and weakness.

To prevent carpal tunnel syndrome:

- Maintain good posture at the computer. Use a chair that provides back support and place the feet flat on the floor or on a footrest.
- Position the screen at eye level and the keyboard so the hands and wrists are straight.
- Take breaks periodically to stretch and flex your wrists and hands to lessen the cumulative effects of stress.

VIOLENCE AND INTENTIONAL INJURIES

According to the Federal Bureau of Investigation (FBI), nearly 1.4 million violent crimes occurred in the United States in 2005. Violence includes assault, sexual assault, homicide, domestic violence, suicide, and child abuse. Compared with rates of violence in other industrialized countries, U.S. rates are unusually high in two areas: homicide and firearm-related deaths.

Assault

Assault is the use of physical force to inflict injury or death on another person. Most assaults occur during arguments or in connection with another crime, such as robbery. Poverty, urban settings, and the use of alcohol and drugs are associated with higher rates of assault. The FBI estimates that more than 16,500 Americans were murdered in 2005. Homicide victims are most likely to be male, between ages 19 and 24, and members of minority groups. Most homicides are committed with a firearm; the murderer and the victim usually know each other.

To protect yourself at home:

- Secure your home with good lighting and effective locks, preferably deadbolts. Make sure that all doors and windows are securely locked.
- Get a dog or post "Beware of Dog" signs.
- Don't hide keys in obvious places, and don't give anyone the chance to duplicate your keys.
- Install a peephole in your front door. Don't open your door to people you don't know.
- If you or a family member owns a weapon, store it securely. Store guns and ammunition separately.
- If you are a woman living alone, use your initials rather than your full name in the phone directory. Don't use a greeting on your answering machine that implies you live alone or are not home.
- Teach everyone in the household how to get emergency assistance.
- Know your neighbors. Work out a system for alerting each other in case of an emergency.
- Establish a neighborhood watch program.

To protect yourself on the street:

- Avoid walking alone, especially at night. Stay where people can see and hear you.
- Walk on the outside of the sidewalk, facing traffic. Walk purposefully. Act alert and confident. If possible, keep at least two arm lengths between yourself and a stranger.
- Know where you are going. Appearing to be lost increases your vulnerability.
- Carry valuables in a fanny pack, pants pocket, or shoulder bag strapped diagonally across the chest.
- Always have your keys ready as you approach your vehicle or home.
- Carry a whistle to blow if you are attacked or harassed. If you feel threatened, run and/or yell. Go into a store or knock on the door of a home. If someone grabs you, yell, "Help!" or "Fire!"

To protect yourself in your car:

- Keep your car in good working condition, carry emergency supplies, and keep the gas tank at least half full.
- When driving, keep doors locked and windows rolled up at least three-quarters of the way.
- Park your car in well-lighted areas or parking garages, preferably those with an attendant or a security guard.
- Lock your car when you leave it, and check the interior before opening the door when you return.

- Don't pick up strangers. Don't stop for vehicles in distress; drive on and call for help.
- Note the location of emergency call boxes along highways and in public facilities. Carry a cell phone.
- If your car breaks down, raise the hood and tie a white cloth to the antenna or door handle. Wait in the car with the doors locked and windows rolled up. If someone approaches to offer help, open a window only a crack and ask the person to call the police or a towing service.
- When you stop at a light or stop sign, leave enough room to maneuver if you need an escape route.
- If you are involved in a minor automobile crash and you think you have been bumped intentionally, don't leave your car. Motion to the other driver to follow you to the nearest police station. If confronted by a person with a weapon, give up your car.

To protect yourself on public transportation:
- While waiting, stand in a populated, well-lighted area.
- Make sure that the bus, subway, or train is bound for your destination before you board it. Sit near the driver or conductor in a single seat or an outside seat.
- If you flag down a taxi, make sure that it's from a legitimate service. When you reach your destination, ask the driver to wait until you are safely inside the building.

To protect yourself on campus:
- Make sure that door and window locks are secure and that halls and stairwells have adequate lighting.
- Don't give dorm or residence keys to anybody.
- Don't leave your door unlocked or allow strangers into your room.
- Avoid solitary late-night trips to the library or laundry room. Take advantage of on-campus escort services.
- Don't exercise outside alone at night. Don't take shortcuts across campus that are unfamiliar or seem unsafe.
- If security guards patrol the campus, know the areas they cover and stay where they can see or hear you.

Sexual Assault—Rape and Date Rape

The use of force and coercion in sexual relationships is one of the most serious problems in human interactions. The most extreme manifestation of sexual coercion—forcing a person to submit to another's sexual desires—is rape. Taking advantage of circumstances that render a person incapable of giving consent (such as when drunk) is also considered sexual assault or rape. Coerced sexual activity in which the victim knows or is dating the rapist is often referred to as date rape.

Nearly 700,000 females are raped annually in the United States, and some males—perhaps 10,000 annually—are raped each year by other males. Rape victims suffer both physical and psychological injury. The psychological pain can be substantial and long-lasting.

To protect yourself against rape:
- Follow the guidelines listed earlier for protecting yourself against assault.
- Trust your gut feeling. If you feel you are in danger, don't hesitate to run and scream.

- Think out in advance what you would do if you were threatened with rape. However, no one knows what he or she will do when scared to death. Trust that you will make the best decision at the time—whether to scream, run, fight, or give in to avoid being injured or killed.

To protect yourself against date rape:
- Believe in your right to control what you do. Set limits and communicate them clearly, firmly, and early. Be assertive; men often interpret passivity as permission.
- If you are unsure of a new acquaintance, go on a group date or double date. If possible, provide your own transportation.
- Remember that some men think flirtatious behavior or sexy clothing indicates an interest in having sex.
- Remember that alcohol and drugs interfere with judgment, perception, and communication about sex. In a bar or at a party, don't leave your drink unattended, and don't accept opened beverages; watch your drinks being poured. At a party or club, check on friends and ask them to check on you.
- Use the statement that has proven most effective in stopping date rape: "This is rape and I'm calling the cops!"

If you are raped:
- Tell what happened to the first friendly person you meet.
- Call the police. Tell them you were raped and give your location.
- Try to remember everything you can about your attacker and write it down.
- Don't wash or douche before the medical exam. Don't change your clothes, but bring a new set with you if you can.
- Be aware that at the hospital you will have a complete exam. Show the physician any bruises or scratches.
- Tell the police exactly what happened. Be honest and stick to your story.
- If you do not want to report the rape to the police, see a physician as soon as possible. Be sure you are checked for pregnancy and STDs.
- Contact an organization with skilled counselors so you can talk about the experience. Look in the telephone directory under "Rape" or "Rape Crisis Center" for a hotline number.

Guidelines for men:
- Be aware of social pressure. It's OK not to score.
- Understand that "No" means "No." Stop making advances when your date says to stop. Remember that she has the right to refuse sex.
- Don't assume that flirtatious behavior or sexy clothing means a woman is interested in having sex, that previous permission for sex applies to the current situation, or that your date's relationships with other men constitute sexual permission for you.
- Remember that alcohol and drugs interfere with judgment, perception, and communication about sex.

Stalking and Cyberstalking

Stalking is characterized by harassing behaviors such as following or spying on a person and making verbal, written, or implied threats. It is estimated that 1 million U.S. women and 400,000 men are stalked each year; most stalkers are men.

Cyberstalking, the use of electronic communications devices to stalk another person, is becoming more common. Cyberstalkers may send harassing or threatening e-mails or chat room messages to the victim, or they may encourage others to harass the victim by posting inflammatory messages and personal information on bulletin boards or chat rooms.

To protect yourself online:
- Never use your real name as an e-mail user name or chat room nickname. Select an age- and gender-neutral identity.
- Avoid filling out profiles for accounts related to e-mail use or chat room activities with information that could be used to identify you.
- Do not share personal information in public spaces anywhere online or give it to strangers.
- Learn how to filter unwanted e-mail messages.
- If you experience harassment online, do not respond to the harasser. Log off or surf elsewhere. Save all communications for evidence. If harassment continues, report it to the harasser's Internet service provider, your Internet service provider, and the local police.
- Don't agree to meet someone you've met online face-to-face unless you feel completely comfortable about it. Schedule a series of phone conversations first. Meet initially in a very public place and bring along a friend to increase your safety.

Coping After Terrorism, Mass Violence, or Natural Disasters

Certain areas of the United States are prone to natural disasters like Hurricane Katrina, which devastated the Gulf Coast in 2005. Other natural disasters include tornadoes, floods, and earthquakes. Less frequent in the United States are episodes of mass violence or terrorist events such as those that occurred in Oklahoma in April 1995 and on September 11, 2001. When such events occur, some people suffer direct physical harm and/or the loss of relatives, friends, or possessions; many others experience emotional distress and are robbed of their sense of security.

Each person reacts differently to traumatic disaster, and it is normal to experience a variety of responses. Reactions may include disbelief and shock, fear, anger and resentment, anxiety about the future, difficulty concentrating or making decisions, mood swings, irritability, sadness and depression, panic, guilt, apathy, feelings of isolation or powerlessness, and many of the behaviorial signs such as headaches or insomnia that are associated with excess stress (see Chapter 10). Reactions may occur immediately or may be delayed until weeks or months after the event.

Taking positive steps can help you cope with powerful emotions. Consider the following strategies:

- Share your experiences and emotions with friends and family members. Be a supportive listener. Reassure children and encourage them to talk about what they are feeling.
- Take care of your mind and body. Choose a healthy diet, exercise regularly, get plenty of sleep, and practice relaxation techniques. Don't turn to unhealthy coping techniques such as using alcohol or other drugs.

- Take a break from media reports and images, and try not to develop nightmare scenarios for possible future events.
- Reestablish your routines at home, school, and work.
- Find ways to help others. Donating money, blood, food, clothes, or time can ease difficult emotions and give you a greater sense of control.

Everyone copes with tragedy in a different way and recovers at a different pace. If you feel overwhelmed by your emotions, seek professional help. Additional information about coping with terrorism and violence is available from the Federal Emergency Management Agency (www.fema.gov), the U.S. Department of Justice (www.usdoj.gov), and the National Mental Health Association (www.nmha.org).

Emergency Preparedness

Most prevention and coping activities related to terrorism, mass violence, and natural disasters occur at the federal, state, and community levels. However, one step individuals can take is to put together an emergency plan and kit for their family or household that can serve for any type of emergency or disaster.

Emergency Supplies   Your kit of emergency supplies should include everything you'll need to make it on your own for at least 3 days. You'll need nonperishable food, water, first aid and sanitation supplies, a battery-powered radio, clothing, a flashlight, cash, keys, copies of important documents, and supplies for sleeping outdoors in any weather. Remember special-needs items for infants, seniors, and pets. Supplies for a basic emergency kit are listed in Figure A.2; add to your kit based on your family situation and the type of problems most likely to occur in your area.

You may want to create several kinds of emergency kits. The primary one would contain supplies for home use. Put together a smaller, lightweight version that you can take with you if you are forced to evacuate your residence. Smaller kits for your car and your workplace are also recommended.

A Family or Household Plan   You and your family or household members should have a plan about where to meet and how to communicate. Choose at least two potential meeting places—one in your neighborhood and one or more in other areas. Your community may also have set locations for community shelters. Where you go may depend on the circumstances of the emergency situation. Use your common sense, and listen to the radio or television to obtain instructions from emergency officials about whether to evacuate or stay in place. In addition, know all the transportation options in the vicinity of your home, school, and workplace; roadways and public transit may be affected, so a sturdy pair of walking shoes is a good item to keep in your emergency kit.

Everyone in the family or household should also have the same emergency contact person to call, preferably someone who lives outside the immediate area and won't be affected by the same local disaster. Local phone service may be significantly disrupted, so long-distance calls may be more likely to go through. Everyone should carry the relevant phone numbers and addresses at all times.

Basic emergency supplies

- Map of the area for locating evacuation routes or shelters
- Cash, coins, and credit cards
- Copies of important documents stored in watertight container
- Emergency contact list and phone numbers
- Extra sets of house and car keys
- Flashlights or lightsticks
- Battery- or solar-powered radio
- Battery-powered alarm clock
- Extra batteries and bulbs
- Cell phone or prepaid phone card

- Signal flares
- Fire extinguisher (small A-B-C type)
- Whistle
- Ladder
- Tube tent and rope
- Sleeping bags or warm blankets
- Foam pads, pillows, baby bed
- Complete change of warm clothing, footwear, outerware (jacket or coat, long pants, long-sleeved shirt, sturdy shoes, hat, gloves, raingear, extra socks and underwear, sunglasses)
- Work gloves

- Shutoff wrench for gas and water supplies
- Shovel, hammer, pliers, screwdriver, and other tools
- Compass
- Matches in a waterproof container
- Aluminum foil
- Plastic storage containers, bucket
- Duct tape, utility knife, and scissors
- Paper, pens, pencils
- Needles and thread

First aid kit

- First aid manual
- Thermometer
- Scissors
- Tweezers
- Safety pins, safety razor blades
- Needle
- Latex or other sterile gloves
- Sterile gauze pads
- Cleansing agents (soap, isopropyl alcohol, antiseptic towelettes)
- Sunscreen

- Insect repellent
- Antibiotic ointment
- Burn ointment
- Petroleum jelly or another lubricant
- Sterile adhesive bandages, several sizes
- Sterile rolled bandages and triangular bandages
- Cotton balls
- Eyewash solution
- Chemical heat and cold packs
- Aspirin or nonaspirin pain reliever

- Anti-diarrhea medication
- Laxative
- Antacid
- Activated charcoal (use if advised by Poison Control Center)
- Potassium iodide (use following radiation exposure if advised by local health authorities)
- Prescription medications and prescribed medical supplies
- List of medications, dosages, and any allergies
- Medicine dropper

Special needs items

- Infant care needs (formula, bottles, diapers, powdered milk, diaper rash ointment)
- Books or toys
- Extra eyeglasses, contact lenses and supplies

- Feminine hygiene supplies
- Denture needs
- Hearing aid or wheelchair batteries; other special equipment

- Pet care supplies, including leash, pet carrier, copy of vaccination history, and tie-out stakes
- Other (list)

Food and related supplies

- Manual (nonelectric) can opener
- Utility knife
- Paper towels

- Eating utensils: Mess kits, or paper cups and plates and utensils
- Plastic garbage bags and resealing bags

- Small cooking stove and cooking fuel (if food must be cooked)
- Water purification tablets

Water: Three-day-supply, at least 1 gallon of water per person per day, stored in plastic containers:

Number of people: _____ x <u>1 gallon</u> x <u>3 days</u> = _____ total minimum gallons of water

Store additional water if you live in a hot climate or if your household includes infants, pregnant women, or people with special health needs. Don't forget to store water for pets. Containers can be sterilized by rinsing them with a diluted bleach solution (one part bleach to ten parts water). Replace your water supply every six months.

Food: At least a three-day supply of nonperishable foods—those requiring no refrigeration, preparation, or cooking and little or no water. Choose foods from the following list and add foods that members of your household will eat. Replace items in your food supply every six months.

- Ready-to-eat canned meats, fruits, soups, and vegetables
- Protein or fruit bars
- Dry cereal or granola
- Peanut butter
- Sugar, salt, pepper

- Dried fruit
- Nuts
- Crackers
- Canned, powdered, or boxed juices
- Nonperishable pasteurized milk or powered milk
- Coffee, tea, sodas

- High-energy foods
- Comfort/stress foods
- MREs (military rations)
- Infant formula and baby foods
- Pet foods

Sanitation

- Plastic garbage bags (and ties)
- Toilet paper
- Moist towelettes or hand soap
- Washcloth and towel

- Personal hygiene items (toothbrush, shampoo, deodorant, comb, shaving cream, and so on)
- Plastic bucket with tight lid

- Household chlorine bleach, disinfectant
- Powdered lime
- Small shovel for digging latrine

For a clean air supply

Face masks or several layers of dense-weave cotton material (handkerchiefs, t-shirts, towels) that fit snugly over your nose and mouth.

Shelter-in-place supplies, to be used in an interior room to create a barrier between you and potentially contaminated air outside: Heavyweight plastic garbage bags or plastic sheeting; duct tape; scissors; and if possible, a portable air purifier with a HEPA filter.

Family emergency plan

Plan places where your family will meet; choose one location near your home and one outside your neighborhood.

Local _____ Outside neighborhood _____

Have one local and one out-of-state contact person for family members to call if separated during a disaster. (It may be easier to make long-distance calls than local calls.)

Local _____ Out-of-state _____

FIGURE A.2 Sample emergency preparedness kit and plan.

It is also important to check into the emergency plans at any location where you or family members spend time, including schools and workplaces. For each location, know the safest place to be for different types of emergencies—for example, near load-bearing interior walls during an earthquake or in the basement during a tornado. Also know how to turn off water, gas, and electricity in case of damaged utility lines; keep the needed tools next to the shutoff valves.

Other steps you can take to help prepare for emergencies include taking a first aid class and setting up an emergency response group in your neighborhood, residential building, or office. Talk with your neighbors: Who has specialized equipment (for example, a power generator) or expertise that might help in a crisis? Do older or disabled neighbors have someone to help them? More complete information about emergency preparedness is available from local government agencies and from the following:

American Academy of Pediatrics (www.aap.org)
American Red Cross (www.redcross.org)
Federal Emergency Management Agency (www.fema.gov)
U.S. Department of Homeland Security (www.ready.gov)

PROVIDING EMERGENCY CARE

You can improve someone else's chances of surviving if you are prepared to provide emergency help. A course in first aid offered by the American Red Cross and on many college campuses can teach you to respond appropriately when someone needs help. Emergency rescue techniques can save the lives of people who have stopped breathing, who are choking, or whose hearts have stopped beating. Pulmonary resuscitation (also known as rescue breathing, artificial respiration, or mouth-to-mouth resuscitation) is used when a person is not breathing (see Figure A.1). Cardiopulmonary resuscitation (CPR) is used when a pulse can't be found. Training is required before a person can perform CPR. Significant changes were made to the guidelines for lay rescue CPR in 2005. Courses are offered by the American Red Cross and the American Heart Association.

When You Have to Provide Emergency Care

Remain calm and act sensibly. The basic pattern for providing emergency care is *check-call-care*:

1. **Check the situation.** Make sure the scene is safe for both you and the injured person. Don't put yourself in danger; if you get hurt too, you will be of little help to the injured person.

2. **Check the victim.** Conduct a quick head-to-toe examination. Assess the victim's signs and symptoms, such as level of responsiveness, pulse, and breathing rate. Look for bleeding and any indications of broken bones or paralysis.

3. **Call for help.** Call 911 or a local emergency number. Identify yourself and give as much information as you can about the condition of the victim and what happened.

4. **Care for the victim.** If the situation requires immediate action (no pulse, shock, etc.), provide first aid if you are trained to do so (see Figure A.1).

SELECTED BIBLIOGRAPHY

Bren, L. 2005. Prevent your child from choking. *FDA Consumer,* September/October.

Central Intelligence Agency. 2007. *The World Factbook.* Washington, D.C.: Central Intelligence Agency.

Federal Bureau of Investigation. 2006. *Hate Crime Statistics, 2005.* Washington, D.C.: U.S. Department of Justice.

Federal Bureau of Investigation. 2007. *Crime in the United States: Preliminary Annual Uniform Crime Reports, 2006.* Washington, D.C.: U.S. Department of Justice.

Insurance Information Institute. 2007. *Road Rage* (http://www.iii.org/individuals/auto/lifesaving/roadrage; retrieved June 14, 2007).

Iudice, A., et al. 2005. Effects of prolonged wakefulness combined with alcohol and hands-free cell phone divided attention tasks on simulated driving. *Human Psychopharmacology* 20(2): 125–132.

National Center for Health Statistics. 2006. Deaths: Preliminary Data for 2004. *National Vital Statistics Reports* 54(19).

National Center for Health Statistics. 2006. *Health, United States, 2006, with Chartbook on Trends in the Health of Americans.* Hyattsville, Md.: National Center for Health Statistics.

National Center for Injury Prevention and Control. 2006. *Intimate Partner Violence Fact Sheet* (http://www.cdc.gov/ncipc/factsheets/ipvfacts.htm; retrieved June 14, 2007).

National Center for Injury Prevention and Control. 2007. *Fire Deaths and Injuries Fact Sheet* (http://www.cdc.gov/ncipc/factsheets/fire.htm; retrieved June 14, 2007).

National Center for Injury Prevention and Control. 2007. *Sexual Violence Fact Sheet* (http://www.cdc.gov/ncipc/factsheets/svfacts.htm; retrieved June 14, 2007).

National Institute on Drug Abuse. 2005. NIDA *InfoFacts: Drugged Driving* (http://www.nida.nih.gov/Infofacts/driving.html; retrieved August 5, 2005).

National Safety Council. 2007. *Injury Facts 2007 Edition Kit.* Itasca, Ill.: National Safety Council.

National Traffic Safety Administration. 2005. *Traffic Safety Facts Research Note: Driver Cell Phone Use in 2004—Overall Results.* Washington, D.C.: National Traffic Safety Administration.

U.S. Department of Homeland Security. 2005. *Ready America* (www.ready.gov/index.html; retrieved March 4, 2005).

B

NUTRITIONAL CONTENT OF COMMON FOODS

For this food composition table, foods are listed within the following groups, corresponding to MyPyramid: (1) breads, cereals, rice, and pasta; (2) vegetables; (3) fruit; (4) milk, yogurt, and cheese; (5) meat, poultry, fish, dry beans, eggs, and nuts; and (6) fats, oils, sweets, and alcoholic beverages.

Data are provided for a variety of nutrients. For planning and easy reference, complete the following chart with your approximate daily goals or limits; refer to Chapter 8 and the Nutrition Resources section that follows Chapter 8. Fill in the daily totals that apply to your approximate daily calorie intake, sex, and age.

TOTAL DAILY GOAL OR LIMIT			
Total energy	_____ calories	Cholesterol	___300___ mg
Protein	_____ grams	Sodium	_____ mg
Carbohydrate	_____ grams	Vitamin A	_____ RE
Dietary fiber	_____ grams	Vitamin C	_____ mg
Total fat	_____ grams	Calcium	_____ mg
Saturated fat	_____ grams	Iron	_____ mg

This appendix contains information on the same nutrients found on most food labels, so you can make easy comparisons. On food labels, percent Daily Values without corresponding units are usually provided for vitamins and minerals. For reference, the Daily Values are as follows: 5000 IU of vitamin A, 60 mg of vitamin C, 1000 mg of calcium, and 18 mg of iron.

BREADS, CEREALS, RICE, AND PASTA
MyPyramid recommends a range of daily servings of grains based on caloric intake; for someone consuming a 2000-calorie diet, 6 ounce-equivalents are recommended, half of them whole grains. Each of the following counts as 1 ounce-equivalent: a slice of bread, a small muffin, 1 cup ready-to-eat cereal flakes, or ½ cup cooked cereal, rice, grains, or pasta.

Name	Amount	Weight g	Energy calories	Protein g	Carb. g	Fiber g	Total fat g	Sat. fat g	Chol. mg	Sod. mg	Vit. A RE	Vit. C mg	Calc. mg	Iron mg
Bagel, plain	1 bagel, 40″ dia.	89	229	8.9	45.0	2.0	1.4	0.4	0	399	0	1	79	5.4
Barley, pearled, cooked	½ cup	79	97	1.8	22.2	3.0	0.4	0.1	0	2	0	0	9	1.0
Bulgur, cooked	½ cup	91	76	2.8	16.9	4.1	0.2	0	0	5	0	0	9	0.9
Biscuit	1 biscuit, 2½″ dia.	35	128	2.2	17.0	0.5	5.8	0.9	0	368	0	0	17	1.2
Bread, corn	1 piece	60	188	4.3	28.9	1.4	6.0	1.6	37	467	26	0	44	1.1
Bread, French	1 slice	64	185	7.5	36.2	1.5	1.2	0.3	0	416	0	0	28	2.3
Bread, oatmeal	1 slice	27	73	2.3	13.1	1.1	1.2	0.2	0	162	1	0	18	0.73
Bread, pita, white	1 pita, 6½″ dia.	60	165	5.5	33.4	1.3	0.7	0.1	0	322	0	0	52	1.6
Bread, pita, whole wheat	1 pita, 6½″ dia.	64	170	6.3	35.2	4.7	1.7	0.3	0	340	0	0	10	2.0
Bread, pumpernickel	1 slice	26	65	2.3	12.4	1.7	0.8	0.1	0	174	0	0	18	0.8
Bread, raisin	1 slice	32	88	2.5	16.7	1.4	1.4	0.3	0	125	0	0	21	0.9
Bread, rye	1 slice	32	83	2.7	15.5	1.9	1.1	0.2	0	211	0	0.1	23	0.9
Bread sticks	2 sticks, 7⅝″ × ⅝″	20	82	2.4	13.7	0.6	1.9	0.3	0	131	0	0	4	0.9
Bread stuffing	½ cup	100	177	3.2	21.7	2.9	8.6	1.7	0	543	118	0	32	1.1
Bread, white	1 slice	30	80	2.3	15.2	0.7	1.0	0.2	0	204	0	0	45	1.1

Name	Amount	Weight g	Energy calories	Protein g	Carb. g	Fiber g	Total fat g	Sat. fat g	Chol. mg	Sod. mg	Vit. A RE	Vit. C mg	Calc. mg	Iron mg
Bread, whole wheat	1 slice	28	69	3.6	11.6	1.9	0.9	0.2	0	132	0	0	30	0.7
Buckwheat groats, cooked	½ cup	84	77	2.8	16.8	2.3	0.5	0.1	0	3	0	0	6	0.7
Cake, angelfood	¹/₁₂ of 10″ cake	50	128	3.1	29.4	0.1	0.2	0	0	254	0	0	42	0.1
Cake, chocolate w/frosting	⅛ of 18 oz cake	64	235	2.6	34.9	1.8	10.5	3.1	27	214	17	0.1	28	1.4
Cake, yellow w/frosting	⅛ of 18 oz cake	64	243	2.4	35.5	1.2	11.1	3.0	35	216	21	0	24	1.3
Cereal, All-Bran	½ cup	31	81	4.1	23.0	9.1	1.5	0.2	0	75	163	6.2	121	5.5
Cereal, Cheerios	1 cup	30	110	3.0	22.8	2.8	1.8	0.4	0	210	150	6.0	100	8.4
Cereal, corn flakes	1 cup	28	101	1.9	24.3	0.7	0	0	0	202	128	6.2	1	8.1
Cereal, Cream of Wheat	½ cup	125.5	65	1.9	13.8	0.6	0.3	0	0	69	0	0	58	5.2
Cereal, Frosted Flakes	¾ cup	31	114	1.0	28.0	1.0	0.2	0.1	0	148	160	6.2	2	4.5
Cereal, granola, low fat	½ cup	55	209	9.5	44.0	3.4	2.8	0.6	0	135	262	2.8	23	2.0
Cereal, raisin bran	1 cup	61	195	5.2	46.5	7.3	1.5	0.3	0	362	155	0.4	29	4.6
Cereal, Total	¾ cup	30	160	2.0	23.1	2.7	0.5	0.1	0	190	150	60.0	1000	18
Cereal, Wheat Chex	1 cup	50	180	5.0	40.55	5.4	1.0	0.1	0	420	150	6.0	100	14.4
Cereal, Wheaties	1 cup	30	110	3.0	24.2	3.0	1.0	0.2	0	210	150	6.0	20	8.4
Coffeecake w/topping	1 piece	56	178	3.1	30.0	0.7	5.4	1.0	27	236	20	0.1	76	0.8
Cookie, chocolate chip	1 medium cookie	15	69	0.5	8.9	0.5	3.4	1.1	0	49	0	0	2	0.4
Cookie, fig bar	1 cookie	16	56	0.6	11.3	0.7	1.2	0.2	0	56	1	0	10	0.5
Cookie, fortune	1 cookie	8	30	0.3	6.7	0.1	0.2	0.1	0	22	0	0	1	0.1
Cookie, oatmeal	1 large cookie	18	81	1.1	12.4	0.5	3.3	0.8	0	69	1	0.1	7	0.5
Cookie, sandwich	1 cookie	10	48	0.5	7.2	0.1	0.2	0.3	0	35	0	0	3	0.2
Corn meal, dry	¼ cup	35	126	2.9	26.8	2.6	0.6	0.1	0	1	0	0	2	1.4
Corn grits, cooked	½ cup	121	71	1.7	15.6	0.4	0.2	0	0	2	0	0	4	0.7
Couscous, cooked	½ cup	79	88	3.0	18.2	1.1	0.1	0	0	4	0	0	0	0.3
Cracker, crispbread, rye	3 crispbreads	30	110	2.4	24.7	5.0	0.4	0	0	79	0	0	9	0.7
Cracker, graham	3 squares	28	119	2.0	21.3	1.0	2.8	0.4	0	185	0	0	22	1.2
Cracker, matzo	1 matzo	28	111	2.8	23.4	0.8	0.4	0.1	0	1	0	0	4	0.9
Cracker, melba toast	6 pieces	30	117	3.6	23.0	1.9	1.0	0.1	0	249	0	0	28	1.1
Cracker, Ritz	5 crackers	16	79	1.2	10.3	0.3	3.7	0.6	0	124	0	0	24	0.6
Cracker, saltine	10 squares	30	128	2.8	21.3	0.9	3.4	0.5	0	322	0	0	20	1.7
Cracker, whole wheat	6 crackers	24	106	2.1	16.5	2.5	4.1	0.8	0	158	0	0	12	0.7
Croissant, butter	1 medium	57	231	4.7	26.1	1.5	12.0	6.6	38	424	117	0.1	21	1.2
Danish pastry, cheese	1 pastry	71	266	5.7	26.4	0.7	15.5	4.8	11	320	25	0.1	25	1.1
Doughnut, glazed	1 medium	45	192	2.3	22.9	0.7	10.3	2.7	14	181	1	0	27	0.5
English muffin, plain	½ muffin	29	67	2.2	13.1	0.8	0.5	0.1	0	132	0	0	50	0.3
French toast	1 slice	65	149	5.0	16.3	0	7.0	1.8	75	311	81	0.2	65	1.1
Macaroni, cooked	½ cup	70	111	4.1	21.6	1.3	0.7	0.1	0	1	0	0	5	1.0
Muffin, blueberry	2″ by 2¾″	57	162	3.71	23.2	0	6.2	1.2	21	251	22	0.9	108	1.3
Muffin, oat bran	1 small	66	178	4.6	31.9	3.0	4.9	0.7	0	259	0	0	42	2.8
Noodles, chow mein	½ cup	23	119	1.9	12.9	0.9	6.9	1.0	0	99	0	0	4	1.1
Noodles, egg, cooked	½ cup	80	110	3.6	20.0	1.0	1.7	0.3	23	4	5	0	10	1.2
Noodles, Japanese soba	½ cup	57	56	2.9	12.2	0	0.1	0	0	34	0	0	2	0.3
Oat bran, raw	¼ cup	24	58	4.1	15.6	3.6	1.7	0.3	0	1	0	0	14	1.3
Oatmeal, instant	1 packet	28	102	3.6	18.8	2.7	2.0	0.3	0	78	330	0	110	8.2
Pancake	4″ pancake	38	74	2.0	13.9	0.5	1.0	0.2	5	239	4	0.1	48	0.6
Pasta, cooked	2 oz.	57	75	2.9	14.2	0	0.6	0.1	19	3	3	0	3	0.7
Popcorn, air-popped	2 cups	16	62	2.0	12.4	2.3	0.7	0.1	0	1	2	0	1	0.5
Popcorn, oil-popped	2 cups	22	110	2.0	12.6	2.2	6.2	1.1	0	194	0	0.1	2	0.6
Pretzels, hard, salted	10 twists	60	228	6.2	47.9	1.8	1.6	0.2	0	814	0	0	11	3.1
Quinoa, uncooked	¼ cup	43	159	5.6	29.3	2.5	2.5	0.3	0	9	0	0	26	3.9
Rice, brown, cooked	½ cup	98	108	2.5	22.4	1.8	0.9	0.2	0	5	0	0	10	0.4
Rice cake	1 cake	9	35	0.7	7.3	0.4	0.3	0	0	29	0	0	1	0.1
Rice, white, cooked	½ cup	79	103	2.1	22.3	0.3	0.2	0	0	1	0	0	8	0.9
Rice, wild, cooked	½ cup	82	83	3.3	17.5	1.5	0.3	0	0	3	0	0	2	0.5
Roll, dinner	1 roll, 2″ square	28	87	3.0	14.6	0.6	1.8	0.4	0	150	0	0	50	1.0
Spaghetti, cooked	½ cup	70	110	4.0	21.4	1.3	0.6	0.1	0	90	0	0	5	0.9
Taco shell	1 medium	13	59	0.9	8.0	0.6	2.7	0.6	0	49	0	0	13	0.2
Tortilla chips	1 oz.	28	137	2.2	18.3	1.5	6.5	0.7	0	119	1	0	49	0.7
Tortilla, corn	1 medium	24	52	1.4	10.7	1.5	0.6	0.1	0	11	0	0	19	0.3
Tortilla, flour	8″ tortilla	51	146	4.4	25.3	0	3.1	0.4	0	249	0	0	97	1.0
Wheat germ, toasted	¼ cup	28	108	8.3	14.1	4.3	3.0	0.5	0	1	1	1.7	13	2.6

VEGETABLES

MyPyramid recommends a range of daily servings of vegetables based on caloric intake; for someone consuming a 2000-calorie diet, 2½ cups are recommended. Each of the following counts as ½ cup or equivalent: ½ cup raw or cooked vegetables, ½ cup vegetable juice, or 1 cup raw leafy salad greens.

Name	Amount	Weight g	Energy calories	Protein g	Carb. g	Fiber g	Total fat g	Sat. fat g	Chol. mg	Sod. mg	Vit. A RE	Vit. C mg	Calc. mg	Iron mg
Alfalfa sprouts	½ cup	17	4	0.7	0.4	0.3	0.1	0	0	1	1	1.4	5	0.2
Artichoke, cooked	1 medium	120	60	4.2	13.4	6.5	0.2	0	0	114	11	12.0	54	1.5
Arugula, raw	1 cup	20	5	0.5	0.7	0.3	0.1	0	0	5	24	3.0	32	0.3
Asparagus, cooked	6 spears	90	20	2.2	3.7	1.8	0.2	0.1	0	13	45	6.9	21	0.8
Bamboo shoots, canned	½ cup	66	12	1.1	2.1	0.9	0.3	0.1	0	5	1	0.7	5	0.2
*Beans, baked (plain)	½ cup	127	119	6.0	26.9	5.2	0.5	0.1	0	428	6	0	43	1.5
*Beans, black, cooked	½ cup	86	114	7.6	20.4	7.5	0.5	0.1	0	1	0	0	23	1.8
*Beans, fava, raw	½ cup	63	55	4.9	11.1	0	0.5	0.1	0	16	11	2.3	23	0.9
Beans, green snap, cooked	½ cup	63	22	1.2	4.9	2.0	0.2	0	0	1	22	6.1	28	0.4
*Beans, kidney, cooked	½ cup	89	112	7.7	20.2	5.7	0.4	0.1	0	1	0	1.1	31	2.0
*Beans, lentils, cooked	½ cup	99	115	8.9	19.9	7.8	0.4	0.1	0	2	0	1.5	19	3.3
*Beans, lima, cooked	½ cup	94	108	7.3	19.6	6.6	0.4	0.1	0	2	0	0	16	2.2
*Beans, navy, cooked	½ cup	91	127	7.5	23.7	9.6	0.5	0.1	0	0	0	0.8	63	2.2
*Beans, pinto, cooked	½ cup	85.5	122	7.7	22.4	7.7	0.6	0.1	0	1	0	0.7	39	1.8
*Beans, refried	½ cup	126	118	6.9	19.6	6.7	1.6	0.6	10	377	0	7.6	44	2.1
Beans, yellow snap, cooked	½ cup	63	22	1.2	4.9	2.1	0.2	0	0	2	2	6.1	29	0.8
Beet greens, cooked	½ cup	72	19	1.9	3.9	2.1	0.1	0	0	174	276	17.9	82	1.4
Beets, cooked	½ cup	85	37	1.4	8.5	1.7	0.2	0	0	65	2	3.1	14	0.7
Broccoli spears, cooked	2 spears	74	21	2.2	3.7	2.4	0.3	0	0	30	73	31.0	30	1.0
Brussels sprouts, cooked	4 sprouts	84	34	2.1	7.3	2.2	0.4	0.1	0	18	33	52.1	30	1.0
Cabbage, cooked	½ cup	75	17	1.0	4.1	1.4	0	0	0	6	3	28.1	36	0.1
Cabbage, raw	½ cup	45	11	0.6	2.6	1.1	0	0	0	8	2	16.3	18	0.2
Carrot, juice	¾ cup	177	71	1.7	16.4	1.4	0.3	0	0	51	1692	15.0	42	0.8
Carrots, cooked	½ cup	78	27	0.6	6.4	2.3	0.1	0	0	236	671	2.8	23	0.3
Carrots, raw	1 medium	61	25	0.6	5.8	1.7	0.2	0	0	42	513	3.6	20	0.2
Cauliflower, cooked	½ cup	62	14	1.1	2.5	1.7	0.3	0	0	9	1	27.5	10	0.2
Celery, raw	8 sticks	32	5	0.2	1.0	0.5	0	0	0	26	7	1.0	13	0.1
Chard, cooked	½ cup	88	18	1.6	3.6	1.8	0.1	0	0	157	268	15.8	51	2.0
Coleslaw, homemade	½ cup	60	47	0.8	7.4	0.9	1.6	0.2	5	14	32	19.6	27	0.4
Collards, cooked	½ cup	95	25	2.0	4.7	2.7	0.3	0	0	9	386	17.3	133	1.1
Corn, yellow, cooked	½ cup	82	89	2.7	20.6	2.3	1.1	0.2	0	14	11	5.1	2	0.5
Cucumber, raw	½ cup	52	8	0.3	1.9	0.3	0.1	0	0	1	3	1.5	8	0.2
Eggplant, cooked	½ cup	50	17	0.4	4.3	1.2	0.1	0	0	0	1	0.6	3	0.1
Endive, raw	½ cup	25	4	0.3	0.8	0.8	0.1	0	0	6	27	1.6	13	0.2
Hominy, canned	½ cup	83	59	1.2	11.8	2.1	0.7	0.1	0	173	0	0	8	0.5
Kale, cooked	½ cup	65	18	1.2	3.6	1.3	0.3	0	0	15	443	26.6	47	0.6
Kohlrabi, cooked	½ cup	83	24	1.5	5.5	0.9	0.1	0	0	17	2	44.5	21	0.3
Leeks, raw	½ cup	45	27	0.7	6.3	0.8	0.1	0	0	9	37	5.3	26	0.9
Lettuce, green leaf, shredded	1 cup	36	5	0.5	1.0	0.5	0.1	0	0	10	133	6.5	13	0.3
Lettuce, iceberg, shredded	1 cup	72	10	0.7	2.1	0.9	0.1	0	0	7	18	2.0	13	0.3
Lettuce, romaine, shredded	1 cup	47	8	0.6	1.5	1.0	0.1	0	0	4	136	11.3	16	0.5
Mushrooms, raw	½ cup	35	8	1.1	1.1	0.3	0.1	0	0	2	0	0.7	1	0.2
Mushrooms, cooked	½ cup	78	22	1.7	4.1	1.7	0.3	0	0	2	0	3.1	5	1.4
Mustard greens, cooked	½ cup	70	10	1.6	1.5	1.4	0.2	0	0	11	221	17.7	52	0.5
Okra, cooked	½ cup	80	18	1.5	3.6	2.0	0.1	0	0	5	11	13.0	62	0.2
Onion, raw	½ cup	80	32	0.9	7.5	1.4	0.1	0	0	3	0	5.9	18	0.2
Parsley, raw	2 tablespoons	8	3	0.2	0.5	0.3	0.1	0	0	4	32	10.1	10	0.5
Parsnip, raw	½ cup	67	50	0.8	12.0	3.3	0.2	0	0	7	0	11.3	24	0.4
*Peas, chickpeas (garbanzos)	½ cup	82	134	7.3	22.5	6.2	2.1	0.2	0	6	1	1.1	40	2.4
Peas, edible, podded	10 pea pods	34	14	1.0	2.6	0.9	0.1	0	0	1	18	20.4	15	0.7
Peas, green	½ cup	80	67	4.3	12.5	4.4	0.2	0	0	2	32	11.4	22	1.2
*Peas, split, cooked	½ cup	98	116	8.2	20.6	8.1	0.4	0.1	0	2	0	0.4	14	1.3
Pepper, green chili, canned	½ cup	70	15	0.5	3.2	1.2	0.2	0	0	276	4	23.8	25	0.9
Pepper, sweet green, raw	1 small	74	15	0.6	3.4	1.3	0.1	0	0	2	13	59.5	7	0.3
Pepper, sweet red, raw	1 small	74	19	0.7	4.5	1.5	0.2	0	0	1	116	140.6	7	0.3

Name	Amount	Weight g	Energy calories	Protein g	Carb. g	Fiber g	Total fat g	Sat. fat g	Chol. mg	Sod. mg	Vit. A RE	Vit. C mg	Calc. mg	Iron mg
Pickle, dill	1 medium	65	8	0.4	1.7	0.7	0.1	0	0	569	6	0.5	27	0.2
Potato, mashed w/milk	½ cup	105	87	2.0	18.4	1.6	0.6	0.3	2	317	4	7.0	25	0.3
Potato salad	½ cup	125	179	3.4	14.0	1.6	10.3	1.8	85	661	40	12.5	24	0.8
Potato, baked w/skin	1 medium	173	161	4.3	36.6	3.8	0.1	0	0	17	2	16.6	26	1.9
Potato, boiled	1 potato, 2 ½" dia.	136	118	2.5	27.4	2.4	0.1	0	0	5	0	17.7	7	0.4
Potato, french fries	10 fries	50	109	1.7	17.0	1.6	4.1	1.9	0	22	0	4.8	5	0.7
Pumpkin, canned	½ cup	123	42	1.3	9.9	3.6	0.3	0.2	0	6	953	5.1	32	1.7
Radish, raw	13 medium	59	9	0.4	2.0	0.9	0	0	0	23	0	8.7	15	0.2
Rutabaga, mashed	½ cup	120	47	1.5	10.5	2.2	0.3	0	0	24	0	22.6	58	0.6
Sauerkraut, canned	½ cup	71	13	0.6	3.0	1.8	0.1	0	0	469	1	10.4	21	1.0
Soybeans, green, boiled	½ cup	90	127	11.1	9.9	3.8	5.8	0.7	0	13	7	15.3	131	2.3
Spinach, raw	1 cup	30	7	0.9	1.1	0.7	0.1	0	0	24	141	8.4	30	0.8
Spinach, cooked	½ cup	90	21	2.7	3.4	2.2	0.2	0	0	63	472	8.8	122	3.2
Squash, summer, raw	½ small squash	59	9	0.7	2.0	0.6	0.1	0	0	1	6	10.0	9	0.2
Squash, summer, cooked	½ cup	90	18	0.8	3.9	1.3	0.3	0	0	1	10	5.0	24	0.3
Squash, winter	½ cup	103	38	0.9	9.1	2.9	0.4	0.1	0	1	268	9.8	23	0.5
Sweet potato, baked	½ cup	100	90	2.0	20.7	3.3	0.2	0	0	36	961	19.6	38	0.7
Sweet potato, canned w/syrup	½ cup	114	101	1.1	23.7	2.9	0.2	0.1	0	50	430	12.0	17	0.9
Tomato, red, raw	1 medium	123	22	1.1	4.8	1.8	0.2	0	0	13	21	16.0	17	0.9
Tomato sauce	½ cup	122	29	1.6	6.6	1.8	0.2	0	0	642	21	8.6	16	1.3
Tomato juice	¾ cup	182	31	1.4	7.7	0.7	0.1	0	0	18	42	33.4	18	0.8
Turnip, cooked, mashed	½ cup	115	25	0.8	5.8	2.3	0.1	0	0	118	0	13.3	38	0.2
Vegetable juice	¾ cup	182	34	1.1	8.3	1.5	0.2	0	0	490	142	50.3	20	0.8
Vegetables, mixed	½ cup	91	59	2.6	11.9	4.0	0.1	0	0	32	195	2.9	23	0.7
Vegetable soup	1 cup	241	72	2.1	12.0	0.5	1.9	0.3	0	822	116	1.4	22	1.1
Waterchestnuts	½ cup	62	60	0.9	14.8	1.9	0.1	0	0	9	0	2.5	7	0

*Dry beans and peas (legumes) can be counted as servings of vegetables or as servings from the meat, poultry, fish, dry beans, eggs, and nuts group. They are listed here and marked with an asterisk.

FRUIT

MyPyramid recommends a range of daily servings of fruit based on caloric intake; for someone consuming a 2000-calorie diet, 2 cups are recommended. Each of the following counts as ½ cup or equivalent: ½ cup fresh, canned, or frozen fruit, ½ cup fruit juice, 1 small whole fruit, or ¼ cup dried fruit.

Name	Amount	Weight g	Energy calories	Protein g	Carb. g	Fiber g	Total fat g	Sat. fat g	Chol. mg	Sod. mg	Vit. A RE	Vit. C mg	Calc. mg	Iron mg
Apple, raw, w/skin	1 medium	138	72	0.4	19.1	3.3	0.2	0	0	1	4	6.3	8	0.2
Apple juice	¾ cup	179	84	0.3	20.7	0.2	0.2	0	0	13	0	44.8	11	0.5
Apple sauce, unsweetened	½ cup	122	52	0.2	13.8	1.5	0.1	0	0	2	1	25.9	4	0.1
Apricots	2 medium	70	34	1.0	7.8	1.4	0.3	0	0	1	67	7.0	10	0.3
Apricots, dried	9 halves	32	76	1.1	19.7	2.3	0.1	0	0	3	57	0.3	17	0.8
Avocado	1 medium	201	322	4.0	17.1	13.5	29.5	4.3	0	14	14	20.1	24	1.1
Banana	1 medium	118	105	1.3	27.0	3.1	0.4	0.1	0	1	4	10.3	6	0.3
Blackberries, raw	½ cup	72	31	1.0	6.9	3.8	0.4	0	0	1	8	15.1	21	0.5
Blueberries	½ cup	74	42	0.6	10.7	1.8	0.2	0	0	1	2	7.2	4	0.2
Cantaloupe	¼ melon, 5" dia.	138	47	1.2	11.3	1.2	0.3	0.1	0	22	233	50.6	12	0.3
Carambola (starfruit)	1 small	70	22	0.7	4.7	1.2	0.2	0	0	1	2	24.1	2	0.1
Cherries, sweet, raw	11 cherries	75	47	0.8	12.0	1.6	0.2	0	0	0	2	5.2	10	0.3
Cherries, canned in syrup	½ cup	127	105	0.8	26.9	1.9	0.2	0	0	4	10	4.6	11	0.4
Cranberries, raw	½ cup	48	22	0.2	6.0	2.2	0.1	0	0	1	1	6.3	4	0.1
Cranberry juice cocktail	¾ cup	190	102	0	25.6	0	0.2	0	0	4	0	80.3	6	0.2
Cranberry sauce	¼ cup	69	105	0.1	26.9	0.7	0.1	0	0	20	1	1.4	3	0.2
Currants, dried	¼ cup	36	102	1.5	26.7	2.4	0.1	0	0	3	1	1.7	31	1.2
Dates, dried	¼ cup	45	125	1.1	33.4	3.6	0.2	0	0	1	0	0.2	17	0.5
Figs, raw	2 medium	100	74	0.8	19.2	2.9	0.3	0.1	0	1	7	2.0	35	0.4
Fruit cocktail, heavy syrup	½ cup	124	91	0.5	23.4	1.2	0.1	0	0	7	12	2.4	7	0.4
Fruit cocktail, light syrup	½ cup	121	69	0.5	18.1	1.2	0.1	0	0	7	12	2.3	7	0.4
Fruit cocktail, juice	½ cup	119	55	0.5	14.1	1.2	0	0	0	5	18	3.2	9	0.3
Grapefruit	½ medium	123	37	0.7	9.2	1.4	0.1	0	0	0	16	45.5	18	0.2
Grapefruit juice	¾ cup	185	72	1.0	17.0	0	0.2	0	0	2	41	70.4	17	0.4
Grapes	10 grapes	49	34	0.4	8.9	0.4	0.1	0	0	1	1	5.3	5	0.2

Name	Amount	Weight g	Energy calories	Protein g	Carb. g	Fiber g	Total fat g	Sat. fat g	Chol. mg	Sod. mg	Vit. A RE	Vit. C mg	Calc. mg	Iron mg
Guava	1 fruit	55	37	1.4	7.9	3.0	0.5	0.2	0	1	17	125.6	10	0.3
Honeydew	1/8 melon, 5 1/4" dia.	125	45	0.7	11.4	1.0	0.1	0	0	22	4	22.5	8	0.2
Kiwifruit	1 large	91	56	0.9	13.5	3.1	0.4	0	0	5	8	68.2	24	0.4
Kumquats	5 fruits	95	67	1.8	15.1	6.2	0.8	0.1	0	10	14	41.7	59	0.8
Lemon, with peel	1 fruit	108	22	1.3	11.6	5.1	0.3	0	0	3	2	83.2	66	0.8
Lemon juice	2 tablespoons	30	6	0.1	1.9	0.1	0.1	0	0	6	0	7.4	3	0
Mango	1/2 medium	103	67	0.5	17.0	1.9	0.3	0.1	0	2	39	28.7	10	0.1
Nectarine	1 fruit	142	62	1.5	15	2.4	0.5	0	0	0	24	7.7	9	0.4
Olives, ripe	10 large	44	51	0.4	2.8	1.4	4.7	0.6	0	384	9	0.4	39	1.5
Orange	1 medium	131	62	1.2	15.4	3.1	0.2	0	0	0	14	69.7	52	0.1
Orange juice	3/4 cup	186	84	1.3	19.3	0.4	0.4	0	0	2	19	93	20	0.4
Papaya	1/2 medium	152	59	0.9	14.9	2.7	0.2	0.1	0	5	84	93.9	36	0.2
Peach, raw	1 medium	150	58	1.4	14.3	2.2	0.4	0	0	0	24	9.9	6	0.4
Peach, canned in juice	1/2 cup	125	55	0.8	14.3	1.6	0	0	0	5	24	4.5	7	0.3
Pear, raw	1 medium	178	103	0.7	27.5	5.5	0.2	0	0	2	2	7.5	16	0.3
Pear, canned	1/2 cup	124	62	0.4	16	2.0	0.1	0	0	5	0	2.0	11	0.4
Persimmon, raw	1 fruit	25	32	0.2	8.4	0	0.1	0	0	0	0	16.5	7	0.6
Pineapple, canned in juice	1/2 cup	125	75	0.5	19.5	1.0	0.1	0	0	1	2	11.8	17	0.3
Pineapple, raw	1 slice, 3 1/2" × 3/4"	84	40	0.5	10.6	1.2	0.1	0	0	1	3	30.4	11	0.2
Plantain, raw	1 medium	179	218	2.3	57.1	4.1	0.6	0.3	0	7	100	32.9	5	1.1
Plums	1 1/2 medium	99	46	0.7	11.3	1.4	0.3	0	0	0	17	9.4	6	0.2
Prune juice	3/4 cup	192	136	1.2	33.5	1.9	0.1	0	0	8	0	7.9	23	2.3
Prunes (dried plums)	5 prunes	48	114	1.0	30.3	3.4	0.2	0	0	1	19	0.3	20	0.4
Raisins	1/4 cup	41	125	1.4	32.8	1.6	0.2	0	0	5	0	1.3	22	0.7
Raspberries	1/2 cup	62	32	0.7	7.3	4.0	0.4	0	0	1	1	16.1	15	0.4
Rhubarb, raw	1 stalk	51	11	0.5	2.3	0.9	0.1	0	0	2	3	4.1	44	0.1
Strawberries	5 large	90	29	0.6	6.9	2.1	0.3	0	0	1	1	52.9	14	0.4
Tangerine	1 medium	88	47	0.7	11.7	1.6	0.3	0	0	2	30	23.5	33	0.1
Watermelon	1/16 melon	283	85	1.7	21.3	1.1	0.4	0	0	3	79	22.9	20	0.7

MILK, YOGURT, AND CHEESE

MyPyramid recommends a range of daily servings of milk products based on caloric intake; for someone consuming a 2000-calorie diet, 3 cups of milk or the equivalent are recommended. Each of the following counts as 1 cup: 1 cup milk or yogurt, 1/2 cup ricotta cheese, 1 1/2 ounces natural cheese, or 2 ounces processed cheese.

Name	Amount	Weight g	Energy calories	Protein g	Carb. g	Fiber g	Total fat g	Sat. fat g	Chol. mg	Sod. mg	Vit. A RE	Vit. C mg	Calc. mg	Iron mg
Buttermilk, lowfat	1 cup	245	98	8.1	11.7	0	2.2	1.3	10	257	17	2.5	284	0.1
Cheese, American	2 oz.	57	188	11.1	4.7	0	13.9	8.7	36	548	90	0	282	0.5
Cheese, blue	1 1/2 oz.	43	150	9.1	1.0	0	12.2	7.9	32	593	84	0	225	0.1
Cheese, cheddar	1 1/2 oz.	43	171	10.6	0.5	0	14.1	9.0	45	264	113	0	307	0.3
Cheese, cottage, creamed	1 cup	210	216	26.2	5.6	0	9.5	6.0	32	850	92	0	126	0.3
Cheese, cottage, lowfat (1%)	1 cup	226	163	28.0	6.1	0	2.3	1.5	9	918	25	0	138	0.3
Cheese, cottage, non-fat	1 cup	145	123	25.0	2.7	0	0.6	0.4	10	19	13	0	46	0.3
Cheese, cream	2 oz.	57	198	4.3	1.5	0	19.8	12.5	62	168	208	0	45	0.7
Cheese, cream, fat free	2 oz.	57	55	8.2	3.3	0	0.8	0.5	5	311	159	0	105	0.1
Cheese, feta	1 1/2 oz.	43	112	6.0	1.7	0	9.0	6.4	38	475	53	0	210	0.3
Cheese, Mexican	1 1/2 oz.	43	151	9.6	1.2	0	12.0	7.6	45	279	23	0	281	0.2
Cheese, Monterey	1 1/2 oz.	43	159	10.4	0.3	0	12.9	8.1	38	228	84	0	317	0.3
Cheese, mozzarella (part skim)	1 1/2 oz.	43	108	10.3	1.2	0	6.8	4.3	27	263	54	0	333	0.1
Cheese, Parmesan, grated	2 tablespoons	10	43	3.9	0.4	0	2.9	1.7	9	153	12	0	111	0.1
Cheese, process spread	2 oz.	56	170	9.1	5.5	0	12.3	8.1	45	839	100	0.1	261	0.1
Cheese, provolone	1 1/2 oz.	43	149	10.9	0.9	0	11.3	7.3	29	373	100	0	321	0.2
Cheese, ricotta, part skim	1/2 cup	123	170	14.0	6.3	0	9.7	6.1	38	154	132	0	335	0.5
Cheese, Swiss	1 1/2 oz.	43	162	11.5	2.3	0	11.8	7.6	39	82	94	0	336	0.1
Ice cream, chocolate	1 cup	132	285	5.0	37.2	1.6	14.2	9.0	45	100	156	0.9	144	1.2
Ice cream, vanilla, rich	1 cup	214	533	7.5	47.7	0	34.7	22.1	197	131	389	0	250	0.7
Ice cream, vanilla, light	1 cup	152	251	7.3	39.2	0.5	7.3	4.4	41	12	195	1.8	245	0.3
Ice cream, vanilla, soft-serve	1 cup	172	382	7.0	38.2	1.2	22.4	12.9	157	105	279	1.4	225	0.4
Milk, chocolate	1 cup	250	208	7.9	25.9	2.0	8.5	5.3	30	150	65	2.2	280	0.6
Milk, fat free (nonfat)	1 cup	245	83	8.3	12.1	0	0.2	0.3	5	103	149	0	306	0.1
Milk, lowfat (1%)	1 cup	244	102	8.2	12.2	0	2.4	1.6	12	107	142	0	290	0.1

Name	Amount	Weight g	Energy calories	Protein g	Carb. g	Fiber g	Total fat g	Sat. fat g	Chol. mg	Sod. mg	Vit. A RE	Vit. C mg	Calc. mg	Iron mg
Milk, reduced fat (2%)	1 cup	244	122	8.1	11.2	0	4.8	3.0	20	122	134	0.5	285	0.1
Milk, whole	1 cup	244	146	7.9	11.0	0	7.9	4.6	24	98	68	0	276	0.1
Pudding, chocolate	½ cup	147	163	4.6	27.6	1.5	4.6	2.7	16	417	38	1.3	150	0.4
Yogurt, frozen, vanilla	1 cup	144	235	5.8	34.9	0	8.1	4.9	3	125	85	1.2	206	0.4
Yogurt, lowfat, plain	8 oz. container	227	143	11.9	16.0	0	3.5	2.3	14	159	32	1.8	415	0.2
Yogurt, lowfat, with fruit	8 oz. container	227	238	11.0	42.2	0	3.2	2.1	14	132	36	1.6	345	0.2
Yogurt, nonfat, plain	8 oz. container	227	127	13.0	17.4	0	0.4	0.3	5	175	5	2.0	452	0.2

MEAT, POULTRY, FISH, DRY BEANS, EGGS, AND NUTS

MyPyramid recommends a range of daily servings of meat and beans based on caloric intake; for someone consuming a 2000-calorie diet, 5.5 ounce-equivalents are recommended. Each of the following counts as 1 ounce-equivalent: 1 ounce cooked lean meat, poultry, or fish; ¼ cup cooked dry beans or tofu; 1 egg; 1 tablespoon peanut butter; or ½ ounce nuts or seeds.

Name	Amount	Weight g	Energy calories	Protein g	Carb. g	Fiber g	Total fat g	Sat. fat g	Chol. mg	Sod. mg	Vit. A RE	Vit. C mg	Calc. mg	Iron mg
Bacon, Canadian	2 slices	47	87	11.3	0.6	0	3.9	1.3	27	727	0	0	5	0.4
Beef, lean, fat trimmed	3 oz.	85	179	25.4	0	0	7.9	3.0	73	56	0	0	7	2.5
Beef, corned	3 oz.	85	213	15.4	0	0	16.1	5.3	83	964	0	0	7	1.6
Beef, ground, 95% lean, broiled	3 oz.	85	145	22.4	0	0	5.6	2.5	65	55	0	0	6	2.4
Beef, ground, 85% lean, broiled	3 oz.	85	212	22.0	0	0	13.2	5.0	76	61	0	0	15	2.2
Beef, ground, 70% lean, broiled	3 oz.	85	232	21.6	0	0	15.5	6.3	70	69	0	0	30	1.9
Beef liver, braised	1 slice	68	130	19.8	0	0	3.6	1.2	269	54	6421	1.3	4	4.5
Beef ribs, broiled	3 oz.	85	309	20.1	0	0	24.8	10.5	71	53	0	0	11	1.8
Chicken breast, w/skin, rst	½ breast	98	193	29.2	0	0	7.6	2.1	82	70	27	0	14	1.0
Chicken, dk mt, w/skin, rst	3 oz.	85	215	22.1	0	0	13.4	3.7	77	74	51	0	13	1.2
Chicken, dk mt, w/o skin, rst	3 oz.	85	205	27.4	0	0	9.7	2.7	93	93	22	0	15	1.3
Chicken, dk mt, w/skin, fried	3 oz.	85	253	18.6	8.0	0	15.8	4.2	76	251	26	0	18	1.2
Chicken, drumstick, w/skin, rst	1 drumstick	52	112	14.1	0	0	5.8	1.6	47	47	16	0	6	0.7
Chicken, lt mt, w/skin, rst	3 oz.	85	189	24.7	0	0	9.2	2.6	71	64	28	0	13	1.0
Chicken, lt mt, w/o skin, rst	3 oz.	85	147	26.3	0	0	3.8	1.1	72	65	8	0	13	0.9
Chicken, lt mt, w/skin, fried	3 oz.	85	235	20.0	8.1	0	13.1	3.5	71	244	20	0	17	1.1
Chicken, thigh, w/skin, rst	1 thigh	62	153	15.5	0	0	9.6	2.7	58	52	31	0	7	0.8
Chicken, wing, w/skin, rst	1 wing	34	99	9.1	0	0	6.6	1.9	29	28	16	0	5	0.4
Chicken liver, pan-fried	3 oz.	100	172	25.8	1.1	0	6.4	1.7	564	92	4296	2.7	10	12.9
Egg white, large	1 egg white	33	17	3.6	0.2	0	0	0	0	55	0	0	2	0
Egg, whole, large	1 egg	50	74	6.3	0.4	0	5.0	1.6	212	70	70	0	26	0.9
Egg yolk, large	1 yolk	17	55	2.7	0.6	0	4.5	1.6	210	8	65	0	22	0.5
Fish, catfish, baked/broiled	3 oz.	85	129	15.9	0	0	6.8	1.5	54	68	13	0.7	8	0.7
Fish, cod, baked/broiled	3 oz.	85	89	19.4	0	0	0.7	0.1	47	66	12	0.8	0.2	0.4
Fish, halibut, baked/broiled	3 oz.	85	119	22.7	0	0	2.5	0.4	35	59	46	0	51	0.9
Fish, salmon, baked/broiled	3 oz.	85	175	18.8	0	0	10.5	2.1	54	52	13	3.1	13	0.3
Fish, salmon, canned, w/o salt	3 oz.	85	130	17.4	0	0	6.2	1.4	37	64	45	0	203	0.9
Fish, salmon, smoked	3 oz.	85	99	15.5	0	0	3.7	0.8	20	666	22	0	9	0.7
Fish, sardine, canned in oil	1 can (3.75 oz.)	92	191	22.7	0	0	10.5	1.4	131	465	29	0	351	2.7
Fish, snapper, baked/broiled	3 oz.	85	109	22.3	0	0	1.5	0.3	40	48	30	1.4	34	0.2
Fish sticks	3 sticks	84	209	9.3	17.8	1.2	11.1	1.7	27	354	26	0	22	0.9
Fish, swordfish, baked/broiled	3 oz.	85	132	21.6	0	0	4.4	1.2	42	98	35	0.9	5	0.9
Fish, trout, baked/broiled	3 oz.	85	162	22.6	0	0	7.2	1.3	63	57	16	0.4	47	1.6
Fish, tuna, canned in oil	3 oz.	85	158	22.6	0	0	6.9	1.2	26	337	4	0	3	0.6
Fish, tuna, canned in water	3 oz.	85	109	20.1	0	0	2.5	0.7	36	320	5	0	12	0.8
Ham, extra lean	3 oz.	85	116	18.0	0.4	0	4.1	1.4	26	965	0	0	5	0.8
Ham, regular	3 oz.	85	137	13.9	3.2	1.1	7.2	2.5	48	1095	0	3.4	20	0.9
Lamb, trimmed	3 oz.	85	218	20.8	0	0	14.3	6.7	74	65	0	0	14	1.6
Lunch meat, beef pastrami, cured	3 oz.	84	123	18.3	0	0	4.9	2.3	57	743	28	1.1	8	1.9
Lunch meat, beef, sliced	3 oz.	85	127	16.2	0.8	0	6.0	2.5	60	1201	0	0	9	1.8
Lunch meat, bologna (beef)	3 slices	84	261	8.6	3.3	0	23.7	9.4	47	907	11	12.8	26	0.9
Lunch meat, bologna (turkey)	3 slices	84	176	9.6	3.9	0.4	13.5	3.7	63	1052	8	11.2	103	2.5
Lunch meat, chicken breast, fat-free	3 oz.	85	67	14.3	1.8	0	0.3	0.1	31	924	0	0	5	0.3
Lunch meat, franks (beef)	1 frank	56	162	7.0	1.2	0	14.4	5.9	38	557	2	11.2	8	1.0
Lunch meat, franks (chicken)	1 frank	45	116	5.8	3.1	0	8.8	2.5	45	616	18	0	43	0.9

Name	Amount	Weight g	Energy calories	Protein g	Carb. g	Fiber g	Total fat g	Sat. fat g	Chol. mg	Sod. mg	Vit. A RE	Vit. C mg	Calc. mg	Iron mg
Lunch meat, liverwurst	3 oz.	85	277	12.0	1.9	0	24.2	9.0	134	731	7066	0	22	5.4
Lunch meat, salami, dry	8 slices	80	326	18.1	1.2	0	27.0	9.5	63	1808	0	0	10	1.0
Lunch meat, turkey, smoked	3 oz.	85	85	15.0	2.0	0	2.0	0.5	36	781	0	0	8	0.6
Luncheon slices, meatless	3 oz.	85	161	15.1	3.8	0	9.4	1.1	0	604	0	0	35	1.5
Meatloaf (80% lean meat)	3 oz.	85	216	21.5	0	0	13.7	5.2	76	57	0	0	20	2.2
Nuts, almonds	⅓ cup	47	273	10.0	9.3	5.6	23.9	1.8	0	0	0	0	117	2.0
Nuts, cashews, dry roasted, w/o salt	⅓ cup	46	262	7.0	14.9	1.4	21.2	4.2	0	7	0	0	21	2.7
Nuts, chestnuts, roasted	⅓ cup	48	117	1.5	25.2	2.4	1.0	0.2	0	1	1	12.4	14	0.4
Nuts, macadamia, dry roasted	⅓ cup	45	321	3.5	6.0	3.6	34.0	5.3	0	2	0	0.3	31	1.2
Nuts, pecans	⅓ cup	36	249	3.3	5.0	3.5	25.9	2.2	0	0	1	0.4	25	0.9
Nuts, pine	⅓ cup	45	300	6.1	5.8	1.6	30.5	2.2	0	1	0	0.4	7	2.5
Nuts, pistachios, dry roasted	⅓ cup	41	234	8.8	11.3	4.2	18.9	2.3	0	4	5	0.9	45	1.7
Nuts, walnuts	⅓ cup	40	261	6.1	5.5	2.7	26.1	2.5	0	1	0	0.5	39	1.2
Peanut butter, chunky	2 tablespoons	32	188	7.7	6.9	2.6	16.0	2.6	0	156	0	0	14	0.6
Peanut butter, smooth	2 tablespoons	32	188	8.0	6.3	1.9	16.1	3.3	0	147	0	0	14	0.6
Peanuts, dry roasted	⅓ cup	48	281	11.4	10.4	3.9	23.9	3.3	0	3	0	0	26	1.1
Pork chop, pan fried	3 oz.	85	205	21.0	0	0	12.8	4.4	70	66	2	0.7	19	0.9
Pork ribs, braised	3 oz.	85	252	20.3	0	0	18.3	6.8	74	50	2	0.6	25	1.0
Pork roast	3 oz.	85	214	22.9	0	0	12.9	4.5	69	41	3	0	5	0.8
Pumpkin seeds, roasted	¼ cup	57	296	18.7	7.6	2.2	23.9	4.5	0	10	22	1.0	24	8.5
Sausage, beef	1 sausage	43	134	6.1	1.0	0	11.6	4.9	29	486	0	0	3	0.8
Sausage, pork	1 link	68	265	15.1	1.4	0	21.6	7.7	46	1020	0	1.4	20	0.8
Sausage, smoked links	3 2″ links	48	150	6.4	0.9	0	13.3	4.7	31	563	0	0	20	0.7
Shellfish, clams, canned	3 oz.	85	126	21.7	4.4	0	1.7	0.2	57	95	154	18.8	78	23.8
Shellfish, clams, steamed	10 clams	95	141	24.3	4.9	0	1.9	0.2	64	106	162	21.0	87	26.6
Shellfish, crab, steamed	3 oz.	85	82	16.4	0	0	1.3	0.1	45	911	8	6.5	50	0.6
Shellfish, oysters, fried	6 medium	88	173	7.7	10.2	0	11.1	2.8	71	367	80	3.3	55	6.1
Shellfish, shrimp, canned	3 oz.	85	85	17.4	0	0	1.2	0.2	214	660	0	3.5	123	1.8
Shellfish, shrimp, fried	4 large	30	73	6.4	3.4	0.1	3.7	0.6	53	103	17	0.5	20	0.4
Sunflower seeds, dry roasted	¼ cup	32	186	6.2	7.7	2.9	15.9	1.7	0	1	0	0.4	22	1.2
Tempeh	½ cup	83	160	15.4	7.8	0	9.0	1.8	0	7	0	0	92	2.2
Tofu, firm	½ cup	126	183	19.9	5.4	2.9	11.0	1.6	0	18	10	0.3	861	3.4
Turkey, dk mt, w/o skin, rst	3 oz.	85	138	24.5	0	0	3.7	1.2	95	67	0	0	22	2.0
Turkey, dk mt, w/skin, rst	3 oz.	85	155	23.5	0	0	6.0	1.8	99	65	0	0	23	2.0
Turkey, lt mt, w/o skin, rst	3 oz.	85	119	25.7	0	0	1.0	0.3	73	48	0	0	13	1.3
Turkey, lt mt, w/skin, rst	3 oz.	85	139	24.5	0	0	3.9	1.1	81	48	0	0	15	1.4
Veal, sirloin, roasted	3 oz.	85	172	21.4	0	0	8.9	3.8	87	71	0	0	11	0.8
Vegetarian bacon, cooked	1 oz.	16	50	1.7	1.0	0.4	4.7	0.7	0	234	1	0	4	0.4
Vegetarian franks	1 link	51	495	12.1	1.5	1.5	7.1	0.7	0	224	0	0	16	1.0
Vegetarian patties (burger)	1 patty	71	117	12.6	10.2	3.1	2.9	0.4	1	370	22	3.1	42	1.6
Vegetarian sausage	1 patty	38	98	7.0	3.7	1.1	6.9	1.1	0	337	0	0	24	1.4

FATS, OILS, SWEETS, AND ALCOHOLIC BEVERAGES

If nutrient-dense forms are selected from each of the basic food groups in MyPyramid, a small amount of additional calories can be consumed from solid fats and added sugars (see Chapter 8). Foods in this category should not replace foods from the other groups because they tend to provide calories but few nutrients.

Name	Amount	Weight g	Energy calories	Protein g	Carb. g	Fiber g	Total fat g	Sat. fat g	Chol. mg	Sod. mg	Vit. A RE	Vit. C mg	Calc. mg	Iron mg
Alcoholic beverage, beer	1 can or bottle	356	153	1.6	12.6	0	0	0	0	14	0	0	14	0.1
Alcoholic beverage, wine	5 oz.	148	124	0.1	4.0	0	0	0	0	7	0	0	12	0.6
Bacon	3 slices	24	133	8.7	0.3	0	10.5	3.4	26	533	3	0	2	0.4
Beverage, fruit punch	1 cup	247	114	0.2	28.8	0.2	0	0	0	10	0	108.2	10	0.2
Beverage, cola	1 can	368	136	0.3	35.2	0	0	0	0	15	0	0	7	0.4
Beverage, lemon-lime soda	1 can	369	148	0.2	37.4	0	0.1	0	0	33	0	0	7	0.4
Beverage, tea, bottled, sweetened	1 bottle	518	186	0	47.1	0	0	0	0	109	0	0	16	0
Butter	1 tablespoon	14	102	0.1	0	0	11.5	7.3	31	82	97	0	3	0
Candy, caramels	1 piece	10	39	0.5	7.8	0	0.8	0.3	1	25	1	0	14	0
Candy, fudge	1 piece	17	70	0.4	13	0.3	1.8	1.0	2	8	7	0	8	0.3

Name	Amount	Weight g	Energy calories	Protein g	Carb. g	Fiber g	Total fat g	Sat. fat g	Chol. mg	Sod. mg	Vit. A RE	Vit. C mg	Calc. mg	Iron mg
Candy, jelly beans	10 large	28	105	0	26.4	0	0.1	0	0	14	0	0	1	0
Candy, milk chocolate	1 bar	44	235	3.4	26.1	1.5	13.1	6.3	10	35	22	0	83	1.0
Chocolate syrup	2 tablespoons	39	109	0.8	25.4	1.0	0.4	0.2	0	28	0	0.1	5	0.8
Cream, half and half	2 tablespoons	30	39	0.9	1.3	0	3.5	2.1	11	12	29	0.3	32	0
Cream, whipped	½ cup	60	207	1.2	1.7	0	22.2	13.8	82	23	247	0.4	39	0
Cream, sour	1 tablespoon	12	26	0.4	0.5	0	2.5	1.6	5	6	21	0.1	14	0
Frosting, chocolate	2 tablespoons	41	163	0.5	25.9	0.4	7.2	2.3	0	75	0	0	3	0.6
Honey	1 tablespoon	21	64	0.1	17.3	0	0	0	0	1	0	0.1	1	0.1
Jam/preserves	1 tablespoon	20	56	0.1	13.8	0.2	0	0	0	6	0	1.8	4	0.1
Juice bar	1 bar	92	80	1.1	18.6	0.9	0.1	0	0	4	1	8.7	5	0.2
Lard	1 tablespoon	13	115	0	0	0	12.8	5.0	12	0	0	0	0	0
Marmalade, orange	1 tablespoon	20	49	0.1	13.3	0	0	0	0	11	1	1.0	8	0
Margarine, regular stick	1 tablespoon	14	101	0.1	0.1	0	11.4	2.0	0	133	115	0	4	0
Margarine, liquid	1 tablespoon	14	102	0.3	0	0	11.4	1.9	0	111	116	0	9	0
Margarine-like spread (40% fat)	1 tablespoon	14	46	0.3	0.3	0	4.9	1.0	0	88	115	0	7	0
Mayonnaise, regular	1 tablespoon	15	57	0.1	3.5	0	4.9	0.7	4	105	3	0	2	0
Mayonnaise, fat free	1 tablespoon	16	11	0	2.0	0.3	0.4	0	2	120	1	0	1	0
Oil, canola	1 tablespoon	14	124	0	0	0	14.0	1.0	0	0	0	0	0	0
Oil, corn	1 tablespoon	14	120	0	0	0	13.6	1.7	0	0	0	0	0	0
Oil, olive	1 tablespoon	14	119	0	0	0	13.5	1.8	0	0	0	0	0	0.1
Salad dressing, blue cheese	2 tablespoons	30	151	1.4	2.2	0	15.7	3.0	5	328	20	0.6	24	0.1
Salad dressing, French	2 tablespoons	32	146	0.3	5.0	0	14.3	1.8	0	268	7	0	8	0.3
Salad dressing, Italian	2 tablespoons	29	86	0.1	3.1	0	8.3	1.3	0	486	1	0	2	0.2
Salad dressing, Italian, reduced fat	2 tablespoons	30	22	0.1	1.4	0	1.9	0.1	0	410	0	0	3	0.2
Sherbet	½ cup	74	107	0.8	22.5	0	1.5	0.9	0	34	7	2.3	40	0.1
Shortening, vegetable	1 tablespoon	13	113	0	0	0	12.8	3.2	0	1	0	0	0	0
Sugar, brown	1 tablespoon	14	52	0	13.4	0	0	0	0	5	0	0	12	0.3
Sugar, white	1 tablespoon	13	49	0	12.6	0	0	0	0	0	0	0	0	0
Syrup, corn	1 tablespoon	20	57	0	15.5	0	0	0	0	0	31	0	0	0.1
Syrup, maple	¼ cup	80	210	0	54.0	0	0.2	0	0	7	0	0	53	1.0

DATA SOURCE: U.S. Department of Agriculture, Agricultural Research Service. 2006. *USDA National Nutrient Database for Standard Reference, Release 19* (http://www.nal.usda.gov/fnic/foodcomp).

Arby's

	Serving size	Calories	Protein	Total fat	Saturated fat	Trans fat	Total carbohydrate	Sugars	Fiber	Cholesterol	Sodium	Vitamin A	Vitamin C	Calcium	Iron	% calories from fat
	g		g	g	g	g	g	g	g	mg	mg	% Daily Value				
Regular roast beef	154	320	21	14	5	-	34	5	2	44	953	0	0	6	20	34
Super roast beef	198	398	21	19	6	-	40	10	2	44	1060	7	10	7	25	44
Junior roast beef	125	272	16	10	4	-	34	5	2	29	740	0	0	6	15	33
Market Fresh® Ultimate BLT	294	779	23	45	11	0.5	75	18	6	51	1571	16	28	17	27	52
Market Fresh® Roast Turkey & Swiss	359	725	45	30	8	0.5	75	17	5	91	1788	13	17	36	29	37
Market Fresh® Low Carbys™ Southwest chicken wrap	254	567	36	29	9	1	42	3	4	88	1451	12	13	24	24	47
Chicken Breast Fillet (grilled)	233	414	32	17	3	-	36	7	3	9	913	13	18	9	15	37
Martha's Vineyard™ salad (w/o dressing)	330	277	26	8	4	0	24	17	4	72	451	61	55	19	9	26
Raspberry vinaigrette	64	194	0	14	2	0	18	16	0	0	387	-	4	-	-	63
Santa Fe™ salad (w/o dressing)	365	477	29	21	6	0.5	42	6	42	53	1131	128	58	36	20	40
Curly fries (medium)	125	397	5	24	4	0	46	0	4	0	928	8	10	5	11	53
Jalapeno Bites®, regular (5)	110	305	5	21	9	1	29	3	2	28	526	14	1	3	5	63
Chocolate shake, regular	397	507	13	13	8	-	83	81	0	34	357	8	9	51	2	24

SOURCE: Arby's © 2007, Arby's, Inc. (http://www.arbysrestaurant.com). Used with permission of Arby's, Inc.

Burger King

	Serving size	Calories	Protein	Total fat	Saturated fat	Trans fat	Total carbohydrate	Sugars	Fiber	Cholesterol	Sodium	Vitamin A	Vitamin C	Calcium	Iron	% calories from fat
	g		g	g	g	g	g	g	g	mg	mg	% Daily Value				
Original Whopper®	290	670	28	39	11	1.5	51	11	3	51	1020	10	15	15	30	32
Original Whopper® w/o mayonnaise	269	510	28	22	9	1	51	11	3	80	880	10	15	15	30	39
Original Double Whopper® w/cheese	398	990	52	64	24	2.5	52	11	3	195	1520	15	15	30	45	59
Original Whopper Jr.®	158	370	15	21	6	0.5	31	6	2	50	570	4	6	8	15	51
Original Chicken Sandwich	219	660	24	40	8	2.5	52	5	4	70	1440	2	2	10	20	55
Chicken Tenders® (8 pieces)	123	340	19	20	5	3	21	1	<1	55	960	2	0	2	6	50
French fries (medium, salted)	116	360	4	220	4.5	4.5	41	1	4	0	590	0	15	2	4	45
Onion rings (medium)	91	320	4	16	4	3.5	40	5	3	0	460	0	0	6	6	45
Tendergrill™ Chicken Garden Salad	292	240	33	9	3.5	0	8	1	4	80	720	200	60	15	15	33
Ken's® Border Ranch Dressing	57	190	1	20	3	0	2	1	0	20	560	2	2	4	2	64
Croissan'wich® w/bacon, egg & cheese	115	300	12	17	6	2	26	5	<1	145	740	10	0	15	15	50
Hershey®'s sundae pie	79	310	3	19	12	0	32	22	1	0	220	2	0	4	6	53
Vanilla shake (medium)	412	560	11	21	13	0.5	79	77	0	85	330	15	6	50	2	34

SOURCE: BURGER KING® nutritional information used with permission from Burger King Brands, Inc.

Domino's Pizza
(1/8 of Pizza)

	Serving size	Calories	Protein	Carbohydrates	Fiber	Sugars	Total fat	Saturated fat	Trans fat	Cholesterol	Vitamin A	Vitamin C	Calcium	Iron	Sodium	Calories from fat
	g	Kcal	g	g	g	g	g	g	g	mg		% Daily Value			mg	Kcal
Medium Hand Tossed Cheese	88	190	8	27	1	2	6	2.5	0	10	6	6	8	10	370	50
Medium Thin Crust Cheese	55	140	5	14	1	1	7	2.5	0	10	6	4	10	2	240	60
Medium Deep Dish Cheese	95	220	8	27	3	1	10	3.5	0	10	8	4	10	10	530	90
Large Hand Tossed Cheese	122	260	11	38	2	3	8	3	0	10	10	8	10	15	510	70
Large Thin Crust Cheese	75	180	7	19	1	2	10	3.5	0	15	10	6	15	2	340	90
Large Deep Dish Cheese	137	320	12	41	5	2	14	5	0	15	10	4	15	15	750	130
Large Hand Tossed Pepperoni	132	310	13	38	2	3	12	5	0	20	10	8	10	15	700	110
Large Hand Tossed Pepperoni & Sausage	145	350	14	39	2	3	16	6	0	30	10	8	15	15	830	140
Large Hand Tossed Ham & Pineapple	145	280	12	40	2	5	8	3.5	0	15	10	10	10	15	620	80
Large Hand Tossed ExtravaganZZa	183	390	18	41	3	3	18	7	0	35	10	15	20	20	970	160
Large Hand Tossed Hawiian Feast	157	310	15	41	2	5	11	5	0	25	10	10	15	15	740	100
Large Hand Tossed Vegi Feast	155	300	13	40	2	3	11	4.5	0	20	10	15	20	15	670	100
Large Hand Tossed MeatZZa	163	380	17	39	2	3	18	7	0	35	10	8	20	15	940	160
Barbeque Buffalo Wings (2 per serving)	87	230	17	6	0	4	14	3.5	0	50	4	2	2	6	410	130
Domino's Pizza Chicken Kickers (2 per serving)	50	100	9	7	1	0	4.5	0.5	0	20	0	0	0	2	280	40
Blue Cheese Dipping Cup (one cup)	43	210	1	2	0	2	22	4	0	20	2	0	2	0	390	200
Breadsticks (1 of 8 average size pieces)	33	120	2	12	0	1	6	1.5	0	0	0	2	0	4	105	60
Brownie Squares	40	160	2	22	1	12	7	1.5	0	15	2	0	2	10	95	38

SOURCE: Domino's Pizza, 2007 (http://www.dominos.com). © Domino's Pizza, 2007. Reproduced with permission from Domino's Pizza LLC.

KFC

	Serving size	Calories	Protein	Total fat	Saturated fat	Trans fat	Total carbohydrate	Sugars	Fiber	Cholesterol	Sodium	Vitamin A	Vitamin C	Calcium	Iron	% calories from fat
	g		g	g	g	g	g	g	g	mg	mg		% Daily Value			
Original Recipe® Chicken breast	161	360	37	21	5	0	7	0	0	115	1020	2	2	8	6	53
Original Recipe® Chicken thigh	126	330	20	24	6	0	8	0	0	110	870	4	2	4	8	67
Extra Crispy™ Chicken breast	162	440	34	27	6	0	15	0	0	105	970	2	2	6	6	57
Extra Crispy™ thigh	114	370	18	28	6	0	12	0	0	85	850	2	0	2	6	68
Tender Roast® sandwich w/sauce	236	430	37	18	3.5	0	29	4	2	80	1180	6	15	8	15	37
Tender Roast® sandwich w/o sauce	217	300	37	4.5	1.5	0	28	3	2	70	1060	6	15	8	15	13
Hot Wings™ (5 pieces)	112	350	20	24	5	0	14	0	2	105	740	4	0	4	8	63
Popcorn chicken (large)	160	550	29	35	6	0	30	0	3	80	1600	4	2	4	10	58
Chicken pot pie	423	770	33	40	15	14	70	2	5	115	1680	200	0	0	20	47
Roasted Caesar Salad w/o dressing and croutons	301	220	30	8	4.5	0	6	3	3	70	830	45	35	25	10	36
KFC® creamy parmesan caesar dressing	57	260	2	26	5	0	4	2	0	15	540	2	0	6	2	88
Corn on the cob (5.5")	162	150	5	3	1	0	26	10	7	0	10	0	10	6	6	17
Mashed potatoes w/gravy	151	140	2	5	1	0.5	20	1	1	0	560	2	2	4	8	32
Baked beans	136	220	8	1	0	0	45	28	7	0	730	6	2	10	15	5
Cole slaw	130	180	1	10	1.5	0	22	18	3	5	270	10	20	4	4	50
Biscuit (1)	57	220	4	11	2.5	3.5	24	2	1	0	640	2	0	4	10	45
Potato salad	128	180	2	9	1.5	0	22	6	2	5	470	2	10	0	2	45

SOURCE: KFC Corporation, 2007. Nutritional information provided by KFC Corporation from its web site (www.kfc.com) as of July 30, 2007 and subject to the conditions listed therein. KFC and related marks are registered trademarks of KFC Corporation. Reproduced with permission from Kentucky Fried Chicken Corporation.

McDonald's

	Serving size (g)	Calories	Protein (g)	Total fat (g)	Saturated fat (g)	Trans fat (g)	Total carbohydrate (g)	Sugars (g)	Fiber (g)	Cholesterol (mg)	Sodium (mg)	Vitamin A (% DV)	Vitamin C (% DV)	Calcium (% DV)	Iron (% DV)	% calories from fat
Hamburger	100	250	12	9	3.5	0.5	31	6	2	25	528	0	2	10	15	40
Quarter Pounder®	169	410	24	19	7	1	37	8	3	65	730	2	4	15	20	41
Quarter Pounder® w/cheese	198	510	29	26	12	1.5	40	9	3	90	1190	10	4	30	25	45
Big Mac®	214	540	25	29	10	1.5	45	9	3	75	1040	6	2	25	25	48
Big N' Tasty®	206	460	24	24	8	1.5	37	8	3	70	720	6	8	15	25	47
Filet-O-Fish®	143	380	15	18	4	1	38	5	2	35	660	2	0	15	10	42
McChicken®	147	360	14	16	3.5	1	40	5	1	40	790	0	2	10	15	42
Medium French Fries	114	380	4	20	4	5	47	0	5	0	220	0	10	2	6	47
Chicken McNuggets® (6 pieces)	96	250	15	15	3	1.5	15	0	0	35	670	2	2	2	4	52
Chicken Select® Premium Breast Strips (5 pieces)	221	630	39	33	6	4.5	46	0	0	90	1550	0	6	4	8	48
Tangy Honey Mustard Sauce	43	70	1	2.5	0	0	13	9	0	5	170	0	0	0	1	29
Bacon Ranch Salad w/Grilled Chicken (w/o dressing)	321	260	33	9	4	0	12	5	3	90	1010	130	50	15	10	35
Caesar Salad w/Crispy Chicken (w/o dressing)	313	300	25	13	4	1.5	22	4	3	55	1020	130	50	20	10	40
Newman's Own® Ranch Dressing (2 oz)	59	170	1	15	2.5	0	9	4	0	20	530	0	0	4	0	76
Egg McMuffin®	139	300	18	12	5	0	30	3	2	260	820	10	2	30	20	37
Sausage Biscuit w/Egg	156	490	17	32	10	5	34	2	1	250	1110	6	0	8	20	57
Hotcakes (2 pats margarine & syrup)	223	610	9	18	4	4	105	47	3	20	680	2	0	15	15	26
Fruit 'n Yogurt Parfait	149	160	4	2	1	0	31	21	1	5	85	0	15	15	4	13
Chocolate Triple Thick® Shake (16 oz)	444	580	13	14	8	1	102	84	1	50	250	20	0	45	10	21

SOURCE: McDonald's Corporation, 2007 (http://www.mcdonalds.com). Used with permission from McDonald's Corporation. For the most current information, visit the McDonald's Web site.

Subway
Based on standard formulas with 6-inch subs on Italian or wheat bread

	Serving size (g)	Calories	Protein (g)	Total fat (g)	Saturated fat (g)	Trans fat (g)	Total carbohydrate (g)	Sugars (g)	Fiber (g)	Cholesterol (mg)	Sodium (mg)	Vitamin A (% DV)	Vitamin C (% DV)	Calcium (% DV)	Iron (% DV)	% calories from fat
6" Italian BMT®	243	450	23	21	8	0	47	8	4	55	1770	10	35	15	25	42
6" Meatball marinara	377	560	24	24	11	1	63	13	7	45	1690	15	60	20	40	39
6" Steak & cheese	278	400	29	12	6	0.5	48	9	5	60	1110	10	40	15	40	27
Subway Melt®	254	380	25	12	5	0	48	8	4	45	1600	10	35	15	25	29
Tuna	250	530	22	31	7	0.5	44	7	4	45	1010	10	35	15	30	53
Sweet onion chicken teriyaki	281	370	26	5	1.5	0	59	19	5	50	1200	8	40	8	25	12
Roast beef	224	290	19	5	2	0	45	8	4	20	900	8	30	5	35	16
Turkey breast	224	280	18	4.5	1.5	0	46	7	4	20	1000	8	35	6	25	14
Veggie Delite®	167	230	9	3	1	0	44	7	4	0	500	8	35	6	25	13
Turkey Breast salad (w/o dressing)	378	110	12	2.5	0.5	0	13	6	4	20	580	60	50	6	10	20
New England style clam chowder	310	150	6	5	1	0	20	2	4	10	990	0	-	4	6	30
Chili con carne	310	290	19	8	3.5	0	35	13	12	25	990	15	20	8	20	25
Chocolate Chip Cookie	45	210	2	10	6	0	30	18	1	15	150	6	0	0	6	43

SOURCE: Subway U.S. Nutrition Info as found on http://www.subway.com, 6/30/2007. Reprinted by permission of Subway.®

Taco Bell

	Serving size (g)	Calories	Protein (g)	Total fat (g)	Saturated fat (g)	Trans fat (g)	Total carbohydrate (g)	Sugars (g)	Fiber (g)	Cholesterol (mg)	Sodium (mg)	Vitamin A	Vitamin C	Calcium	Iron	% calories from fat
												% Daily Value				
Crunchy Taco	78	170	8	10	3.5	0	13	1	3	25	350	4	2	8	6	47
Crunchy Taco Supreme®	113	210	9	13	6	0	15	2	3	40	370	10	6	10	6	57
Soft taco, beef	99	200	10	9	4	0	21	2	3	25	630	4	2	10	10	40
Gordita Supreme®, steak	153	290	15	13	5	0	28	6	2	40	530	6	6	10	15	41
Grilled steak soft taco, Fresco style	128	160	10	4.5	1.5	0	20	3	2	20	550	4	10	8	10	25
Gordita Baja®, chicken	153	320	17	16	3.5	0	28	6	3	40	800	8	6	10	10	44
Chalupa Supreme, beef	153	380	14	23	7	0.5	30	4	3	40	620	8	6	15	15	55
Chalupa Supreme, chicken	153	380	17	20	5	0	29	4	2	45	650	6	8	10	15	49
1/2 lb. Beef combo burrito	241	430	21	18	8	1	51	4	8	45	1630	15	6	20	30	38
Bean burrito	198	340	13	9	3.5	0.5	54	3	8	5	1190	10	8	20	25	24
Burrito Supreme®, chicken	248	390	20	13	6	0.5	49	5	6	45	1380	15	15	20	25	31
Grilled stuffed burrito, beef	325	680	27	30	10	1	76	6	9	55	2120	15	4	30	40	40
Tostada	170	230	11	10	3.5	0.5	27	2	7	15	730	10	8	20	10	39
Zesty Chicken Border Bowl™ w/dressing	418	640	22	35	6	1	60	4	10	30	1800	15	15	15	25	37
Express taco salad	479	610	25	32	10	1.5	56	8	14	65	1420	20	20	30	25	48
Steak quesadilla	184	520	26	28	13	1	39	4	3	70	1300	10	0	45	20	50
Nachos Supreme	195	450	12	25	7	1.5	41	3	7	35	800	8	8	10	10	51
Nachos BellGrande®	308	770	19	44	9	3	77	5	12	12	1280	8	8	20	20	50
Pintos 'n cheese	128	150	9	6	3	0.5	19	1	7	15	670	10	6	15	8	33
Mexican rice	131	170	6	7	3	0	23	1	1	15	740	15	6	10	8	35

SOURCE: Taco Bell Corporation, 2007 (http://www.tacobell.com). Reproduced courtesy of Taco Bell Corporation.

Wendy's

	Serving size (g)	Calories	Protein (g)	Total fat (g)	Saturated fat (g)	Trans fat (g)	Total carbohydrate (g)	Sugars (g)	Fiber (g)	Cholesterol (mg)	Sodium (mg)	Vitamin A	Vitamin C	Calcium	Iron	% calories from fat
												% Daily Value				
Classic Single® w/everything	218	430	25	20	7	1	37	9	2	65	900	8	8	4	25	42
Jr. Hamburger	117	280	15	9	3.5	0.5	34	7	1	30	590	0	0	2	20	29
Jr. Bacon Cheeseburger	161	370	19	18	7	0.5	34	6	1	50	790	10	6	10	20	46
Ultimate Chicken Grill Sandwich	227	370	28	7	1.5	0	36	8	2	70	950	6	10	4	20	19
Spicy Chicken Fillet Sandwich	231	440	28	16	2.5	0	46	6	3	60	1320	6	8	4	15	32
Homestyle Chicken Fillet Sandwich	228	430	25	16	2.5	0	48	6	2	45	1140	6	8	4	15	31
Homestyle Chicken Strips	159	410	28	21	3.5	0	33	0	0	60	1470	0	0	2	6	39
Caesar Side Salad (no toppings or dressing)	99	80	6	4.5	2	0	6	1	2	10	240	100	35	10	6	57
Mandarin Chicken® Salad (no toppings or dressing)	348	170	21	2.5	0.5	0	16	12	3	60	520	70	50	6	10	9
Southwest Taco Salad (no toppings or dressing)	501	430	30	22	12	1	30	9	8	80	1090	80	35	45	20	45
Creamy ranch dressing	64	200	1	20	3.5	0	4	2	0	15	400	0	0	4	2	87
Reduced fat creamy ranch dressing	64	90	1	7	1.5	0	6	3	1	10	400	0	0	6	2	70
Large French Fries	190	520	7	24	3.5	1	69	0	7	0	560	4	15	2	10	44
Sour Cream & Chive Baked Potato	312	320	9	4	2.5	0	63	4	7	10	55	4	60	8	15	11
Low Fat Strawberry Flavored Yogurt w/Granola	163	250	8	6	1.5	0	42	30	1	5	90	2	2	22	6	33
Chili, small, plain	227	220	17	6	2.5	0	23	6	5	35	780	4	4	8	15	27
Crispy Chicken Nuggets™ (5)	75	230	12	15	3	0	12	0	0	35	520	0	0	0	2	59
Barbecue sauce (1 packet)	28	45	1	0	0	0	10	8	0	0	170	0	0	0	4	0
Frosty,™ medium	298	430	10	11	7	0	74	55	0	45	200	20	0	40	20	23

SOURCE: Wendy's International, Inc., 2007 (http://www.wendys.com). Reproduced with permission from Wendy's International, Inc. The information contained in Wendy's International Information is effective as of May 2007. Wendy's International, Inc., its subsidiaries, affiliates, franchises, and employees do not assume responsibility for a particular sensitivity or allergy (including peanuts, nuts or other allergies) to any food product provided in our restaurants. We encourage anyone with food sensitivities, allergies, or special dietary needs to check on a regular basis with Wendy's Consumer Relations Department to obtain the most up-to-date information.

Information on additional foods and restaurants is available online; see the Web sites listed in this appendix and the following additional sites: **Hardees:** http://www.hardees.com; **White Castle:** http://www.whitecastle.com

MONITORING YOUR PROGRESS

NAME _____ SECTION _____ DATE _____

As you completed the labs listed below, you entered the results in the Preprogram Assessment column of this lab. Now that you have been involved in a fitness and wellness program for some time, do the labs again and enter your new results in the Postprogram Assessment column. You will probably notice improvement in several areas. Congratulations! If you are not satisfied with your progress thus far, refer to the tips for successful behavior change in Chapter 1 and throughout this book. Remember—fitness and wellness are forever. The time you invest now in developing a comprehensive, individualized program will pay off in a richer, more vital life in the years to come.

	Preprogram Assessment	Postprogram Assessment
LAB 2.3 Pedometer	Daily steps: _____	Daily steps: _____
LAB 3.1 Cardiorespiratory Endurance		
1-mile walk test	$\dot{V}O_{2max}$: _____ Rating: _____	$\dot{V}O_{2max}$: _____ Rating: _____
3-minute step test	$\dot{V}O_{2max}$: _____ Rating: _____	$\dot{V}O_{2max}$: _____ Rating: _____
1.5-mile run-walk test	$\dot{V}O_{2max}$: _____ Rating: _____	$\dot{V}O_{2max}$: _____ Rating: _____
LAB 4.1 Muscular Strength		
Maximum bench press test	Weight: _____ lb Rating: _____	Weight: _____ lb Rating: _____
LAB 4.2 Muscular Endurance		
Curl-up test	Number: _____ Rating: _____	Number: _____ Rating: _____
Push-up test	Number: _____ Rating: _____	Number: _____ Rating: _____
Squat endurance test	Number: _____ Rating: _____	Number: _____ Rating: _____
LAB 5.1 Flexibility		
Sit-and-reach test	Score: _____ cm Rating: _____	Score: _____ cm Rating: _____
LAB 5.3 Low-Back Muscular Endurance		
Side bridge endurance test	Right: _____ sec Rating: _____	Right: _____ sec Rating: _____
	Left: _____ sec Rating: _____	Left: _____ sec Rating: _____
Trunk flexors endurance test	Trunk flexors: _____ sec Rating: _____	Trunk flexors: _____ sec Rating: _____
Back extensors endurance test	Back extensors: _____ sec Rating: _____	Back extensors: _____ sec Rating: _____

	Preprogram Assessment	Postprogram Assessment
LAB 6.1 Body Composition		
Body mass index	BMI: _____ kg/m² Rating: _____	BMI: _____ kg/m² Rating: _____
Skinfold measurements (or other method for determining percent body fat)	Sum of 3 skinfolds: _____ mm	Sum of 3 skinfolds: _____ mm
	% body fat: _____ % Rating: _____	% body fat: _____ % Rating: _____
Waist circumference	Circumf.: _____ Rating: _____	Circumf.: _____ Rating: _____
Waist-to-hip-circumference ratio	Ratio: _____ Rating: _____	Ratio: _____ Rating: _____
LAB 8.1 Daily Diet		
Number of oz-eq	Grains: _____	Grains: _____
Number of cups	Vegetables: _____	Vegetables: _____
Number of cups	Fruits: _____	Fruits: _____
Number of cups	Milk: _____	Milk: _____
Number of oz-eq	Meat and beans: _____	Meat and beans: _____
Number of tsp	Oils: _____	Oils: _____
Number of g	Solid fats: _____	Solid fats: _____
Number of g or tsp	Added sugars: _____	Added sugars: _____
LAB 8.2 Dietary Analysis		
Percentage of calories	From protein: _____ %	From protein: _____ %
Percentage of calories	From fat: _____ %	From fat: _____ %
Percentage of calories	From saturated fat: _____ %	From saturated fat: _____ %
Percentage of calories	From carbohydrate: _____ %	From carbohydrate: _____ %
LAB 9.1 Daily Energy Needs	Daily energy needs: _____ cal/day	Daily energy needs: _____ cal/day
LAB 10.1 Identifying Stressors	Average weekly stress score: _____	Average weekly stress score: _____
LAB 11.1 Cardiovascular Health		
CVD risk assessment	Score: _____ Estimated risk: _____	Score: _____ Estimated risk: _____
Hostility assessment	Score: _____ Rating: _____	Score: _____ Rating: _____
LAB 12.1 Cancer Prevention		
Diet: Number of servings	Fruits/vegetables: _____	Fruits/vegetables: _____
Skin cancer	Score: _____ Risk: _____	Score: _____ Risk: _____

INDEX

Boldface numbers indicate pages on which glossary definitions appear.

abdominal curl, 102
abdominal machines, 119
Acceptable Macronutrient Distribution Ranges (AMDRs), 224, 227, 228, 231, 239
ACE (American Council on Exercise), 45, 46
acquired immunodeficiency syndrome (AIDS). *See* HIV/AIDS
across-the-body stretches, 143
ACSM (American College of Sports Medicine), 29–31, 40–42, 45, 46, 100, 139, 203, 204, 248–249, 250
action stage of behavior change, 14, 15
active stretching, **141**
activities, for fitness program, 194–196
activity, 31, 51–52, 72. *See also* physical activity
adaptability, 38
additives, 252
adenosine triphosphate (ATP), **61,** 64
Adequate Intake (AI), 236, 263–265
Adipex-P, 108
adipose tissue, **170**
adolescents, 203
advertising. *See also* consumer guidelines
  dietary supplements, 106
  exercise equipment, 196
AED (automatic external defibrillator), 46, A–4
aerobic, 46, 57, **62,** 235, 257
aerobic (oxidative) energy system, **62**
aerobic exercise, 46, 57, 235
Aerobics and Fitness Association of America (AFAA), 46
African Americans. *See also* ethnicity
  diabetes for, 173
  health disparities for, 8, 173
age
  body composition by, 177
  nutrition and, 245
  target heart rate range v., 71

aggressive driving, A–2–A–3
aging
  body composition and, 177
  exercise for, 34, 54, 65, 138, 203
  muscular strength for, 94–95
  nutrition for, 235–237, 248, 265
  physical fitness and, 34
  strength training for, 94–95
agonist muscles, **101**
AI (Adequate Intake), 236, 263–265
AIDS. *See* acquired immunodeficiency syndrome; HIV/AIDS
air bags, A–1
air passages, 58
air quality, 78
alcohol, nutrition and, 222, 235, 242, 245, B–7
alcohol use. *See also* blood alcohol concentration
  death from, 5, 6, 9
  nutrition and, 222, 235, 242, 245, B–7
  self-assessment of, 25
allergies, 261
alternate leg stretcher, 145, 151
altitude, 82
alveoli, 60, **61**
Alzheimer's disease, 5, 242
AMA (American Medical Association), 204, 255
AMDRs (Acceptable Macronutrient Distribution Ranges), 224, 227, 228, 231, 239
amenorrhea, 174, 175, 248
American College of Sports Medicine (ACSM)
  on cardiorespiratory training, 29–30, 40
  certification by, 45, 46
  on dietary recommendations, 248–249, 250
  on flexibility training, 139
  physical activity guidelines from, 29–31, 40–42
  on strength training, 100, 103, 203, 204
American Council on Exercise (ACE), 45, 46

American Diabetes Association, 173
American Dietetic Association, 248
American Heart Association, A–4
American Indians. *See* Native Americans
American Medical Association (AMA), 204, 255
American Red Cross, A–4, A–10
amino acids, 107, 108, 224, **225**
amphetamines, 107
anabolic steroids, 107
anaerobic, **62**
anaerobic (nonoxidative) energy system, 61, **62**
androstenedione, 106, 107
anecdotal evidence, 107–108
anemia, **235**
ankle dorsiflexion/plantar flexion, 161
antagonist muscles, **101**
antioxidants, 229, **232,** 236, 238, 253, 258
anxiety, 67
aorta, **58,** 59
Apidex-P, 108
appetite suppressants, 108
arteries, **58,** 59–60
arthritis, 200
assault, A–6–A–7
assessment. *See also* laboratory activities; self-assessment
  of body composition, 174–179, 183–188
  of body mass index, 174, 175
  of cardiorespiratory endurance, 67–69, 85–88
  of flexibility, 157–168
  of muscular strength and endurance, 96, 103, 123–134
  of nutrition, 267–272
  of posture, 167, 168
  preprogram/postprogram, D–1–D–2
  in strength training, 103
assisted dip, 118
assisted pull-up, 116
asthma, 191, 200
athletes. *See also* exercise; sports
  nutrition for, 175, 231, 248–250
ATP (adenosine triphosphate), **61,** 64

whole grain, **229,** 230, 240, 243–244

wind chill, **78**

women. *See also* fetal/infant health risks; gender; pregnancy

athletes, 175

body composition for, 174

gestational diabetes in, 173

menstruation for, 82, 237, 248, 264

muscular strength and endurance for, 91

nutrition for, 223, 227, 228, 235, 237, 242, 247, 248, 250, 253, 256

pregnancy for, 203, 237, 256, 263–265

sports for, 175

workout cards. *See* laboratory activities

workplace, A–6

World Health Organization (WHO), 4, 21, 231, 255

yoga, 142, 150

zinc, 234, 247